# VOLUME ONE
## KNOWLEDGE & COMPREHENSION OF SCIENCE

James L. Flowers, M.D., M.P.H.

# A COMPLETE PREPARATION FOR THE MCAT *

**\* MEDICAL COLLEGE ADMISSION TEST**

● **Review Materials in Science**

    Biology
    General Chemistry
    Organic Chemistry
    Physics

● **Includes STUDY TIMETABLE and TEST TAKING TIPS**

**BETZ PUBLISHING COMPANY, INC.**
**BETHESDA, MARYLAND,** *Publisher*

CONTENTS

## LIST OF FIGURES

1. Introduction to Science Knowledge

2. Review of Biology

3.    Review of General Chemistry

4.    Review of Organic Chemistry

5.    Review of Physics

This book is dedicated to my parents,

especially my mother, Ozie,

and to other parents like them whose ambitions, dreams, and potentials may never be realized, but whose lives have been dedicated to seeing that their childrens' are.

It is also my privilege to acknowledge the special contributions of William C. Wallace, University of Illinois College of Medicine, formerly Director of the Harvard Health Careers Summer Program, Harvard School of Medicine, whose constant encouragement and support greatly enhanced this work, and also to acknowledge the Office of Health Resources Opportunity, Department of Health and Human Services, whose support gave incentive to this effort and helped assure its completion as a service to students who aspire to a career in medicine.

James L. Flowers, M.D.
Milwaukee, Wisconsin

June, 1985

# PREFACE

This edition of Dr. Flowers' book, A COMPLETE PREPARATION FOR THE MCAT, is the second complete revision of the workbook and study guide originally published in 1978. The 1985 edition of this volume, which is subtitled Knowledge and Comprehension of Science, also has a companion volume, Skills Development in Reading and Quantitative, written by Beryl B. Blain, Drew M. Love, and Philip F. Kelleher, and revised in 1985 by Angelica Braestrup and Aftab Hassan.

These volumes together are a comprehensive preparation for the Medical College Admission Test. Knowledge and Comprehension of Science, the volume you are now reading, includes course content and review materials in biology, general and organic chemistry, and physics. The 1985 edition includes current content revisions in its coverage of the three science areas tested on the MCAT. Illustrations and exercises in this edition have been further augmented, and the same internal structure that enhanced the recognized value of the original edition has been retained.

Knowledge and Comprehension of Science is now a proven review for the science topics included on the MCAT. It remains more comprehensive than a first-year biology course review might provide and aids MCAT candidates in selecting the specific review topics from chemistry and physics first-year courses to be covered on the MCAT.

Writing, reading, and quantitative skills study sections are available separately in Volume II, Skills Development in Reading and Quantitative. Revisions have been made in both the reading and mathematics sections, and, reflecting recent MCAT changes, an essay module is included. This second volume provides instruction in writing, analytical reading skills, and practice with reading passages similar to those on the MCAT. In mathematics and quantitative analysis, the book provides the content material needed for an understanding of those quantitative procedures that are essential to a complete preparation for the MCAT.

Among the many individuals whose able contributions assisted Dr. Flowers in the original development of this book and its first revision are James L. Angel and the following reviewers: James J. Watrous, Department Chairman and Associate Professor of Biology, and William A. Kriner, Associate Professor of Chemistry, both of St. Joseph's University, and Mark A. Sartor, physics.

Production of the manuscript for the second revision of this book is the work of staff members at Betz Publishing Company, which assumed responsibility for its publication in 1982.

Editor

# CHAPTER 1:

## INTRODUCTION

### TO

## SCIENCE KNOWLEDGE

## 1.1     The Role of the MCAT in the Admission Process

The primary use of the old MCAT in the medical school admission process prior to 1977 was as a screening device in combination with college grades. These objective measures could be reviewed and compared rapidly to the more lengthy recommendations and personal letters. After the initial screening, the MCAT probably played a lesser role as grade point average, letters of recommendation, major, undergraduate college, and so forth, became more important considerations. It is fair to say that a low MCAT probably did not weigh too unfavorably against high grades and good recommendations, and that a high MCAT probably helped in the instances of average grades. Numerous studies showed no correlation between MCAT scores and success in the clinical phase of medical school or competence as a practicing physician. There was a positive correlation between MCAT scores (especially the Science subtest) and the success in the basic sciences (or preclinical phase of medical school). So despite the apparent lack of validity, at least in the pre-1977 MCAT, medical schools have used and will continue to use this device as an entrance requirement for medical school.

As described above, the MCAT is only one part of the complex requirements and considerations inherent in the process of admission to medical school. Grade point average, recommendations, undergraduate major, types and quality of courses taken, extracurricular activities, the interview, personality and other noncognitive factors, all play an important role. Attention should not be paid to the MCAT review to the exclusion of these other important factors. Books/manuals/pamphlets on the admission process to medical school should be available from your bookstore, premedical advisor, or premedical association.

The exact role of the new MCAT in the admissions process remains to be determined as this test is distinctly different from its pre-1977 counterpart.

## 1.2     Structure of the New MCAT

The following information is found in The MCAT Student Manual*, which is at most college bookstores or may be obtained from:

Association of American Medical Colleges
One Dupont Circle, NW
Washington, D. C.  20036

There is also an interpretation manual available to educators. Information for registration, on the other hand, should be obtainable from your premed advisor or equivalent, or from:

MCAT Registration
The American College Testing Program
P. O. Box 414
Iowa City, IA  52243

---

     *The MCAT Student Manual, third edition, 1984, published by the Association of American Medical Colleges. References to the manual in this text are to the third edition.

The MCAT is a day-long test divided into a morning session and an afternoon session. The morning session test includes science knowledge, science problems, and a written essay (see fig. 1.1). The afternoon session includes reading and quantitative skills analysis. The workbook you are now using roughly corresponds to the content of the morning session with the exception of the essay module, which may be found in the companion Volume II. The Science Knowledge part of the MCAT involves separate tests in biology, chemistry (organic and general), and physics of approximately 40 questions each. These questions are directed both to the content of your knowledge in the stated subject areas and to your understanding of the principles at the core of this knowledge. The Science Problems part consists of approximately 60 questions. The questions apply the knowledge and principles learned in biology, chemistry, and physics to specific examples that are presented in short paragraphs, as a chemical structure, as an experiment, a chart or graph, for example. The questions on any one example may be drawn from any combination of the physical sciences. To reemphasize, the questions are direct applications to specific examples of what you have learned in physics, biology, and chemistry. You need no new knowledge to do this section, but only the science knowledge you have already learned, integrated with your analytical skills.

As of April 1985 the MCAT will include an essay module to be written after Science Problems and before lunch. The writing score for students who take the exam in 1985 will be available for use by institutions in 1986. (Refer to Volume II for specific details about preparation for the essay module.)

The Reading subtest and Quantitative subtest each has 68 questions. The companion volume to this workbook is entitled A COMPLETE PREPARATION FOR THE MCAT (Volume II): Skills Development in Reading and Quantitative and provides a thorough guide to prepare students for these portions of the examination. The test contains reading selections drawn from medical and health related topics, the natural sciences, and social science passages from psychology, history, anthropology, economics, and so forth. The questions test comprehension of the material presented in the selection and your ability to draw logical conclusions. These require no prior knowledge. The Quantitative examples present information in the form of graphs, tables, charts, maps, and equations. Once again, you are required to interpret and draw valid conclusions. The MCAT Student Manual explores each of these subtests in detail and provides examples. (The 1984 edition includes no information on the new essay portion.)

## 1.3     How to Prepare for the MCAT in High School and College

The MCAT accentuates the importance of developing good reading and data interpretive skills. These are skills that take a long time to acquire and cannot be crammed into a month or so of preparation. For this reason, what you do in college, in high school, and even before, will help prepare you for the MCAT (and the medical profession) as much as any review manual or review course. If you feel your reading/study/interpretive skills are weak and your school or college offers a course specifically directed at this, then take it. If you can select your own courses, select those courses which demand interpretive reading (such as literature, philosophy, or history courses). And select those science courses that require you to understand and apply principles and to interpret data, rather than those that demand only memorization.

Speed reading will not help you unless you are already getting the right answers. When you read newspapers, journals, magazines, or watch TV news shows, for example, force yourself to draw conclusions about what is being presented, interpret the graphs and charts, predict trends in data, and assay the limitations and errors present in the data or opinions. By constantly forcing yourself to do these types of things, the skills necessary to do well on the Skills Analysis sections will be developed and sharpened.

By taking the required courses for admission into medical school, you will have covered most of the information on the Science Knowledge sections. The following courses are suggested in addition to the basic requirements (if you have the time to take them, they will not only make the test easier, but they will also ease the shock of med school):

    Preferred:  Physiology, Biochemistry, Microbiology
    Useful:     Genetics, Anatomy (of any type), Embryology
    Luxury:     Human Anatomy, Histology

But understand that these courses are not needed before you take the test if your basic biology, chemistry and physics preparations are good.

In addition to the above long-term preparations, short-term "crash" courses are available. MCAT review courses are useful, they do raise scores; they tend to be expensive, but provide motivation to follow through. MCAT manuals other than the ones mentioned above vary in their effectiveness. Some have good questions, whereas others are nearly irrelevant. None, to date, provides a systematic review of topics as they are presented in the workbook you are using. The MCAT Student Manual is a valuable adjunct because it provides sample tests that are probably as close to the real test as you will find. The Manual is the main reason space has not been allocated in this science volume to practice tests and extra reading. You can review the material in this book and use the Student Manual test for practice in science to see how well you have learned the material.

## 1.4    Rationale and Structure of Volume I

The main purpose of this book is to provide a concise and thorough review and preparation for the MCAT. Science Knowledge subtests (biology, chemistry, and physics) and the Science Problems subtest will be adequately prepared for by studying chapters 2, 3, 4, and 5 of Volume I, which you are now using. The math required for the Science Problems subtest and Quantitative Analysis subtest is presented in Volume II, Skills Development in Reading and Quantitative. Volume II also contains preparation for the writing and reading subtests. To prepare chapters 2 through 5 of this book, the outlines presented in The MCAT Student Manual were used as a guide. This material is presented in more or less the same order as it exists in the Manual. The actual content of any section in chapters 2 through 5 reflects the author's interpretation of material that is relevant to the stated topic. The material to be presented here should in no way be construed as the only material to be presented on the exam, nor should it be inferred that the exam at some other time will include all the material discussed herein.

It is assumed that students will have taken the appropriate premedical courses before attempting to review this book. The author assumes that most students will have seen most (not necessarily all) of the material presented, so that studying this book will be a true review. It is probably possible that a student who has not had a major science course can use the material presented here as a primary text, but this will require considerable time and effort. This text can reasonably be used in a course to review for the MCAT. It may be used along with the appropriate coursework as a text for a pre-course or a prep-course in any of the areas presented (such as Chapter 2 on Biology during a biology course), and for a variety of other similar purposes.

The numbering of sections in this volume is based on the following system: the last number in a series separated by periods represents a division of the number (or section) prior to it. The first number is also the chapter number. The second number is the major section within each chapter. The third number represents divisions or subsections within each of those sections, as in:

3.2.5

This series represents the fifth subsection of the second major section of the third chapter. The value of this system is that it allows for an infinite number of divisions of any level (such as chapter or section) without running out of symbols or having to change symbols such as letters, numbers, or Roman numerals.

Each of the major sections of any given chapter (as an example, Atomic Structure, 3.1) is subdivided in a stereotyped way. In 3.1.1, a review of the topic is presented. This, again, is the author's interpretation of the relevant material and it is presented in a way to give it maximum meaning yet simplicity of review. Many statements are presented as facts without much explanatory material because students generally have covered this in their primary course. But difficult concepts and key concepts are usually presented in slightly greater detail to make comprehension easier. In 3.1.2, questions are given for review of the material discussed. These questions are arranged in a specific sequence. The first questions may be answered by rote and merely ask the student to recall what was read. Their purpose is to emphasize important facts to remember and help assess comprehension. They will, in general, cover the whole section. The second group of questions is problematic in nature. Their purpose is to allow the student to apply principles or concepts discussed in the section, and they emphasize what the student should be able to do with the information presented. Depending on the specific topic, the number of rote or problematic questions will vary. Some sections have no problematic questions. Notice that rote questions are similar to the Science Knowledge subtest questions and problematic questions are similar to those on the Science Problems subtest. (Remember that "similar" means "like," not "identical.")

The questions are not as difficult as the questions on the actual test. The questions in this manual are intended to review the material presented and not mimic a true test situation. The third subsection, 3.1.3, lists all the answers to the questions given. The fourth subsection, 3.1.4, is a discussion of the answers to the questions. The rote questions are not discussed because they are explained in the section. The problematic questions, however, are discussed in detail.  The fifth subsection, 3.1.5, is a vocabulary checklist.  This is a listing of all the terminology  in the section you should try to master.  The sixth subsection, 3.1.6, which may be combined with the fifth in some sections, is a checklist of concepts and principles.   It attempts to list the concepts you should understand and the types of problems you should be able to do.  In summary, the structure of this book is designed to deliver a maximum of relevant information in a concise manner and to provide a means of learning it well.

## 1.5     Suggestions on How to Use Volume I Effectively

As explained previously, the book you are now using was written to a uniform format designed to maximize speed of review and learning. Use of the book may be approached in many different ways based upon this format.  One way is simply to review it cover to cover if it is felt that a comprehensive review is required.  But if a student feels confident in a given subject, or specific topic within that subject, it is reasonable to skim or even pass over it.  This is done best by going over the checklists or questions before reading the review itself and deciding if complete study of the section is required.

This book can also be used along with the corresponding college course (for example, the physics chapter with a physics course). It should be observed that much less information is required for the MCAT than is required for the course. But the value of using the book is in knowing what to focus on for the test. Of course, do not focus in on the MCAT to the point that grades are jeopardized and course perspective is lost.

If the explanation on a given topic is not adequate, don't hesitate to refer to a general text for a more detailed explanation.

Take notes as you study.  You may want to refer to **Volume II:  Skills Development in Reading and Quantitative** for a system and practice in notetaking.   The page layout of this workbook was designed with notetaking in mind, as the right-hand column headings on each page of this chapter show.

## 1.6     Preparation for the New MCAT

It is important to reemphasize that the best preparation for the MCAT is good high school and college preparation. But even if this is lacking, a good, well-planned review can improve your performance on this exam.   Arbitrarily, three phases of preparation and testtaking may be delineated.  The first should precede the test by months and should be concerned with the work of hard study.   The second phase may be the weeks- to month-long period or so before the test and should be concerned with a final systematic review and relaxation.  Taking the test is the third phase.  A rough timetable should be established by each student to fit individual needs.

For the first phase, the following are important considerations:

(1)   the student should determine his/her weaknesses and strengths by subject or sub-subject areas;

(2)   more time should be spent on weak subjects, but enough time should be spent on strong subjects to keep them strong;

(3)   based on the above considerations, a loose timetable should be established for a systematic and thorough review of the following subjects:

    (a)   Biology
    (b)   General Chemistry
    (c)   Organic Chemistry
    (d)   Physics
    (e)   Quantitative Skills
    (f)   Reading Skills
    (g)   Practice Tests in The MCAT Student Manual and How To Prepare for the MCAT, or others;

(4)   make the approximate timetable by estimating the number of sections of the manual which can be done each week and the total number of sections which need to be studied-- for example, if a student decides to do three sections per week and intends to review 54 sections, this will require 18 weeks; time required for the other activities will have to be added to this;

(5)   as the review progresses, note questions and points in the section which will need to be reviewed again and plan on some time to review them--for example, 4 weeks to review again what has already been studied;

(6)   during the semester the MCAT is to be taken, register for a reasonable course load to allow time for review;

(7)   course texts should be consulted for points which need additional discussion;

(8)   an example of a timetable is the following:

| | |
|---|---|
| Time to review 54 sections at a rate of 3 per week | 18 weeks |
| Time to study reading and quantitative study materials in **Volume II** | 12 weeks |
| Time to study and take practice tests | 2 weeks |
| Time to review materials again | 4 weeks |
| Total time to prepare | 36 weeks |

As can be seen, an adequate review takes many months.


## WEEKS/DAYS BEFORE THE TEST DATE

The second phase covers the week and days just prior to the test.

Relaxation and last-minute reviews are indicated. Relaxation does not mean inebriation, however. It means sufficient rest and activities to keep anxiety and tension at a healthy level--there is usually no way that these can be eliminated. If a solid preparation has been made as outlined above, there is no need for a last-minute panic that not enough is known for the test. Knowledge will not fade away so rapidly. To alleviate some of this stress, unhurried but relaxed reviews of certain areas that are of concern may be useful.

These reviews should not be at the expense of rest. The night before the test, a good night's sleep is essential. Drugs of any type should be avoided unless medically indicated. Also, the last week is a good time to take additional practice tests and review testtaking techniques and strategy. The checklists and notes made in the margins of this workbook are a valuable means of rapid review during this time, and relaxation tapes may reduce further stress.

## TAKING THE TEST

The third phase is the test itself. Certain principles are basic to the development of testtaking skills:

(1)   knowledge of the subject is fundamental; a good preparation will pay many dividends;

(2)   there is a finite amount of time to answer a finite number of questions;

(3)   no one (repeat, no one) will answer all of the questions correctly and no one will answer all the questions wrong.

Suggestions during the test:

(1)   Take time to skim the total number and, briefly, the types of questions. Look over the answer sheet to be certain of its format. From this, a little relief in tension may occur and an estimate of how fast to progress through the questions may be made. All this can take 1 minute at the most.

(2)   Estimate what question to be on about one-quarter, one-half, and three-quarters through the time period, and when the 'first pass' should be completed. Remember, time should be left available to go over missed answers. For example, suppose a section has 45 questions and the time limit is 30 minutes. The "first pass" through the test may require 20 minutes. Then by 10 minutes into the test, 22-23 questions should be completed. The final 10 minutes (of the total 30 minutes) may be spent going over the more difficult questions which were skipped. The time allocation is highly individual and should be established through practice.

(3)   During the first pass, all questions should be answered which are definitely known (greater than 80% certain) or definitely not known (greater than 80% unsure). There

will be many questions which will be known immediately--answer them and then forget them. By the same token, learn to recognize questions which there is no chance of answering and spend no more than 5-10 seconds on them. These should be marked on the same letter each time so that the maximum probability of getting them right is obtained.

(4)  **No answer should be filled in on the answer sheet, on the first pass, that has any chance of being changed later.** The answer sheet should be used as a means of rapid assessment of those questions which need to be gone over. This also ensures that all questions are answered--which they should be. See #3 above and #5 below.

(5)  After spending approximately 30 seconds on any one question, it should be passed over and that space on the answer sheet left blank. If this much time is spent on a question, there should be some chance of getting it right. If there are options which are definitely wrong, they should be crossed out. This means when the question is gone over again, time is not wasted on those options. Enhancement of the probability of getting the question right and increasing the time efficiency of going over the question the second time are key objectives of this approach.

(6)  If arithmetic operations or problem solving questions pose particular difficulties, and these types of questions do not form a large part of the subtest, it is reasonable to go over the other questions first. Don't get bogged down on one problem because it seems like you should be able to solve it. Save this for last and go on to other questions. Set up arithmetic operations (adding, dividing, etc.) on scrap paper to be sure no stupid mistake is made in arithmetic after setting up the problem correctly.

(7)  **Make sure the question is being answered as it is stated and that a different question has not been consciously or unconsciously imposed upon it.** This requires constant, diligent checking by the testtaker.

(8)  There is no prize for finishing early. Take enough time to go through the test.

Just before the test or during breaks, make sure physiological needs are satisfied. Time lost during the test for bladder, bowel, hunger or thirst is unfortunate.

All of the above points should be practiced while reviewing specific sections of this workbook. Set time limits and practice the required techniques discussed above.

**1.7     Correlation of Volume I and II Content and the Actual MCAT**

The MCAT Student Manual published by the Association of American Medical Colleges does not yet (1986) reflect the new changes incorporated into the test in the Science Knowledge, Science Problems, and Writing sections. Those changes are explained below in figure 1.1. Actual exam time exceeds 6½ hours (see below).

Questions on the sample MCAT in the manual were analyzed for the Biology, Physics, Chemistry, and Science Problems subtests only. If a question on the sample test was found verbatim or nearly verbatim in this book, that question was labeled as direct. If a question on the sample test could be answered directly from a concept or something explained in this book, then it was labeled as indirect. A question in the sample MCAT that was not covered in this book was labeled as not in book. However, many of these questions could be answered from information present in the question itself. Figure 1.1 illustrates the correlation between the sample questions and the material covered in this book. The data in figure 1.1 mean that if this book is studied and all the information in it is correctly applied, an average of 80-90 percent of all questions on the actual MCAT could be answered.

**AAMC PRACTICE MCAT:   SAMPLE TEST (6.5 hours)**

| Subtest | Total Number of Questions | Number of Direct Questions | Number of Indirect Questions | Number of Questions Not in Book | Percent Covered* in this edition A COMPLETE PREP |
|---|---|---|---|---|---|
| BIOLOGY | 38 | 28 | 8 | 2 | 95% |
| CHEMISTRY | 49 | 22 | 19 | 8 | 84% |
| PHYSICS | 38 | 26 | 10 | 2 | 95% |
| SCIENCE PROBLEMS | 66 | - - - | 20 | - - - | 30% |
| | 191 | | | | |

*Note: "Percent Covered" equals Number of Direct Questions plus Number of Indirect Questions, divided by Total Number of Questions, times 100; or, the sum of the questions (Direct plus Indirect) that can by gotten correct by studying this book, divided by the total questions, times 100.

**AAMC ACTUAL MCAT (6.8 hours)**

| Subtest | Number of Questions | Time Allocated** |
|---|---|---|
| SCIENCE KNOWLEDGE | Biol- 38 } Chem- 38 } 109 Phys- 33 | 115 min. |
| Rest Period: | - - - | 10 min. |
| SCIENCE PROBLEMS | 60 (20 sets: Biol 6, Chem 10, Phys 4) | 78 min. |
| WRITING | 1 essay | 45 min. |
| Lunch Break: | - - - | 60 min. |
| READING SKILLS | 68 | 85 min. |
| Rest Period: | - - - | 10 min. |
| QUANTITATIVE SKILLS | 68 | 85 min. |

**Note: Actual exam time exceeds six and one-half hours. Total MCAT time equals 408 minutes; total break time equals 80 minutes.

Fig. 1.1 - Correlation of this book with "Sample Test" from The MCAT Student Manual

# CHAPTER 2:

# REVIEW

# OF

# BIOLOGY

## 2.1    Enzymes

### 2.1.1    REVIEW OF ENZYMES

Enzymes are the means by which organisms make (anabolism) needed molecules, break down (catabolism) unneeded molecules, produce energy, and, in general, maintain homeostasis (e.g., by regulating entry and exit of molecules and ions).  A key aspect of their function is that they can be regulated to function as needed.

The total enzyme (holoenzyme) may be composed of a protein (apoenzyme) part with or without an associated molecule called a prosthetic group (nonprotein organic molecule) also called a cofactor or coenzyme or a metal ion.  The enzyme molecule catalyzes (by lowering the activation energy) chemical reactions at the conditions found in living organisms--conditions under which these reactions would not ordinarily occur.  Note that the protein part passes through the reaction unchanged (like a true catalyst), but the prosthetic groups, etc., which function as donors or acceptors of chemical groups, may or may not pass through the reaction unchanged.  Some enzymes exist as zymogens and need to be activated by the cleaving of certain peptide bonds.  A portion of the molecule may or may not be lost, but a conformational change usually occurs to expose the active site of the enzyme.  An example is the conversion of trypsinogen to trypsin by enterokinase.

A key feature of enzyme function is their specificity.  This means that enzymes are able to recognize certain molecules and not others due to minor chemical differences between them.  A microenvironment is created by the tertiary structure of the protein that creates distinctive requirements of spatial and electrical organization (distribution of positive/negative charges or polar groups) that a molecule must possess in order to be bound by the molecule.  This microenvironment need not be rigid as in the lock (enzyme) and key (molecule or substrate) idea, but may be inducible in the enzyme by the substrate as in the "induced fit hypothesis" of Koshland. Specificity may be absolute (only one molecule acceptable to the enzyme) or relative (a series of molecules acceptable, but some more than others).  Note that since enzyme reactions are reversible, an enzyme can still have absolute specificity by reacting with one molecule in one direction and with another molecule in the opposite direction.  The bonding is of a non-covalent type (hydrogen, ionic, van der Waals, hydrophobic).

Another key aspect of enzyme function is the active site idea.  The substrate (molecule) is bound as discussed under specificity above. The appropriate chemical reaction is then catalyzed by structures in this active site.  Note that for a reaction to occur the molecule bound must be able to undergo the reaction catalyzable by the enzyme. It is doubtful that the active site functions by causing mechanical bond strain in appropriate bonds, such that they are broken and new ones are made.  Rather, the active site has the appropriate side groups of the amino acids, appropriate prosthetic groups, etc., and a microenvironment all conducive to lowering the activation energy of the reaction.  The combination required varies with the type of reaction being catalyzed.  For example, a reaction that involves a hydrolysis reaction of an ester may have serine (with its -OH group) to displace the alcoholic part of the ester, aspartic acid (with its $-CO_2H$) and/or histidine (acts as acid or base) for acid-base catalysis, and a hydrophilic microenvironment (versus a hydrophobic one) because ions are produced during the reaction.

Enzymes are controlled in a number of ways. Feedback inhibition (FI) is a basic and effective method of enzyme control. In FI, the product of the enzyme reaction feeds back and blocks the enzyme from converting more substrate to product. In this manner, excessive product is not produced. Similarly, when the product is present in low amounts, there is no enzyme inhibition and the enzyme is converting substrate to product.  Graphically:

Enzyme Reaction:  Substrate(S) $\xrightarrow{\text{Enzyme (E)}}$ Product(P)

Excess Product:  (1) Excess product present: S $\xrightarrow{E}$ P

(2) Enzyme binds product:  E ······· P

(3) Reaction is blocked:  S $\xrightarrow{E\cdots P}\!\!/\!\!/\!\!\rightarrow$

Insufficient Product:  (1) Low amounts of product: S $\xrightarrow{E}$ P

(2) Enzyme does not bind product

(3) Reaction proceeds:  S $\xrightarrow{E}$ P

## 2.1.2    QUESTIONS TO REVIEW ENZYMES

(1)  Enzymes probably play a direct role in all of the following except:

  (a)   maintenance of resting membrane potential by extrusion of $Na^+$ from cells
  (b)   synthesis of mRNA from DNA
  (c)   storage of hereditary information ─ ✓
  (d)   production of ATP

(2)  Since enzymes are proteins, they are affected by the same factors that affect proteins.  An enzyme is "designed" to function under a certain set of conditions.  Which of the following conditions would be most conducive to the normal function of a human cellular enzyme?

  (a)   Temperature = 25°C     (b)   Temperature = 37°C ✓ ✓
  (c)   pH = 1.0               (d)   pH = 10.0

(3)  $NAD^+$ is a non-covalently bound coenzyme for the enzyme $\alpha$-glycerol-phosphate dehydrogenase.  $NAD^+$ picks up an $H^{-1}$ (hydride) and becomes NADH; the enzyme is not affected by the reaction.  The activation energy was lowered by the system.

  (a)   This is not true catalysis because the $NAD^+$ was changed in the reaction.
  (b)   This is true catalysis because the $NAD^+$ was not covalently bound to the enzyme.
  (c)   This is true catalysis because the activation energy of the reaction was lowered by the enzyme which was unchanged in the reaction.
  (d)   None of the above.

(4)  Succinate dehydrogenase catalyzes the following reaction:

succinate $\rightleftharpoons$ fumarate.

This is the only reaction it catalyzes.

(a)    The specificity of the enzyme is relative because it binds more than one substrate.
(b)    The specificity of the enzyme is absolute because it catalyzes only one reaction of one pair of substrates.
(c)    The specificity of the enzyme is absolute because it has only one substrate, succinate.
(d)    None of the above.

(5)    D-amino acid oxidase catalyzes the following reaction:

$$\underset{\underset{HNR'}{|}}{\overset{(1)(2)}{R\text{-}CH\text{-}CO_2H}} + \tfrac{1}{2}O_2 \longrightarrow \underset{\overset{\|}{O}}{R\text{-}C\text{-}CO_2H} + R'NH_2.$$

Following are some relative rates of reaction of various substrates with this enzyme.

| Substrate | Relative Rate | R | R' |
|---|---|---|---|
| D-Tyrosine | 13.6 | ⬡–OH | H |
| D-Alanine | 4.6 | $-CH_3$ | H |
| D-Isoleucine | 1.6 | $-\overset{\overset{CH_3}{|}}{C}-CH_2-CH_3$ | H |
| D-Leucine | 1.0 | $-CH_2-CH\overset{CH_3}{_{CH_3}}$ | H |
| L-Tyrosine | 0 | ⬡–OH | H |
| L-Leucine | 0 | $-CH_2-CH\overset{CH_3}{_{CH_3}}$ | H |
| D-Leucylalanyltyrosine | 0 | ⬡–OH | $-\overset{\overset{O}{\|}}{C}-\overset{\overset{H}{\|}}{C}-\overset{\overset{H}{\|}}{N}-\overset{\overset{O}{\|}}{C}-\overset{\overset{NH_2}{\|}}{C}-H$ |

The above information implies that

(a)    the specificity of D-amino acid oxidase is absolute because D-tyrosine has a much higher rate of reaction than other substrates;
(b)    the configuration of carbon #1 is not important for the reaction to occur;
(c)    from the data given, the group at R has more effect on the outcome of the reaction than the group at R';
(d)    the specificity of the enzyme is relative because several molecules may react with the enzyme.

(6)    Enzymes usually combine readily with substrates in order for a reaction to occur.  When the reaction is over, the product (derived from the substrate) usually readily dissociates from the enzyme.  This is in spite of only minor changes in the substrate.  A reason for this might be (the best of those given):

(a)    Although the site of attachment for the substrate has not changed, the overall conformation of the enzyme may be made unfavorable to the product by the reaction.

14

(b) Minor differences in spatial or electrical organization of a molecule are all that are required to make a molecule unacceptable to the enzyme.

(c) The enzyme is forced into an unnatural conformation and this causes it to forceably expel the product.

(d) The substrate is covalently bound to the enzyme because of the enzyme's specificity, whereas the product is not.

(7) Malonate blocks (inhibits) the catalysis of the following reaction by succinate dehydrogenase:

    succinate          fumarate           malonate

Diethyl malonate will not block the reaction. Nor will the diethyl esters of succinate or fumarate undergo the reaction. The above information implies that

(I)    inhibition of the enzyme may be brought about by molecules that resemble the substrate but cannot undergo the reaction;

(II)   the active site of the enzyme may contain positive ions or at least require the presence of $-CO_2^-$ on the substrate;

(III)  monoethyl malonate will not inhibit the reaction.

    (a)  (I) only              (b)  (II) and (III) only
    (c)  (I) and (II) only     (d)  all are implied by the data

2.1.3        ANSWERS TO QUESTIONS IN SECTION 2.1.2

(1) c    (2) b    (3) c    (4) b    (5) d    (6) b    (7) c

2.1.4        DISCUSSION OF ANSWERS TO QUESTIONS IN SECTION 2.1.2


QUESTION #1  (Answer:  c)  The storage of hereditary information is a function of DNA, enzymes play no direct role in this. All of the other processes require direct involvement of enzymes.

QUESTION #2  (Answer:  b)  The function of a cellular enzyme should be maximal at those conditions found in the internal milieu of a cell or a particular compartment of a cell. This would generally be conditions similar to the whole organism. The temperature of 37°C is the normal human body temperature and the normal pH of blood is 7.40. The other conditions are extreme, but there are enzymes that can function at or near most of these--some in the human, some not.

QUESTION #3  (Answer:  c)  True catalysis occurs when the activation energy is lowered and this lowering is accomplished by the enzyme's active site environment. Coenzymes serve the accessory function of transferring chemical groups.

QUESTION #4  (Answer:  b)  Nearly all enzymatic reactions are truly reversible. The product occupies the same site occupied by the substrate, so the enzyme can recognize it, and the substrate-product can be considered as a pair.

QUESTION #5 (Answer: d) The relative specificity of the enzyme should be clear from the several different substrates undergoing the reaction. A case might be made for the "absolute" specificity for D-amino acids which is supported by the data. The configuration of carbon #1 is essential to the reactivity of the substrate because this is the carbon about which the D or L configuration is determined (see $\propto$ -amino acids in Section 4.13.1). The R group represents the side chains of the various amino acids, if the configuration is D at the $\propto$ -carbon (#1 in diagram), the reaction can still occur although variable. The R' could represent a second amino acid (or more), as in D-leucylalanyltyrosine, which does not react at all. Hence, with the limited information given, the presence of a group (other than H) appears critical in the reaction.

QUESTION #6 (Answer: b) Although the other options may sound reasonable, the simplest reason is as in (b) which serves to emphasize that only small differences in substrate structure can affect enzyme recognition and reaction.

QUESTION #7 (Answer: c) The structures not given are

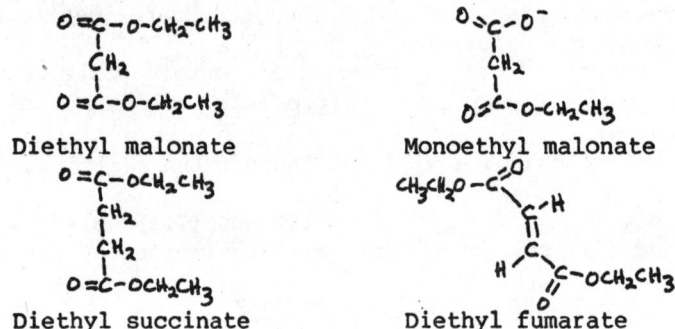

Diethyl malonate          Monoethyl malonate

Diethyl succinate          Diethyl fumarate

Statement (I) is reasonable given that malonate and succinate are similar and since specificity is based upon similarity in structure. Also this reaction requires the group,

for the reaction to occur and malonate does not have this. So, malonate will bind at the active site and block succinate; but it will just sit there and not react. It appears that only molecules with two (or one?) $-CO_2^-$ (which is negative) are attracted to the active site. There is no evidence one way or the other about a molecule with one $-CO_2^-$ and one $-CO_2CH_2CH_3$.

2.1.5          VOCABULARY CHECKLIST FOR ENZYMES

√ __ anabolism —          √ __ prosthetic group
√ __ catabolism —         √ __ cofactor
√ __ holoenzyme —         √ __ coenzyme
√ __ apoenzyme  p 20      √ __ catalysis

16

2.1.6          CONCEPTS, PRINCIPLES, ETC. CHECKLIST FOR ENZYMES

&check; general role of enzymes
&check; specificity of enzymes
&check; Active Site Concept
&check; feedback inhibition


2.2          Bioenergetics


2.2.1          REVIEW OF BIOENERGETICS


Energy production involves the step-wise degradation of organic
molecules from more reduced to more oxidized states (reduced means
abundance of hydrogen atoms and lack of, or few, oxygen atoms).  The
process may be aerobic (in the presence of oxygen) or anaerobic
(without the presence of oxygen).  Fermentation is a type of
anaerobic respiration where the final acceptor of electrons is an
organic molecule.  In aerobic respiration, $O_2$ is the final acceptor
of electrons producing $H_2O$ (fate of hydrogens in organic molecules
being oxidized) and $CO_2$ is also produced (the fate of carbon).  (See
Section 2.11.1 for the fate of nitrogen.)


Key organic molecules in energy production are:

(1)    ATP (adenosine  triphosphate).      The  bonds  between  the
       phosphates are high energy (P$\sim$P), and when hydrolyzed (split
       by adding water), this energy (about 7-8 kcals/mole) is
       released.  ATP is the main short term energy storage molecule.


(2)    $NAD^+$ and  $NADP^+$ (nicotinamide  adenine  dinucleotide  and
       nicotinamide adenine dinucleotide phosphate).  These carry two
       electrons and one hydrogen to form, respectively, NADH and
       NADPH.  NADH transfers its electrons to the electron transport
       system.  NADPH is used for synthetic purposes and is the major
       product of the Pentose Shunt in which glucose-6-phosphate
       dehydrogenase is a key enzyme.  Niacin is a part of $NAD^+$ and
       $NADP^+$.


(3)    FAD (Flavin adenine dinucleotide).  FAD carries two electrons
       and two hydrogens as $FADH_2$ to the electron transport chain.
       Its most important role is in the breakdown of fatty acids.
       Riboflavin is a component of FAD.


(4)    Cytochromes (b,c,a).      They transfer electrons (which are
       attached to iron) and they are part of the electron transport
       chain. The iron is in a porphyrin ring (together called heme)
       which is bound by a protein.


The four key processes of energy production are glycolysis, the
citric acid cycle (Kreb's cycle, Tricarboxylic Acid Cycle or TCA

17

cycle), the electron transport system (ETS), and oxidative phosphorylation. Glycolysis (Fig. 2.1) takes glucose ($C_6$) and converts it to two pyruvates ($C_3$). This produces 2ATPs and 2NADHs. If no oxygen is around, the NADH converts pyruvate to lactic acid (as in exercise) which may be converted to alcohol (as in a type of fermentation). The latter process is anaerobic glycolysis. In the presence of oxygen, the pyruvate ($C_3$) is converted to acetyl CoA ($C_2$) and $CO_2$ with 2NADHs produced per original glucose. CoA (Coenzyme A) is an acyl carrier and the vitamin pantothenic acid is a key component. Acetyl CoA may also arise from fatty acid and amino acid breakdown. The acetyl CoA ($C_2$) enters the citric acid cycle (Fig. 2.2) by combining with oxaloacetic acid ($C_4$) to form citrate ($C_6$). This is degraded step-wise to oxaloacetic acid again producing 3NADHs, 1FADH$_2$, and 1ATP (from GTP) for each cycle (must double to get production per original glucose) as well as $CO_2$ and $H_2O$. The NADH and FADH$_2$ enter the ETS in this sequence:

$$(1) \qquad\qquad\qquad (2) \qquad\qquad (3)$$
$$NAD \longrightarrow FAD \longrightarrow ubiquinone\ (CoQ) \longrightarrow Cyt\ b \longrightarrow Cyt\ c \longrightarrow Cyt\ a \longrightarrow O_2$$

Each intermediate is first reduced (receives electrons from) by the preceding and oxidized (gives electrons to) by the following, with oxygen as the final acceptor being converted to water. ATPs are produced at 1, 2, and 3 by the process called oxidative phosphorylation. Each NADH produces 3ATPs and each FADH$_2$ produces 2ATPs. Malonate is a potent inhibitor of the citric acid cycle. Cyanide is a potent inhibitor of the ETS at Cyt a.

Anaerobic glycolysis yields a net of 2ATPs per glucose. Aerobic glycolysis (because it proceeds to the citric acid cycle and ETS) yields a total of 38ATPs per glucose as follows:

| STEP | Molecules Produced | ATP Yield |
|---|---|---|
| Glycolysis | 2ATP | 2ATP |
|  | 2NADH | 6ATP |
| Pyruvate to acetyl CoA | 2NADH | 6ATP |
| Citric Acid Cycle (2 turns) | 2ATP | 2ATP |
|  | 6NADH | 18ATP |
|  | 2FADH$_2$ | 4ATP |
|  |  | 38ATP |

Of the 686 kcals (for glucose $\longrightarrow CO_2 + H_2O$), aerobic processes store 308 kcals (for 45% efficiency) as ATP; anaerobic efficiency is much less.

Fats store the most energy (9.1 kcals/gm), whereas proteins (about 4.1) and carbohydrate (approximately 4) are about the same.

Glycolysis occurs in the cell cytoplasm. The citric acid cycle occurs in the matrix of the mitochondrion. Electron transport and oxidative phosphorylation occur on the inner membrane of the mitochondrion.

Glycogen

Glucose-1-phosphate ($C_6$)

(1) $\downarrow$ (1) $\leftarrow ATP$

Glucose ($C_6$) $\rightarrow$ Glucose-6-phosphate ($C_6$)

$\downarrow$ (2)

Fructose-6-phosphate ($C_6$)

$\downarrow$ (3) $\leftarrow ATP$

Fructose 1-6 diphosphate ($C_6$)

$\downarrow$ (4)

Glycerol $\leftarrow\leftarrow$ 2 Triose phosphate ($C_3$)

$\downarrow$ (5) $\rightarrow 2NADH + ATP$

2 Phosphoenolpyruvate ($C_3$)

$\downarrow$ (6) $\rightarrow ATP$ $CO_2$

Amino Acids $\rightarrow$ 2 Pyruvate ($C_3$) $\rightarrow$ Acetyl CoA

Lactate $\leftarrow$ (7)   (8) $\nearrow$

Amino   Fatty
Acids   Acids

(1),(3) require 1ATP each
(5) net yield 2NADH, 2ATP per glucose
(6) net 2ATP per glucose
(7) 2NADH used per glucose in the absence of $O_2$
(8) yield 2NADH per glucose

**Fig. 2.1 – Glycolysis** _____

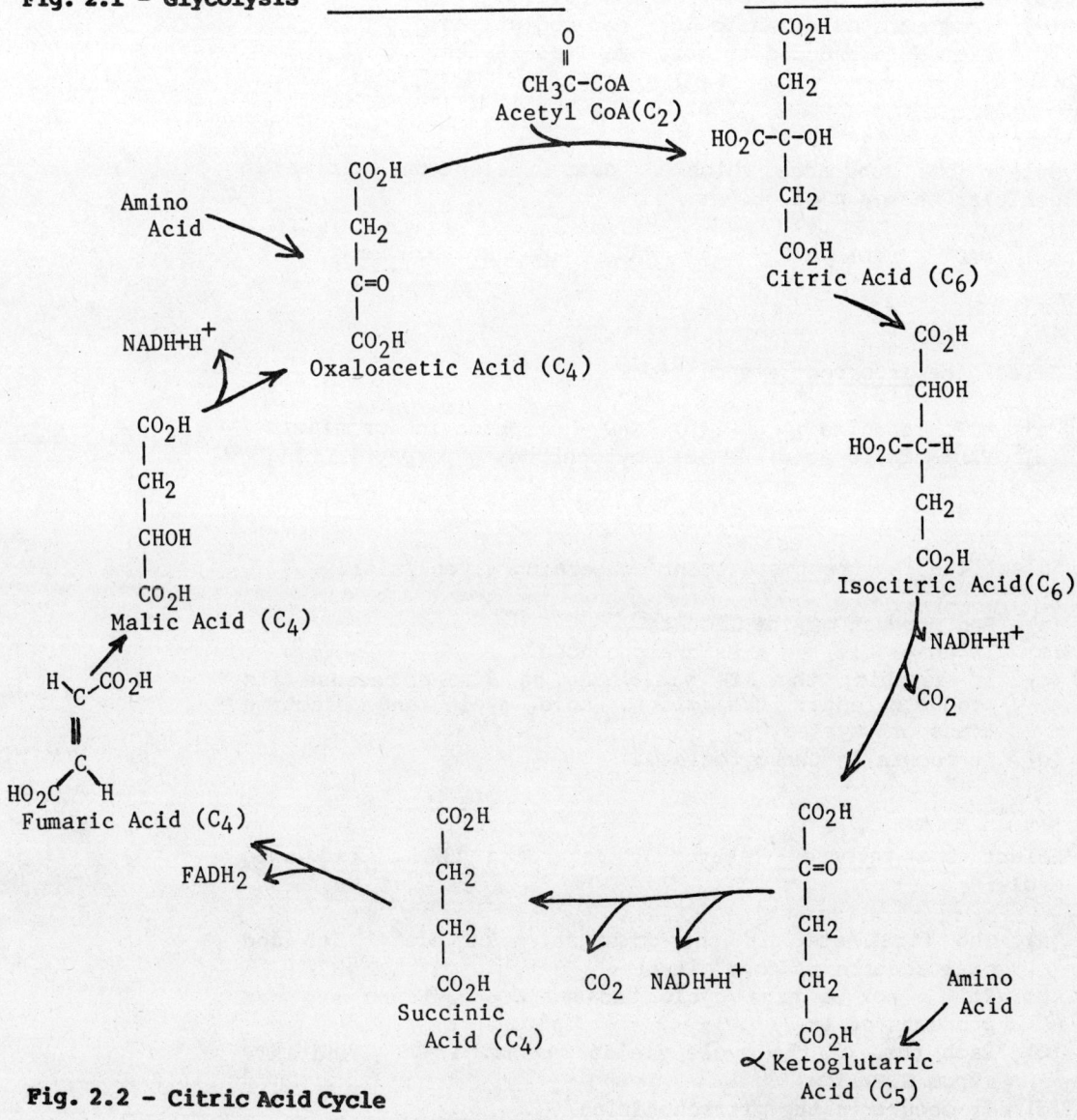

$$\underset{\text{Acetyl CoA}(C_2)}{CH_3\overset{\overset{O}{\|}}{C}-CoA}$$

Amino Acid $\rightarrow$

$CO_2H$
|
$CH_2$
|
$C=O$
|
$CO_2H$
Oxaloacetic Acid ($C_4$)

$CO_2H$
|
$CH_2$
|
$HO_2C-C-OH$
|
$CH_2$
|
$CO_2H$
Citric Acid ($C_6$)

$CO_2H$
|
$CHOH$
|
$HO_2C-C-H$
|
$CH_2$
|
$CO_2H$
Isocitric Acid ($C_6$)

NADH+H$^+$ $\uparrow$

$CO_2H$
|
$CH_2$
|
$CHOH$
|
$CO_2H$
Malic Acid ($C_4$)

$\downarrow$ NADH+H$^+$
$\downarrow$ $CO_2$

$$\underset{\text{Fumaric Acid }(C_4)}{\overset{H\diagdown C-CO_2H}{\underset{HO_2C\diagup C\diagdown H}{\|}}}$$

FADH$_2$ $\leftarrow$

$CO_2H$
|
$CH_2$
|
$CH_2$
|
$CO_2H$
Succinic Acid ($C_4$)

$CO_2$   NADH+H$^+$

$CO_2H$
|
$C=O$
|
$CH_2$
|
$CH_2$
|
$CO_2H$
$\alpha$ Ketoglutaric Acid ($C_5$)

Amino Acid $\nearrow$

**Fig. 2.2 – Citric Acid Cycle** _____

19

(1)    Which substance has the highest energy content per gram?

   (a)  proteins    (b)  fats    (c)  carbohydrates    (d)  phospholipids


(2)    The cytochromes are involved in:

   (a)  citric acid cycle       (b)  oxidative phosphorylation
   (c)  glycolysis              (d)  electron transport system


(3)    In the biological production of energy from chemical molecules, the step-wise degradation is

   (a)  by addition of hydrogens to molecules;
   (b)  by removal of oxygen from molecules;
   (c)  from more oxidized to more reduced states;
   (d)  from more reduced to more oxidized states.


(4)    Select the substance which is not an electron carrier in cellular energy production:

   (a)  $NAD^+$    (b)  ATP    (c)  FAD    (d)  ubiquinone


(5)    Select the incorrect association:

   (a)  ATP - adenine        (b)  NAD - nicotinamide or niacin
   (c)  FAD - folic acid     (d)  cytochromes - porphyrin ring


(6)    Select the incorrect statement concerning glycolysis:

   (a)  End product may be lactate.
   (b)  If anaerobic, no ATPs are produced.
   (c)  If aerobic, the ATP yield can be 38ATPs because its products enter the citric acid cycle and electron transport system.
   (d)  It occurs in the cytoplasm.


(7)    Select the incorrect statement regarding the citric acid cycle:

   (a)  The first step is the combination of acetyl CoA and oxaloacetate to form citrate.
   (b)  It is not a true cycle because $CO_2$ and $H_2O$ are net products of it.
   (c)  Each turn of the cycle yields 3NADHs, 1$FADH_2$, and 1ATP (from GTP).
   (d)  It occurs in the mitrochondrion.

(8)  Select the incorrect statement:

  (a)  The final receptor of electrons in the electron transport
       system is oxygen.
  (b)  Oxidative phosphorylation (production of ATPs) occurs
       only at certain steps in the electron transport system.
  (c)  The electron transport system can produce ATPs without
       oxidative phosphorylation occurring.
  (d)  Both electron transport and oxidative phosphorylation
       occur on the inner membrane of the mitochondrion.

(9)  Cyanide blocks cellular production of energy at which stage?

  (a)  glycolysis                (b)  citric acid cycle
  (c)  electron transport system (d)  oxidative phosphorylation

(10) Below are structures of a typical fatty acid and a hexose:

Fatty Acid

Hexose

If both were degraded bioenergetically to $CO_2$ and $H_2O$, equal
weights of fatty acid would yield

  (a)  more energy because it is more reduced than the hexose;
  (b)  less energy because it is more oxidized than the hexose;
  (c)  less energy because it is more reduced than the hexose;
  (d)  more energy because it is more oxidized than the hexose.

2.2.3      ANSWERS TO QUESTIONS IN SECTION 2.2.2

(1)  b      (2)  d      (3)  d      (4)  b      (5)  c
(6)  b      (7)  b      (8)  c      (9)  c      (10) a

2.2.4      DISCUSSION OF ANSWERS TO QUESTIONS IN SECTION 2.2.2

QUESTION #1-9  Answers found or discussed in reading.

QUESTION #10  (Answer: a)  A reduced compound has all (or mostly)
hydrogens and not oxygens.  The fatty acid has many more hydrogens
and fewer oxygens so it is more reduced.  The more reduced a
compound, the higher the energy that can be released when it is
oxidized to $CO_2$ and $H_2O$.  The factor of the number of atoms in each
molecule is eliminated by considering the substances on a weight
basis.

## 2.2.5 VOCABULARY CHECKLIST FOR BIOENERGETICS

- aerobic
- anaerobic
- fermentation
- ATP
- high energy bonds
- acetyl CoA

- $NAD^+$, $NADP^+$
- FAD
- cytochromes
- pyruvate
- glucose

## 2.2.6 CONCEPTS, PRINCIPLES, ETC. CHECKLIST FOR BIOENERGETICS

- energy content of reduced vs. oxidized organic molecules
- molecules that serve as electron acceptors
- glycolysis
- citric acid cycle
- electron transport system
- oxidative phosphorylation
- localization of the processes of energy production in the cell
- interrelationships of the pathways above
- energy production (ATPs) by the various pathways from glucose
- relative energy content of proteins, fats, carbohydrates

## 2.3 Nucleic Acids

### 2.3.1 REVIEW OF NUCLEIC ACIDS

Nitrogen bases (NB) combine with five carbon sugars (S) to form
<u>nucleosides</u> which combine with <u>inorganic phosphate</u> (P) to form
<u>nucleotides</u> which polymerize to form <u>nucleic acids</u> (Fig. 2.3).

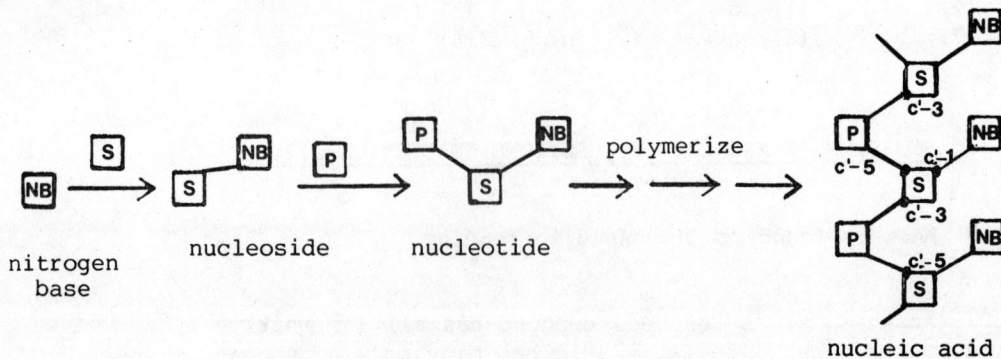

**Fig. 2.3 – Relation of Nucleotides, Nucleosides, and Nucleic Acids**

An example of a nucleotide is deoxyadenylic acid:

AMP (Adenosine monophosphate)

The <u>nitrogen bases</u> are the substituted <u>purines</u> (two rings) and <u>pyrimidines</u> (one ring), see Fig. 2.4. <u>Guanine (G)</u> and <u>adenine (A)</u> are purines. <u>Thymine (T)</u>, <u>cytosine (C)</u>, and <u>uracil (U)</u> are pyrimidines.

purine          pyrimidine          D-ribose          D-2-deoxyribose

**Fig. 2.4 – Components of Nucleotides**

The sugars are <u>ribose</u> and <u>2-deoxyribose</u> (Fig. 2.4.) The nitrogen bases bond at C'-1 to form nucleosides. Then one, two, or three phosphates attach at C'-5 of the sugar and nucleotides result (Figs. 2.3, 2.4).

The triphosphate nucleotides then polymerize to form nucleic acids by eliminating two phosphates in the process. The phosphate of one nucleotide is bound to the C'-3 hydroxyl of the sugar of the next. If the sugar is ribose, then the nucleic acid is <u>ribonucleic acid</u> <u>(RNA)</u>. If the sugar is deoxyribose, then the nucleic acid is <u>deoxyribonucleic acid (DNA)</u>. A further restriction is that DNA contains thymine and RNA contains uracil; they both contain adenine, guanine and cytosine.

DNA has a <u>helical structure</u> with sugar-phosphates as the backbone with the nitrogen bases sticking off at more-or-less right angles (Fig. 2.5). It is composed of two strands of nucleic acids running in antiparallel fashion (i.e., one strand goes 5'⟶ 3' and the other 3'⟶ 5' ). The nitrogen bases pair by hydrogen bonding and this holds the strands together. The nitrogen bases which pair are dictated by the matching up of hydrogen bonding sites and by space limitations in the double helix (proposed by Watson-Crick) which require a purine (two rings) and pyrimidine (one ring) to bond to each other. Adenine and thymine pair forming two hydrogen bonds. Guanine and cytosine pair forming three hydrogen bonds. Uracil replaces thymine in RNA which may occasionally have pairing of strands. The more hydrogen bonds, the more stable the nucleic acid. Hydrophobic bonds between the stacked nitrogen bases also stabilize the double helix.

DNA is <u>duplicated</u> in a semi-conservative fashion. That is, each strand serves as the template upon which a new complementary strand is made (Fig. 2.6). Note that the actual process is very complicated and may occur at multiple sites along the DNA strand simultaneously.

----- = hydrogen bond

**Fig. 2.5 – Base Pairing**

Double Helix    new strands(ns) made by using old(os)    completed duplication

**Fig. 2.6 – Semiconservative Duplication**

### 2.3.2    QUESTIONS TO REVIEW NUCLEIC ACIDS

(1)    Which of the pairs below do not normally hydrogen bond in nucleic acids?

    (a)    adenine-thymine    (b)    adenine-guanine
    (c)    guanine-cytosine    (d)    adenine-uracil

(2)    Both DNA and RNA contain all the nitrogen bases except:

    (a)    guanine    (b)    adenine    (c)    cytosine    (d)    thymine

(3)    The sugar found in DNA is:

    (a)    deoxyribose    (b)    ribose    (c)    dextrose    (d)    deoxyglucose

(4)    Nucleic acids are composed of repeating units of:

    (a)    nucleotides    (b)    nucleosides
    (c)    nitrogen bases    (d)    adenines

(5)    Which is not a pyrimidine?

    (a)    guanine    (b)    thymine    (c)    cytosine    (d)    uracil

(6)    DNA always differs from RNA by

    (a)    forming hydrogen bonds between strands;
    (b)    having thymine and not uracil;
    (c)    being found only in the nucleus;
    (d)    having a sugar-phosphate backbone.

(7)   The following is one strand of a double helix of DNA (showing only nitrogen bases).   What is the structure of its complementary strand? (A=adenine, G=guanine, T=thymine, C=cytosine, U=uracil )

(8)   Given the following data, which organism probably has the most heat stable DNA?

| Organism | (A+T)/(G+C) ratio |
| --- | --- |
| Mycobacterium phlei | 0.49 |
| Escherichia coli | 1.02 |
| Calf Thymus | 1.29 |
| Bacteriophage T2 | 1.90 |

(a)  Mycobacterium phlei        (b)  Escherichia coli
(c)  Calf thymus                (d)  Bacteriophage T2

(9)   Methods to differentiate between DNA and RNA might involve all of the following except

(a)   reaction of ribose with orcinol under suitable conditions;
(b)   ultraviolet absorption by nitrogen bases at 260nm;
(c)   chromatography to separate the different nitrogen bases;
(d)   $^{14}C$ labeled uracil.


2.3.3        ANSWERS TO QUESTIONS IN SECTION 2.3.2

(1) b   (2) d   (3) a   (4) a   (5) a   (6) b   (7) c
(8) a   (9) b


2.3.4        DISCUSSION OF ANSWERS TO QUESTIONS IN SECTION 2.3.2


QUESTIONS #1-6  Discussion in Section 2.3.1.

QUESTION #7  (Answer: c) The complementary DNA strand is the opposite of the given strand and must be 3' ⟶ 5' .  The base pairing is as discussed in the reference.

25

QUESTION #8  (Answer: a)  The higher the percentage of G+C pairs, the higher the heat stability because more hydrogen bonds (three per G+C pair vs. two per A+T pair) are present making it more difficult to disrupt the double helix.  This means the smaller the ratio $\frac{A+T}{G+C}$, the larger the G+C so the answer is (a).

QUESTION #9  (Answer: b)  One must look for chemical differences between DNA and RNA and exploit them.  (a) uses the fact that RNA contains ribose and DNA contains deoxyribose.  (c) and (d) use the fact that RNA contains uracil and DNA doesn't.  The selection (b) measures nitrogen bases, in general, and does not distinguish between them and, therefore, could not distinguish between RNA and DNA.  This method does distinguish between proteins and nucleic acids.

2.3.5          VOCABULARY CHECKLIST FOR NUCLEIC ACIDS

| | | |
|---|---|---|
| ✓ nitrogen bases | ✓ nucleic acid | ✓ guanine |
| ✓ cytosine | ✓ nucleoside | ✓ purine |
| ✓ adenine | ✓ uracil | ✓ nucleotide |
| ✓ pyrimidine | ✓ thymine | ✓ ribose |
| ✓ deoxyribose | ✓ DNA | ✓ RNA |

2.3.6          CONCEPTS, PRINCIPLES, ETC.  CHECKLIST FOR NUCLEIC ACIDS

✓ structure of DNA
✓ replication of DNA
✓ composition of DNA vs. RNA
✓ pairing of the nucleotides

2.4          **Biosynthesis**

2.4.1          REVIEW OF BIOSYNTHESIS

DNA has the information which is the key of life.  This information codes for the sequence of amino acids in proteins and is the sequence of nucleotides (see Section 2.3.1) in DNA.  The genetic code (triplet code) is 64 sets of sequences of three nucleotides each.  Sixty-one of these code for amino acids and three are punctuation marks (terminate protein chains).  Some amino acids have only one triplet (methionine, tryptophan) while one has six (leucine).

The genetic code is universal (all living organisms have the same code).  A gene or cistron is the sequence of triplets that codes for a single polypeptide chain.  DNA is duplicated semiconservatively (using each strand as a template for the new DNA strand) by DNA polymerase from 3' to the 5' end (see Section 2.3.1).  Information on DNA is passed to mRNA (messenger RNA) by the process called transcription. Only one of the DNA chains is used, the enzyme is called RNA polymerase, and the direction of synthesis is 3' to 5'. The mRNA is then used as a guide to make proteins by a process called translation.

Once the mRNA is synthesized from DNA, it moves out of the nucleus (eucaryotes) through pores and into the cytoplasm. There it attaches to the small subunit of the ribosome (composed of rRNA and protein). The large subunit is then attached and a complete ribosome is formed. Meanwhile, an amino acid in the cytoplasm is being activated by phosphorylation with ATP by an activating enzyme (there is one enzyme for each amino acid). Another type of RNA called tRNA (transfer RNA), specific for the amino acid (AA) and activating enzyme is first bound by the enzyme, and then the amino acid is transferred to it by enzymatic action (Fig. 2.7). The tRNA~AA dissociates from the enzyme and moves to a specific position on the large subunit. Another position on the large subunit is occupied by the last tRNA to attach and which binds the carboxyl end of the growing peptide chain. The tRNA molecule has at least three recognition regions, one for the activating enzyme, and, hence, the AA, one for the ribosome, and a sequence of three nucleotides called the anticodon which pairs (hydrogen bonds) with the codon of the mRNA. So, the anticodon of tRNA pairs with the codon of mRNA and the next AA is in position for peptide bond formation which causes a transfer of the growing peptide to this new tRNA. After the peptide bond is formed, a translocation occurs moving the newly attached tRNA peptide into the position previously occupied by the old tRNA-peptide. This latter tRNA is now displaced. A new codon is exposed on the mRNA for another tRNA-AA to attach and the process is repeated. The protein is made from the free amino end to the free carboxyl end. More than one ribosome may "read" a mRNA at a time--this creates polyribosomes (polysomes). Synthesis stops when one of the punctuation mark codons is reached. Note that a gene (three nucleotides in this case) is on DNA, a codon is on mRNA and an anticodon is on tRNA (Fig. 2.8, next page).

$$AA + AE \longrightarrow AE - AA{\sim}Pi \xrightarrow{\text{+RNA}} AE \overset{AA{\sim}Pi}{\underset{tRNA}{<}} \xrightarrow{\text{-AE}} t\text{-}RNA{\sim}AA$$

~ = energy bond

**Fig. 2.7 – Activation of Amino Acid (AA) by Activating Enzyme (AE)**

**Fig. 2.8 – Protein Synthesis on Ribosome**

## 2.4.2    QUESTIONS TO REVIEW BIOSYNTHESIS

(1)   The genetic code is composed of sequences of:

    (a)   three nucleotides     (b)   three nucleosides
    (b)   three amino acids     (d)   two amino acids

(2)   The genetic code (triplet code) consists of 64 sets of three nucleotides each. Which statement is <u>incorrect</u> concerning the triplet code?

    (a)   The code is universal (i.e., all living organisms have the same code).
    (b)   All 64 triplets code for amino acids.
    (c)   More than one triplet can code for the same amino acid.
    (d)   A triplet may code for only one amino acid or termination codon.

(3) Select the  correct association:

    (a) duplication-synthesis of DNA using DNA as a template;
    (b) transcription-synthesis of RNA using DNA as a template;
    (c) translation-synthesis of proteins using information on RNA;
    (d) all are correct.

(4) Translation of the genetic code does not directly require:

    (a) activated tRNA~AA      (b) ribosomes
    (c) mRNA                 (d) DNA

(5) Select the incorrect association:

    (a) DNA-codon          (b) mRNA-anticodon
    (c) tRNA-gene           (d) all are incorrect

(6) Translation is the synthesis of proteins using mRNA as a guide.  All are correct concerning translation except

    (a) mRNA initially binds to the small ribosomal subunit;
    (b) the codon of tRNA pairs with the anticodon of mRNA;
    (c) protein synthesis is from the free amino to the free carboxyl end of the protein chain;
    (d) more than one ribosome may read a given mRNA at a time.

(7) All of the following processes occur on the ribosome except

    (a) binding of mRNA to be "read" by tRNAs;
    (b) activation of tRNA and its amino acid;
    (c) peptide bond formation;
    (d) all of the above occur on the ribosome.


2.4.3      ANSWERS TO QUESTIONS IN SECTION 2.4.2


(1) a    (2) b    (3) d    (4) d    (5) d    (6) b    (7) b


2.4.4      DISCUSSION OF ANSWERS TO QUESTIONS IN SECTION 2.4.2


All are adequately discussed in the Section.


2.4.5      VOCABULARY CHECKLIST FOR BIOSYNTHESIS


_____ gene                     _____ tRNA
_____ cistron                _____ rRNA
_____ ribosome subunits     _____ codon
_____ activating enzymes    _____ anticodon
_____ mRNA                    _____ translation

genetic code
duplication of DNA
production of RNA from DNA - transcription
process of translation (overall)
ribosomal role in translation
types of RNA and roles

## 2.5      Eukaryotic Cell

### 2.5.1     REVIEW OF THE EUKARYOTIC CELL

Eukaryotes differ from prokaryotes (see Section 2.6.1) primarily by virtue of membrane bound structures in the former.  The eukaryote is, thus, conveniently divided into a cell membrane, cytoplasmic region, and nuclear region.  The special characteristics of fungi are considered separately.

### 2.5.1.1     The Cell Membrane and Transport

Cell membranes are composed of phospholipid and proteins.  Two major propositions for the structure of the cell membrane are the unit membrane model and the fluid mosaic model (Singer and Nicolson).  The unit membrane model proposes a bilayered structure with two internal lipid layers surrounded by protein layers.  "Pores" (ill-defined) are supposed to be present for movements of large and/or non-lipid molecules (Figure 2.9).  The fluid mosaic model proposes a continuous lipid bilayer with the phosphate ends of the phospholipids in contact with water and their hydrophobic (lipid) tails internally.  Globular proteins are thought to "float" in this sea of lipids.  Some of these proteins may stretch from the outside to the inside of the membrane (Fig. 2.10).

**Fig. 2.9 - Unit Membrane Model    Fig. 2.10 - Fluid Mosaic Model**

Substances move through the membrane by diffusion, osmosis, facilitated diffusion, active transport, phagocytosis, or pinocytosis.  Diffusion is the random movement of free molecules or ions or particles in solution or suspension under the influence of thermal motion toward a uniform distribution throughout the available volume. This can occur through cell membranes if the substance diffuses through the cell "pores." In diffusion, the net movement of solute is from the region of higher concentration to that of lower concentration. Small organic molecules (ethanol, glycerol) and some ions ($Cl^-$) and $H_2O$ are moved by diffusion.

Osmosis is diffusion through a semi-permeable membrane. In osmosis, a solute cannot cross the membrane in order to equalize its concentration on both sides. This then creates a concentration difference for water across the membrane and the water diffuses in response to this to the side with the lower concentration of water (which is the side with the highest concentration of solute). Tonicity refers to relative concentrations of solute in two solutions. Isotonic means the two are equal. A hypertonic solution has more solute per unit volume than the reference. Osmosis (flow of solvent) occurs from hypotonic to hypertonic solution. If an RBC is placed in a solution less concentrated than itself, it swells until it hemolyzes (bursts). If it is placed in a solution more concentrated than itself, it crenates (shrinks). Osmotic pressure is the hydrostatic pressure needed to oppose the movement of the solvent.

Facilitated diffusion is a process by which substances insoluble in a membrane are carried across the membrane with the concentration gradient by means of a carrier substance. Saturation kinetics are observed; that is, as the substrate concentration rises relative to the number of carrier molecules, the rate of transport levels off. Some sugars and amino acids are transported in this fashion.

Active transport is the process of moving molecules uphill against an electrochemical gradient. A carrier molecule is involved as well as the expenditure of energy (ATP). This system exhibits saturation kinetics and inhibition by inhibitors of energy production (e.g., cyanide or 2,4-DNP). An important active transport system is the Na-K pump which is responsible for maintaining the electrical gradient of neurons. Other locations of active transport include the gut (for sugars and amino acids) and the kidney tubules (for secretion and reabsorption of ions and small molecules).

Phagocytosis is a process by which particulate matter adhering to the cell membrane cause the membrane to invaginate around the particle forming a vesicle which is released to the interior of the cell. The vesicle then combines with a lysosome whose enzymes digest its contents.

Pinocytosis is similar to phagocytosis but occurs in response to proteins or strong solutions of electrolytes. It involves the uptake of liquids and for this reason is also called "cell drinking."

2.5.1.2      The Cytoplasm and Cytoplasmic Organelles

The cytoplasm is composed of a matrix containing membrane bound organelles and various other structures such as microtubules. (See Fig. 2.11)

The underlined endoplasmic reticulum (ER) is a double membrane system running throughout the cell. It probably breaks up and reforms and is continuous with the cell membrane and nuclear envelope. In this way it is probably a precursor for other membrane systems and peroxisomes. Rough (granular) ER contains ribosomes on its surface and is concerned with protein synthesis. Smooth ER (SER) is devoid of ribosomes and may serve several functions, a primary one being steroid synthesis. In the liver, SER plays an important role in the metabolism of endogenous small organic molecules, exogenous drugs, and toxins. In muscle, SER is called the sarcoplasmic reticulum and plays a role in impulse conduction and muscle contraction. It may also serve a storage function--starch in plants, glycogen in animals.

The Golgi complex is a collection of smooth membranes probably continuous with the SER. Its primary function is in packaging and secretion of proteins and polysaccharides. It also plays a role in synthesis of complex polysaccharides.

Mitochondria are double membraned organelles which produce ATP. The inner membrane is folded into cristae which contain the enzyme systems of electron transport and oxidative phosphorylation. The matrix contains a circular DNA molecule, procaryotic type ribosomes, elementary bodies (ionic crystals), and enzymes of the Kreb's Cycle. Mitochondria replicate independently of the cell.

Chloroplasts carry out photosynthesis and photophosphorylation. They have a double membrane. The inner membrane is highly folded into grana which contain chlorophyll. DNA and prokaryotic-like ribosomes are also present. Found in green plants.

Lysosomes are single membraned organelles containing acid hydrolases (digestive enzymes). Functions of lysosomes include digestion of the cell at death (autolysis), digestion of substances within the cell, and digestion of substances taken in by phagocytosis (heterolysis). Storage diseases result when one or more of the hydrolytic enzymes are absent or defective. Lysosomes are produced from the rough ER.

Peroxisomes are single membraned, are part of a group of organelles called microbodies and contain enzymes for the metabolism of oxygen and/or hydrogen peroxide.

Cilia have the structure of centrioles (see Section 2.5.1.3), and are at the cell surface bound to the cell by a basal body (kinetosome). Cilia may function in locomotion but more commonly are used to move fluids and particulates past the cell surface.

Flagella are longer than cilia, are used for locomotion, and are composed of a cylinder of nine paired tubules with two unpaired centrally.

Microfilaments are aggregated proteins with no lumen and may be important for maintenance of cell structure and cytoplasmic streaming.

Microtubules are aggregated proteins with a lumen, may be important for intracellular transport and structure, and are inhibited by colchicine.

Ribosomes are important in protein synthesis, composed of rRNA and protein, and are divisible into a large subunit and a small subunit (see Section 2.4.1).

Fig. 2.11 - The Composite Cell

### 2.5.1.3    The Nucleus and Cell Division (Mitosis)

The nucleus is surrounded by a double layered membrane interrupted regularly by pores.  Inside the nucleus is DNA in a form called chromatin (DNA, histones, non-histone protein) which becomes visible as chromosomes during cell division.  A specific region of the chromatin is called the nucleolus where rRNA is made.

Mitosis occurs to maintain an optimal nucleocytoplasmic to volume ratio, allow growth, differentiation, and specialization of cells in a multicellular organism.  There is one division of the cell into two identical diploid (2n, n=number of different chromosomes in a set) daughter cells from one parent cell (assuming these were diploid also).

This cell division involves the processes of cytokinesis (division of the cytoplasm, not discussed) and karyokinesis (division of the nucleus).  When a cell becomes specialized, it generally loses its ability to divide or reproduce itself (nerve cells, muscle cells, red blood cells, e.g.).  Therefore, most cell division occurs in "stem cells" which are highly undifferentiated, multipotential cells with a high rate of cell division (e.g., bone marrow stem cells, crypt cells of the gut).

The cell cycle is divided into four phases.  $G_1$ (Gap) is the first period of cell growth.  It immediately follows cell division and precedes DNA duplication (Phase S).  $G_2$ follows DNA replication and precedes cell division; further growth occurs.  M (mitosis) is the period of cell division.  The cycle is thus:

Interphase comprises $G_1$, S, and $G_2$.  Prophase, metaphase, anaphase, and telophase are part of the M period.  Prophase - the DNA coils tightly and becomes visible as chromosomes, and the nuclear envelope disappears.  The centrioles (structure is a cylinder of nine sets of three tubules each, found near the nucleus in a region called the centrosome; the centrosome contains a pair of centrioles at right angles to each other) have moved to opposite poles of the nucleus and spindle fibers (microtubule structure) are forming from them. Metaphase - the chromosomes arrange radially along the equatorial plane of the cell and the spindle fibers are attached to the centromeres of each chromosome (now being composed of two chromatids, each of which becomes a new chromosome after the centromere divides).  Anaphase - individual chromosomes divide at their centromeres and each new resulting chromosome migrates to the opposite pole being guided by the spindle fibers.  Note that each chromatid of the chromosome at metaphase gives rise to a complete new chromosome after the centromeres divide.  Telophase - the chromosomes uncoil, the nuclear membrane reforms, cytokinesis occurs, and the centrioles replicate themselves.  The cell now enters interphase.  See Section 2.18.1.2 to contrast mitosis and meiosis.  The above concepts are diagrammed in Fig. 2.12.

Interphase-
chromosomes
duplicated

Prophase-
chromosomes form
membranes dissolve
spindles forming

Metaphase-
each duplicated
chromosome lines up

Telophase-
membranes reform
cytokinesis

Anaphase-
centromeres divide
chromosomes migrate

**Fig. 2.12 - Mitosis**

2.5.1.4     General Characteristics of Fungi and Their Life Cycle

Fungi are composed of eukaryotic cells, are plant-like, but contain no chlorophyll.  They are unicellular (e.g., yeast) or multicellular (e.g. molds, mushrooms) with little differentiation into tissue types.  They are parasitic (survive upon living organisms) or saprophytic (survive upon dead organic matter), and they can digest food extracellularly by the excretion of digestive enzymes before absorbing them or can absorb already digested foods.  Multicellular

fungi tend to be filamentous with individual filaments called
hyphae. Masses of hyphae are called mycelia. Fungi are important as
causes of disease, in spoilage of food and materials, as decomposers
of dead organic matter, as sources of food (mushrooms), in food
production (bread yeast, cheese molds), and in alcohol production.

Reproduction is by sexual and/or asexual means with the latter
predominating. The specific cycles vary among the different groups
of fungi. Various sexual stages include ascus formation (has
haploid spores), basidium (2n) formation, or just fusion of special
cells to form zygotes (2n). Asexual structures or stages include the
spores (n), the sporangium (n), and the conidia (n). These are
either spores or give rise to spores. The sporangium and conidia
arise from specialized hyphae. A general scheme for the life cycle
of a typical fungus is in Fig. 2.13.

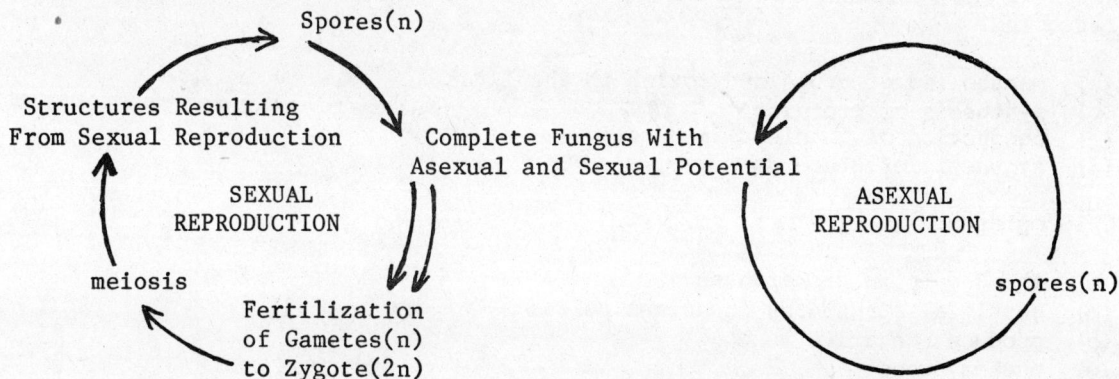

(Note that spores can result from sexual or asexual reproduction.)

**Fig. 2.13 – Life Cycle of a Typical Fungus**

2.5.2      QUESTIONS TO REVIEW THE EUKARYOTIC CELL

(1)   The correct sequence of steps in mitosis is:

      (a)  Prophase, Metaphase, Interphase, Anaphase, Telophase
      (b)  Interphase, Anaphase, Metaphase, Prophase, Telophase
      (c)  Interphase, Prophase, Metaphase, Anaphase, Telophase ✓
      (d)  Anaphase, Prophase, Interphase, Metaphase, Telophase

(2)   Which is not a feature of the unit membrane model of the cell
      membrane?

      (a)  continuous lipid bilayer present
      (b)  globular proteins floating in lipids ✓
      (c)  hydrophobic ends of lipids not in contact with water
      (d)  continuous protein bilayers outside lipid layer

(3)   "Cell Drinking:"

      (a)  phagocytosis          (b)  pinocytosis ✓
      (c)  both                   (d)  neither

35

(4) The substance below not ordinarily found in cell membranes is(are):

(a) globular proteins
(b) phospholipids
(c) DNA ✓
(d) all are found in cell membranes

(5) Active Transport:

(a) diffusion
(b) with the concentration gradient
(b) phagocytosis
(d) Na-K-ATPase ✓

(6) Which of the following is not a function of smooth endoplasmic reticulum?

(a) metabolism of drugs and toxins in the liver
(b) synthesis of proteins ✓
(c) conduction of impulses in muscle
(d) synthesis of steroids

(7) Chloroplasts:

(a) found only in prokaryotes
(b) vestigial structures in animal cells
(c) produce negative ions
(d) photosynthesis ✓

(8) Mitochondria (best answer):

(a) transport of molecules
(b) protein synthesis
(c) cell replication
(d) energy production ✓

(9) Synthesis of Proteins:

(a) lysosomes
(b) Golgi bodies
(c) mitochondria
(d) rough endoplasmic ✓ reticulum

(10) Centrioles:

(a) found in the nucleus
(b) found on chromosomes
(c) make microvilli
(d) form spindle fibers during cell division

(11) Which is not true about the cell cycle?

(a) there are typically four phases $G_1$, $G_2$, S, and M
(b) interphase corresponds with the M phase ✓
(c) S is the phase of DNA synthesis
(d) M is the phase of cell division

(12) Which is not true about mitosis?

(a) It can maintain an optimal nucleocytoplasmic to volume ratio.
(b) It can allow growth of organisms.
(c) It has phases of karyokinesis and cytokinesis.
(d) It results in haploid daughter cells. ✓

(13)  The chromosomes become coiled and visible and the nuclear
      membrane disintegrates.   This is what phase of mitosis?

      (a)  interphase  (b)  prophase  (c)  metaphase  (d)  telophase


(14)  Facilitated diffusion:

      (a)  carrier substances carry molecules across the membrane
      (b)  can go against a concentration gradient
      (c)  requires energy
      (d)  saturation kinetics is not observed

(15)  Fungi:

      (a)  are prokaryotic      (b)  may be unicellular
      (c)  contain chlorophyll  (d)  hyphae are unicellular stages

(16)  In the Fungus

      (a)  the haploid phase tends to dominate;
      (b)  the diploid phase tends to dominate;
      (c)  there is only asexual reproduction;
      (d)  spores are sexual structures only.

(17)  All are associated with reproductive functions in fungi
      except:

      (a)  conidia              (b)  sporangium
      (c)  basidium             (d)  mesenchymal

(18)  A key difference in the mechanism of mitosis and meiosis is

      (a)  mitosis has crossing over of homologous chromosomes
           during prophase;
      (b)  meiosis has a second duplication of DNA during interphase
           I;
      (c)  meiosis has alignment of homologous chromosomes in
           metaphase I and separation of homologous chromosomes in
           anaphase I;
      (d)  mitosis has a reductional division.

(19)  The main difference in the outcome of mitosis versus meiosis
      is

      (a)  meiosis produces identical daughter cells and mitosis
           produces different daughter cells;
      (b)  mitosis occurs only in vertebrates;
      (c)  meiosis produces somatic cells;
      (d)  meiosis results in haploid cells and mitosis results in
           diploid cells.

(20)  If container A has a higher concentration of a solute than
      container B, and they are separated by a semipermeable (to
      solute) membrane, then:

      (a)  nothing happens because membrane is only semipermeable;
      (b)  solute particles move from B to A;
      (c)  solvent moves from B to A; ✓
      (d)  solvent moves from A to B.

37

(21) What probably limits the size a cell may attain?

    (a) surface area
    (b) volume of a cell
    (c) balance of surface area and volume
    (d) specialization of the cell

(22) Which structure below is found in eukaryotes but not prokaryotes?

    (a) ribosomes          (b) mesosomes
    (c) cell walls         (d) mitochondria

(23) Which structure or molecule is <u>not</u> found or made in the nucleus of eukaryotes?

    (a) nucleolus    (b) microsomes    (c) tRNA    (d) chromatin

(24) If red blood cells are put into a hypertonic solution, they will:

    (a) remain the same size      (b) hemolyze
    (c) swell up               (d) shrink

(25) Which structure does not play a part in motion of cells?

    (a) microvilli    (b) cilia    (c) flagella    (d) pseudopods

(26) Which of the following substances probably would not cross a membrane by simple diffusion?

    (a) ethanol    (b) chloride ion    (c) glucose    (d) water

## 2.5.3      ANSWERS TO QUESTIONS IN SECTION 2.5.2

| | | | | | | | | | | | | | |
|---|---|---|---|---|---|---|---|---|---|---|---|---|---|
| (1) | c | (2) | b | (3) | b | (4) | c | (5) | d | (6) | b | (7) | d |
| (8) | d | (9) | d | (10) | d | (11) | b | (12) | d | (13) | b | (14) | a |
| (15) | b | (16) | a | (17) | d | (18) | c | (19) | d | (20) | c | (21) | c |
| (22) | d | (23) | b | (24) | d | (25) | a | (26) | c | | | | |

## 2.5.4      DISCUSSION OF ANSWERS TO QUESTIONS IN SECTION 2.5.2

<u>QUESTIONS #1 - #17</u> Discussed adequately in Section.

<u>QUESTIONS #18, #19</u> Answers obtained by comparing Section 2.5.1.3 (Nucleus and Cell Division) and Section 2.18.1.3 (Meiosis). These differences should be understood well.

<u>QUESTION #20</u> (Answer: c) The solvent moves across the semipermeable membrane from the side <u>it</u> is more concentrated, and the solute is less concentrated (which is side B), to the side where it is less concentrated (and the solute is more concentrated) which is side A. This is osmosis.

<u>QUESTION #21</u> (Answer: c) This is not discussed in the Section.

The reasoning is as follows: the nutritional and energy requirements and waste production are proportional to the volume of the cell. The volume of a cell is proportional to a linear dimension (l=length) cubed, i.e. $l^3$. The flux (i.e., the exchange rates) of materials in (nutrients) and out (wastes) is proportional to the surface area of a cell. The surface area is proportional to a linear dimension squared, i.e. $l^2$. As the cell increases in size (as volume increases), the requirements, given by $l^3$, increase much more rapidly than supply and waste removal, given by $l^2$. Hence, a balance between surface area and volume is required such that supply (and waste removal) can keep in balance with cell requirements.

QUESTION #22 (Answer: d) Membrane bound organelles are not found in prokaryotes, e.g. the mitochondrion. The cell walls (also in plants) and mesosomes (invaginations of cell membrane) are found in prokaryotes. Ribosomes are found in both, although the structures are different.

QUESTION #23 (Answer: b) Microsomes are artifacts produced from the endoplasmic reticulum during cell homogenization and centrifugation. Nucleolus and chromatin are parts of DNA. All RNA, including tRNA, are made from the DNA template in the nucleus.

QUESTION #24 (Answer: d) This is discussed in the Section. The solvent (water) flows from the hypotonic (red cells) to the hypertonic solution by osmosis.

QUESTION #25 (Answer: a) Microvilli and pseudopods were not discussed in the Section. The latter are cytoplasmic extensions that aid in motion as found in amoeba. Microvilli are evaginations (out pouches) of the cell membrane which increase its surface area. Its function is to permit more area for flux of materials in and out of cells, as in the gut.

QUESTION #26 (Answer: c) This is alluded to in the Section. Some ions, lipid soluble substances, and very small molecules (such as ethanol, glycerol, urea) can diffuse through membranes. Polar molecules, ions (especially cations), and larger molecules must enter by other processes.

## 2.5.5 VOCABULARY CHECKLIST FOR EUKARYOTIC CELL

| | | |
|---|---|---|
| unit membrane model | Golgi complex | nucleolus |
| fluid mosaic model | mitochondria | cytokinesis |
| osmotic pressure | lysosomes | karyokinesis |
| diffusion | peroxisomes | cell cycle |
| osmosis | cilia | interphase |
| tonicity | flagella | prophase |
| facilitated diffusion | microfilaments | centrioles |
| active transport | microtubules | metaphase |
| phagocytosis | ribosomes | anaphase |
| pinocytosis | chromatin | telophase |
| endoplasmic reticulum | chromosomes | hyphae |

**2.5.6**     CONCEPTS, PRINCIPLES, ETC.   CHECKLIST FOR EUKARYOTIC
CELL

___✓___ differences between prokaryotes and eukaryotes
___✓___ models of cell membrane structure
___✓___ functions of cell organelles
___✓___ mechanism  of mitosis
___✓___ characteristics of Fungi and Life Cycle


**2.6**       **Viruses and Bacteria (Prokaryotes)**


**2.6.1**     REVIEW OF VIRUSES AND BACTERIA


Prokaryotes (bacteria and blue-green algae) differ from eukaryotes
(Section 2.5) by the latter having (1) genetic material in a nucleus
and DNA conjugated with proteins, (2) organelles bound within
membranes, (3) subcellular structural units to carry out specific
functions (ATP production, photosynthesis, e.g.), and (4) presence
of cell walls made of cellulose or chitin versus murein (amino sugars
and amino acids) as in prokaryotes.  The DNA of prokaryotes is found
in a non-membrane region called the nucleoid.   Enzymes for
metabolism and energy production are either free in the cytoplasm or
bound to the cell membrane, and the ribosomes are smaller than in
eukaryotes.    Viruses are not prokaryotes or eukaryotes but
constitute a group unto themselves.


**2.6.1.1**     Viruses


Viruses are usually called "non-living" and differ from bacteria and
other "living" organisms because they, (1) don't contain both DNA
and RNA, (2) have no metabolic machinery for energy production or
protein synthesis, (3) do not arise directly from other viruses but
depend on the host's metabolic machinery to synthesize them, and (4)
have no membranes to regulate exit and entry.  Structurally, most
viruses consist of a protein coat surrounding a core (center) of
either DNA or RNA.

There are many variations of the basic life cycle of a virus given
below.  A cell may have a special receptor or region that is
recognized by the virus.  The virus attaches and may enter via a
process similar to phagocytosis.  In the cell, the central core of
DNA or RNA and occasionally special enzymes or proteins take over the
host's metabolic machinery to produce new coat proteins and new
viral DNA or RNA.  This may occur in the nucleus or the cytoplasm or
both.  The viral coat and viral core (DNA or RNA) then combine to
form complete viral particles.  At a certain point, the host cell
lyses (bursts) and releases the new viral particles as well as
uncombined viral coats and viral cores.   Sometimes the viral
particles exit by a process similar to reverse phagocytosis and
incorporate  part of the host's cell membrane onto their protein

coat in doing so. The above is typical of a virus that attacks an animal or plant cell.

Viruses that attack bacteria are called bacteriophages. Bacteriophages, in general, consist of head made of a protein coat and a core as before, and they also contain a tail made of protein which is specialized for attaching to bacteria. A bacteriophage attaches to the surface of a bacteria, the core of RNA or DNA is injected into the bacteria, and the protein coat remains on the surface. Then the cycle may proceed as described for viruses above and is called lytic or virulent. However, the bacteriophage nucleic acid may become combined with the bacterial nucleic acid and remain as such for long periods before new bacteriophages are produced and cell rupture occurs. In this case, the bacteriophage is called lysogenic or temperate. The nucleic acid from the bacteriophage is called a prophage. Newly released bacteriophages may contain some bacterial nucleic acid which may be passed onto other bacteria when they are attacked by these bacteriophages. This is the mechanism of transduction.

## 2.6.1.2     Bacteria

The general characteristics of bacterial structure are discussed above under prokaryotes. More specifically, from outside in, a bacteria may have a capsule which is usually made of a polysaccharide mucoid-like material and protects the bacteria from phagocytosis. Inside the capsule is the cell wall, and this prevents the hypertonic  bacteria from bursting. Inside the cell wall is the cell membrane which may contain invaginations called mesosomes where localization of enzymes concerned with similar functions may be found. The cytoplasm and nucleoid are as described above. The DNA is circular and is haploid. Some bacteria contain flagella or cilia for locomotion--these are structurally different from their eucaryotic counterparts.

Bacteria have three common shapes: Cocci (spherical or ovoid), bacilli (cylindrical or rod-like), and spirillia (helically coiled). The cocci are often found in clusters: diplococci (two bacteria together), streptococci (linear chains of cocci), or staphylococci (grape-like clusters of cocci). All of these are made up of individual bacteria with distinct cell walls.

Metabolically, bacteria are aerobic or anaerobic. Anaerobic bacteria may use fermentation (where an organic molecule such as pyruvate or lactate is the final electron acceptor) or inorganic substances as final electron receptors (such as $S \longrightarrow H_2S$). An obligate anaerobe is one that is killed if exposed to oxygen. This is usually because they cannot handle the peroxides (very toxic) produced in oxidative metabolism. A facultative anaerobe can survive in the presence or absence of oxygen. Bacteria may use a great variety of molecules as nutrients. Some are photosynthetic, others heterotrophic (using organic molecules made by other organisms) and others are chemosynthetic (making organic molecules and energy from inorganic precursors). The last group are important in fixation of nitrogen for use by all organisms. The variety of metabolic nutrients required and products produced are extremely important in studying basic questions of genetics, as well as

41

biochemistry, and also in differentiating between the different types of bacteria.

Most bacteria reproduce asexually by the process of binary fission which produces two identical haploid daughter cells by the simple process of mitosis. Genetic recombination, (e.g., transfer and rearrangement of genetic information) may occur by three distinct means: transformation, transduction, and conjugation. Transformation involves a bacterium picking up free DNA from a medium; the free DNA being from a different bacterium. Transduction is the transfer of parts of DNA between bacteria by bacteriophages. In conjugation there is pairing of "male" and "female" forms. DNA is passed sequentially between them via structures called pili. All or a fraction of the DNA may be passed in this way. The above three genetic mechanisms allow extraordinary adaptability and variability of bacteria. Since bacteria can reproduce in a span as short as twenty minutes, a new trait such as drug resistance can spread rapidly in a given population.

2.6.2    QUESTIONS TO REVIEW VIRUSES AND BACTERIA

(1)    Bacteriophages:

   (a)  cause disease in humans      (b)  are viruses
   (c)  are bacteria                 (d)  can reproduce by binary
                                          fission

(2)    Select the substance not ordinarily found in viruses:

   (a)  carbohydrates    (b)  proteins    (c)  RNA    (d)  DNA

(3)    Viruses:

   (a)  are considered to be living organisms
   (b)  consist of protein, lipids, and carbohydrates only
   (c)  do not arise from other viruses directly
   (d)  have an incomplete metabolic machinery for energy
        production

(4)    Eukaryotes are characterized by all except:

   (a)  genetic material in a nucleus
   (b)  organelles bound within membranes
   (c)  presence of cell walls made of murein
   (d)  subcellular structural units to carry out specific
        functions

(5)    "Contains DNA or RNA, no means of energy production, cannot
       reproduce self directly" would be a description of a(an):

   (a)  animal cell  (b)  plant cell  (c)  bacteria  (d)  virus

(6)    In the replication of a virus in a host cell,

       (a)  the virus directs the metabolic machinery of the host;
       (b)  the host directs synthesis of new viral particles;
       (c)  viral particles are made as a single unit (i.e., coat and
            core);
       (d)  coat and core structures are released from the host and
            then combined.


(7)    Structurally, bacteriophages differ from the usual virus by

       (a)  having a protein coat;
       (b)  having a core of DNA or RNA;
       (c)  being able to replicate independently of a host cell;
       (d)  having a tail region made of protein for attaching to
            cells.


(8)    The part of the cycle of a bacteriophage that may be different
       from that of a typical virus is

       (a)  taking over of host cell's metabolic machinery;
       (b)  incorporation of its nucleic acid into the host cell's
            nucleic acid;
       (c)  lysis of host cell;
       (d)  synthesis by host cell of coat and core separately and
            then combining to form complete particle.


(9)    Which structure may protect a bacteria from phagocytosis by
       white blood cells?

       (a)  mesosome    (b)  capsule    (c)  nucleoid    (d)  cell wall


(10)   Select the incorrect association:

       (a)  cocci-spherical
       (b)  bacilli-rod-like
       (c)  diplococci-two cocci
       (d)  staphylococci-linear combinations of cocci


(11)   The process whereby a bacterium picks up DNA from a medium and
       incorporates it into it's own DNA is called:

       (a)  binary fission          (b)  conjugation
       (c)  transformation          (d)  transduction


(12)   Bacteria transfer (exchange) genetic information between
       themselves by all except:

       (a)  transformation          (b)  transduction
       (c)  budding                 (d)  conjugation

(13) Methods used to distinguish between bacteria may include all of the following except:

(a) shape                 (b) nutrient requirements

(c) products of metabolism     (d) all are possible

(14) A form of hepatitis (inflamation of the liver) is caused by a virus. The serum of patients with hepatitis may contain antigens from the virus, $HB_SAg$ (hepatitis B surface antigen) and $HB_CAg$ (hepatitis B core antigen). (An antigen is a substance foreign to the body capable of eliciting an immune response.) Select the correct statement:

(a) This information is inconsistent with what is known about modes of viral replication.
(b) The $HB_CAg$ is probably a lipid.
(c) The $HB_SAg$ is probably a protein.
(d) Enzymes found in liver cells probably do not increase in The serum during the acute disease.

(15) Which of the following would interfere most with the replication of a virus? Assume all agents can only affect the host cell and its contents.

(a) an agent that blocks synthesis of lipids
(b) an agent that blocks synthesis of carbohydrates
(c) an agent that blocks synthesis of proteins
(d) all of the above

(16) In the treatment of viral infections, a drug is discovered that directly blocks the synthesis of the viral protein coat. This drug

(a) probably adversely affects protein synthesis by the host cell and hence may cause side affects in the host;
(b) probably does not affect host protein synthesis.

(17) Given a bacterial population without resistance to a certain drug, all of the following may cause introduction of bacterial resistance except (excluding mutations):

(a) transformation          (b) binary fission
(c) transduction            (d) conjugation

2.6.3       ANSWERS TO QUESTIONS IN SECTION 2.6.2

(1) b    (2) a    (3) c    (4) c    (5) d    (6) a    (7) d
(8) b    (9) b    (10) d   (11) c   (12) c   (13) d   (14) c
(15) c   (16) a   (17) b

2.6.4       DISCUSSION OF ANSWERS TO QUESTIONS IN SECTION 2.6.2

QUESTIONS #1-#13   Adequately discussed in Section.

QUESTION #14 (Answer: c) From the knowledge about viral replication, the coat (protein) and core (nucleic acid) are synthesized separately and then combined. When cell lysis occurs, complete viral particles as well as coat (e.g. $HB_SAg$) and core ($HB_CAg$) may be released. Since, the cells do lyse, their contents would also appear (e.g., the liver enzymes). And, since the antigens are found in the serum, it is not unreasonable to expect the liver enzymes to be there also. In fact, a rise in certain liver enzymes are key to the diagnosis of hepatitis. Also, since incomplete viral particles are liberated into the serum, it might be expected that other viral products might also appear as antigens. Some do, for example the "e"-antigen and viral DNA-polymerase.

QUESTION #15 (Answer: c) Viruses need the synthesis of proteins by the host cell machinery to make their protein coats as well as enzymes necessary to make nucleic acids.

QUESTION #16 (Answer: a) It is the host's metabolic machinery that makes virual protein. Therefore, if the synthesis of viral coat protein is blocked, it is likely, not absolutely necessary, that this is due to a blockage of host protein synthesis.

QUESTION #17 (Answer: b) Without new mutations, binary fission can only produce identical non-resistant daughter cells. The other mechanisms allow the introduction of new nucleic acid which may contain drug resistant genes.

2.6.5    VOCABULARY CHECKLIST FOR VIRUSES AND BACTERIA

_____ bacteriophage                    _____ lytic
_____ virulent                         _____ lysogenic
_____ temperate                        _____ prophage
_____ transduction                     _____ capsule
_____ mesosomes                        _____ cocci
_____ bacilli                          _____ spirillia
_____ diplococci                       _____ streptococci
_____ staphylococci                    _____ obligate anaerobe
_____ facultative anaerobe             _____ binary fission
_____ transformation                   _____ transduction
_____ conjugation

2.6.6    CONCEPTS, PRINCIPLES, ETC. CHECKLIST FOR VIRUSES AND BACTERIA

_____ differences between prokaryotes and eukaryotes
_____ difference of viruses from other organisms
_____ structure of a virus
_____ life cycle of a virus
_____ difference between viruses and bacteriophages in structure and life cycle
_____ structure of a bacterium
_____ shapes of bacteria
_____ metabolism of bacteria
_____ reproduction of bacteria

**2.7**      **Embryology**

*Review*

**2.7.1**      <u>REVIEW OF EMBRYOLOGY</u>


<u>Fusion of the gametes</u> produced by meiosis (see Section 2.18.1 for details) involves first the penetration of the ovum by the sperm. The acrosome (part of sperm that contains hydrolytic enzymes) dissolves the <u>corona radiata</u> (collection of follicle cells and zona pellucida around ovulated ovum), and only the head of the sperm (contains the DNA) penetrates the ovum. Upon penetration, a reaction in the ovum occurs preventing additional sperm from entering. The ovum now completes meiosis II (see Section 2.18.1.3). Then the male and female pronuclei fuse and cleavage of the fertilized egg (zygote) begins.



<u>Growth, differentiation, and morphogenesis</u> occur together after the first few cleavages. The amount of <u>yolk</u> in the egg is an important determinator of the cleavage pattern but will not be discussed. Note, though, that the egg has polarity (i.e., is asymmetrical) by virtue of the yolk distribution. The first few cleavages (4-5) result in a grape-like cluster of cells called the <u>morula</u>. These divisions occurred without cell growth, and, hence, the morula is not much larger than the zygote. The morula develops into a <u>blastula</u> which is a hollow sphere one-cell thick with a cavity called the blastocoel. From this point <u>morphogenesis</u> (movements of cells to delineate shape and function) begins with the invagination of the blastula. What results is a two-layered structure with a new cavity called the <u>archenteron</u> that opens to the outside via the <u>blastopore</u> (site of invagination); this structure is the <u>gastrula</u>. Cells from the lip of the blastopore migrate between the two layers of cells to form a third layer. The gastrula then becomes a three—layered structure composed of <u>ectoderm</u> (outside), <u>mesoderm</u> (middle), and <u>endoderm</u> (inside). The blastopore cells induce the overlying ectoderm to form a neural groove and the embryo is now called a <u>neurula</u>. The neural groove forms the <u>neural tube</u>. At the margins of the neural tube detachment are a group of cells called the <u>neural crest</u> cells which form the adrenal medulla, melanocytes, and myelin sheaths among other tissues. The neural tube develops into the central nervous system (spinal cord and brain). Ventral to the neural tube, mesodermal tissue forms somites which gives rise to the vertebral column (formed on, but not from, the notochord) and associated muscles. The <u>ectoderm develops into</u> the nervous system, the epidermis of the skin and its derivatives, the lens of the eye, and the linings of the mouth and anus. The <u>endoderm will develop into</u> the gut (esophagus, stomach, intestines), associated organs (liver, gallbladder, pancreas), the lung, and the thyroid gland. <u>The mesoderm develops into</u> the skeleton, muscles, kidney, circulatory system (heart and vessels), blood, and dermis of skin. A schematic summary of the sequence above is in Fig. 2.14, following.

**Fig. 2.14 - Early Development of the Embryo**

The question of how a single egg develops into a complex organism is not completely answered. The concepts of differentiation, determination and induction are integral to understanding the changes which occur. <u>Differentiation</u> is the process whereby a cell can change into more specialized cells to become a tissue. A <u>tissue</u> is a set of similar cells which carries out a specific function, such as muscle. The magnitude of this process is appreciated when one realizes that all the varied cells of the human body (muscle, bone, skin, nerve, etc.) arise from the same zygote. What is it about the zygote that allows this differentiation to occur? It is generally accepted that <u>all cells in an organism contain the same genetic information</u> (sequences of genes on DNA). What probably makes one cell different from another is which of these genes is activated. The <u>set of activated genes is responsible for each cell's characteristics</u>--the structural components, metabolic machinery, and general composition of the cell. So, in some way, as the zygote divides (cleavages), different sets of its <u>daughter cells must have different sets of genes activated</u>. Differentiation is not brought about by the daughter cells having different genes (i.e., different sets of genetic material), in general. If the cytoplasm of the zygote was totally homogeneous, then each daughter cell, resulting from the cleavage, would be identical with regard to the nucleus and the cytoplasm and would remain undifferentiated. But, if there were an asymmetrical distribution of cytoplasmic constituents, and the cleavage results in daughter cells with different distributions of these constituents, then the daughter cells would be different. That is, a small amount of cytoplasmic differentiation would have occurred. If these cytoplasmic differences led to the activation of different sets of genes in their respective nuclei, differences between the cells would be perpetuated in their daughter cells, and some degree of true differentiation (production of daughters different from parent cells) will have occurred. So, asymmetrical distribution of cytoplasmic constituents is one way differentiation may be brought about. Then, in general, if a factor can affect the cells' cytoplasmic composition (which can affect the set of activated genes) or if it can affect the nucleus directly to activate (or inactivate) genes, and this effect is unevenly distributed among the cells, differentiation of the cells along different lines can be brought about. Other factors which cause cells to differentiate are: (1) <u>Neighboring cells</u> (by contact inhibition of growth by secreting a diffusible chemical that stimulates or inhibits the cytoplasm or nucleus). An example is <u>tissue induction</u> in which a given tissue can induce cells in contact with it to develop along a certain line. For example, the dorsal lip of the blastopore induces the overlying ectoderm to become neural tissue as mentioned above.

(2) Physical environment (by differences in light, temperature, pressure, humidity, pH, etc.). As the embryo develops, some cells are internal, some are on the surface, some have lots of yolk, some a little yolk, etc., so more opportunities occur for agents to act on cells in a differential manner. In general, the more specialized a cell becomes (i.e., the more differentiated), the less likely it is to differentiate to perform other functions or even divide. Certain cells remain at low levels of differentiation such that they may differentiate as they are needed. Examples are the mesenchymal cell found throughout the body and the bone marrow stem cell which can give rise to all the blood elements. Occasionally, a cell may dedifferentiate (i.e., revert to a less differentiated form), and, thus, its potential to divide increases. This is what happens in many cancers.

The concept of determination is related to that of differentiation in that, as a cell differentiates, fewer options become available. That is, at certain points a cell or tissue may be "determined" to become one of a certain set of cells and not others. For example, the surface cells of the gastrula are "determined" to become ectodermal structures and not endodermal or mesodermal structures. So, although in the blastula all the cells were surface cells and, apparently (!), had the option of becoming ectodermal cells, only those that did not invaginate became so. The mechanism of determination is probably also related to the environmental differences of cells and their interaction with preset sequences of gene activation and inactivation. Occasionally, the cells resulting from cleavage of a zygote are not "determined" until after 3 divisions (8 cells). Up to this point each cell can develop into a complete organism. After this point, only incomplete organisms would develop from each cell. Cleavages up to this point are called indeterminate because each cell still has all the options available. The next cleavage is called determinate because the daughter cells no longer have all options available. In some instances the first cleavage may be determinate.

2.7.2     QUESTIONS TO REVIEW EMBRYOLOGY

(1)   The blastula is generally preceded by the:

      (a)  gastrula              (b)  morula
      (c)  neurula               (d)  both (a) and (b)

(2)   The three germ layers--the ectoderm, the mesoderm and the endoderm--are found at which stage?

      (a)  morula  (b)  gastrula  (c)  blastula  (d)  neurula

(3)   Select the one that is not derived from the ectoderm germinal layer:

      (a)  nerve                 (b)  muscle
      (c)  lens of eye           (d)  epidermis of skin

(4)   Select the organ/tissue not derived from the mesodermal germinal layer:

      (a)  muscle  (b)  kidney  (c)  intestines  (d)  bones

48

(5)   Select the organ/tissue not derived from the endodermal germinal layer:

(a) nerve   (b) liver   (c) intestines   (d) lung

(6)   The individual cells resulting from the cleavage of a fertilized egg may occasionally give rise to complete organisms up to the <u>third</u> cleavage.   Select the correct statement.

(a) Cleavages prior to the <u>third</u> were determinate cleavages.
(b) The number of cells resulting from the third cleavage is 16.
(c) Determinate cleavages cannot occur, in general, prior to the third cleavage.
(d) The cells resulting after the next cleavage are probably different in the set of activated genes and/or cytoplasmic composition.

(7)   Once the sperm head penetrates the _____, a reaction ensues that _____

(a) corona radiata; causes the pronuclei to fuse.
(b) corona radiata; prevents the penetration of additional sperm.
(c) ovum; causes the pronuclei to fuse.
(d) ovum; prevents the penetration of additional sperm.

(8)   All of the following processes occur during the process of fertilization of the egg by the sperm except

(a) acrosome dissolves the corona radiata;
(b) only the head of the sperm enters the ovum;
(c) the sperm nucleus completes its second meiotic division;
(d) the ovum nucleus completes its second meiotic division.

(9)   The correct sequence of the early stages of development is:

(a) morula, gastrula, blastula, neurula
(b) morula, blastula, gastrula, neurula
(c) blastula, morula, gastrula, neurula
(d) neurula, blastula, gastrula, morula

(10)  Which of the following stages is essentially the same size as the zygote?

(a) gastrula                 (b) blastula
(c) morula                   (d) all are larger

(11)  The first stage of development in which a cavity appears is the:

(a) neurula   (b) morula   (c) gastrula   (d) blastula

(12)  Morphogenesis begins at which stage?

(a) morula   (b) blastula   (c) gastrula   (d) neurula

49

(13) Factors important in the differentiation of cells include:

   (a) cytoplasmic composition and distribution of constituents;
   (b) characteristics of neighboring cells;
   (c) physical environmental agents;
   (d) all of the above.

(14) As a cell becomes more specialized for a particular function, the opportunity for it to become specialized for other functions:

   (a) decreases    (b) increases    (c) remains the same

(15) A cell found in the middle layer of the three-layered gastrula has probably lost the option to become:

   (a) epidermis  (b) kidney  (c) muscle  (d) blood

(16) Select the following situation(s) that have the best likelihood of leading to differentiated daughter cells after a cleavage occurs:

I. Blastula (all cells similar) pH of medium = 7.4

II. Zygote — cleavage line, yolk

III. Zygote — cleavage line, yolk

IV. Surface layer Layers #1 and #2 with similar cells — light, #1, #2, cleavage of layers #1 and #2

V. Rim of similar cells — symmetrical release of a chemical

VI. pH = 7.4, yolk

   (a) III, IV, VI                 (b) II, IV, V, VI
   (c) II, III, IV, V, VI          (d) all of them

(17) Which of the following cells or cell types is the most differentiated?

   (a) mesenchymal cell        (b) nerve cell
   (c) cancer cell             (d) bone marrow stem cell

2.7.3      ANSWERS TO QUESTIONS IN SECTION 2.7.2

(1) b  (2) b  (3) b  (4) c  (5) a  (6) d
(7) d  (8) c  (9) b  (10) c  (11) d  (12) b
(13) d  (14) a  (15) a  (16) a  (17) b

QUESTIONS #1-#5, #7-#15, #17: All discussed adequately in reference.

QUESTION #6 (Answer: d) This is discussed in the Section. The implication of the question being that the divisions after the third are determinate and result in cells that are somewhat differentiated. The cells resulting from the $n^{th}$ cleavage is $2^n$ assuming at each cleavage all cells divide (not always true). Then $2^3 = 2 \cdot 2 \cdot 2 = 8$ and not 16 as in option (b).

QUESTION #16 (Answer: a) The point stressed in the Section was that differentiation is possible if a factor can affect a group of similar cells in an unsymmetrical or unequal manner. In (I), the pH affects all the similar cells equally. In (II), the cleavage results in two cells with similar yolk distributions. In (III), the cleavage results in different yolk distributions so the daughter cells are different cytoplasmically and this can lead to differentiation. In (IV), the light may either affect the surface layer only or affect the surface layer (#1) more strongly than the underlying layer (#2). This can potentially affect gene activation and can lead to differentiation between the cell layers. In (V), the rim of similar cells are probably affected similarly by the symmetrically diffusing chemicals, and the daughter cells will probably be similar. In (VI), although the pH is constant, this can have different effects on cells with and without yolks, and, hence, result in potentially differentiated daughter cells.

2.7.5    VOCABULARY CHECKLIST FOR EMBRYOLOGY

| | | |
|---|---|---|
| ____ acrosome | ____ corona radiata | ____ cleavages |
| ____ morula | ____ blastula | ____ blastocoel |
| ____ archenteron | ____ blastopore | ____ gastrula |
| ____ ectoderm | ____ mesoderm | ____ endoderm |
| ____ neurula | ____ neural tube | ____ neural crest |
| ____ tissue induction | | |

2.7.6    CONCEPTS, PRINCIPLES, ETC. CHECKLIST FOR EMBRYOLOGY

____ fertilization of the ovum and related changes in the egg
____ sequences of stages of development
____ development of the ectoderm, mesoderm, endoderm into organs and/or organ systems
____ morphogenesis
____ concept of determination
____ concept of differentiation
____ concept of induction

2.8.1        REVIEW OF RESPIRATORY SYSTEM

In humans, air enters through the mouth or nose where it is cleaned,
warmed and moistened.  It then passes down the trachea to two main
bronchi and then to bronchioles then to alveoli.  Gas exchange occurs
in the alveoli.   Incomplete cartilage rings hold the trachea,
bronchi, and bronchioles open.  Mucus traps particles which are then
moved out of the respiratory tract by ciliary action of the lining
cells.  Coughing is a reflex action mediated by the medulla.  The
reflex is initiated by a stimulation (e.g. by particles) of the
tracheobronchial tree, followed by expulsion of these particles and
mucus as sputum (or phlegm).  Sneezing is a reflex mediated by the
medulla also, but the initial stimulation is in the nose followed by
forceful expulsion of the irritating substance and naso-oral
secretions.

The act of inspiration is accomplished by the contraction of the
diaphragm (via impulses from the phrenic nerve) which moves downward
and/or by certain rib muscles lifting the rib cage up.   These
mechanisms create a negative pressure inside the chest cavity which
causes the lungs to expand and pull in air.  Expiration is a passive
process due to the elastic recoil of the chest wall and lung tissue
itself.   Respiration is largely involuntary, but some voluntary
control is possible over the rate and depth of respiration.   The
control center of respiration is in the medulla of the brainstem.  It
causes an increase in the rate of respiration when there is a fall in
pH (e.g., more acidic), an increase in $CO_2$ tension (which causes a
drop in pH), or a decrease in oxygen tension in the blood.   Also
impulses from the cerebrum can affect ventilatory rate, as in
anxiety, when the rate increases.

A  key  substance  for  the  function  of  lungs  is  surfactant
(dipalmitoyl lecithin--a phospholipid).  This substance coats the
alveoli and creates a variable surface tension in them.   As the
alveoli  get  smaller,  the  surface  tension  decreases  due  to
surfactant.   This prevents the alveoli from collapsing during
expiration, because high surface tension would cause alveoli to
collapse.  In the absence of surfactant, collapsed alveoli require
fairly high inspiratory forces to re-expand them.  This is what
happens in RDS (Respiratory Distress Syndrome) of the newborn in
whom there is an absence of surfactant.  The infant is not strong
enough to re-expand the collapsed alveoli.

In summary, the respiratory system functions mechanically to move
air in and out of the lungs (highest $O_2$ and lowest $CO_2$ tension) and
to allow diffusion of gases in and out of the body.  Oxygen moves
into the blood (lower $O_2$ tension and highest $CO_2$ tension) where it is
taken up and utilized.  In the tissues, carbon dioxide ($CO_2$) is
produced by oxidation of nutrients.  The $CO_2$ then diffuses into the
blood where it dissolves in the serum, is converted to carbonic acid
($CO_2 + H_2O \longrightarrow H_2CO_3$) and then to bicarbonate ($HCO_3^-$), or combines with
hemoglobin.   Next it circulates to the lungs where the above
reactions are reversed and the $CO_2$ is expired.  Note that in all

cases the gases go from higher tensions (pressures) to lower. By regulating the amount of carbonic acid and bicarbonate in the serum, the lungs are important in the regulation of acid-base balance in the body.


2.8.2        QUESTIONS TO REVIEW THE RESPIRATORY SYSTEM


(1)    The path of air into the lungs of man is:

       (a)   alveoli, trachea, bronchi, bronchioles;
       (b)   trachea, bronchi, bronchioles, alveoli;
       (c)   bronchi, bronchioles, trachea, alveoli;
       (d)   trachea, bronchioles, bronchi, alveoli.

(2)    Expiration of air from the lungs

       (a)   is a passive process;
       (b)   causes negative pressure in the chest cavity;
       (c)   requires contraction of the diaphragm;
       (d)   both (b) and (c).

(3)    During inspiration of air into the lungs

       (a)   the chest cavity has a positive pressure;
       (b)   the diaphragm moves upward;
       (c)   the diaphragm contracts;
       (d)   the rib cage moves down.

(4)    What structure(s) is(are) used to prevent the bronchi from collapsing?

       (a)  cartilage rings          (b)  bony rings
       (c)  fibrous tissue           (d)  none of the above

(5)    Surfactant:

       (a)  dipalmitoyl lecithin     (b)  decreases surface
                                           tension
       (c)  deficiency may result    (d)  all of the above
            in RDS

(6)    Which reflex moves secretions out of the tracheobronchial tree?

       (a)  cough  (b)  sneeze  (c)  baroceptor  (d)  pH

(7)    The control center of respiration is in the:

       (a)  cerebrum  (b)  cerebellum  (c)  medulla  (d)  thalamus

(8)    All of the following may cause an increase in respiratory rate except:

       (a)  increased hydrogen ion    (b)  increased carbon
            concentration                  dioxide tension
       (c)  increased oxygen tension  (d)  anxiety

(9) Carbon dioxide may be present in all the following forms except:

(a) dissolved in the blood      (b) bound to hemoglobin
(c) as dimers                (d) as bicarbonate


2.8.3      <u>ANSWERS TO QUESTIONS IN SECTION 2.8.2</u>


(1) b (2) a (3) c (4) a (5) d (6) a (7) c (8) c (9) c


2.8.4      <u>DISCUSSION OF ANSWERS TO QUESTIONS IN SECTION 2.8.2</u>


All questions are adequately discussed in the Section.


2.8.5      <u>VOCABULARY CHECKLIST FOR THE RESPIRATORY SYSTEM</u>

- trachea
- alveoli
- sneeze
- ciliary action

- bronchi
- mucus
- cartilage rings
- phrenic nerve

- bronchioles
- cough
- surfactant
- control center of respiration


2.8.6      <u>CONCEPTS, PRINCIPLES, ETC. CHECKLIST FOR THE RESPIRATORY SYSTEM</u>

- structure/function of the respiratory system
- mechanism of inspiration and expiration
- factors that affect rate of respiration
- role of surfactant in lung function
- functions of lung in $O_2$ and $CO_2$ homeostasis


## 2.9      Circulatory System


2.9.1      <u>REVIEW OF THE CIRCULATORY SYSTEM</u>


The elements of the circulatory system in humans are the heart, the blood vessels, blood and the lymphatics (Section 2.10.1).

2.9.1.1      <u>The Heart</u>


The <u>heart</u> consists of two <u>atria</u> (left-LA and right-RA) and two <u>ventricles</u> (LV and RV). Between the RA and RV is the <u>tricuspid valve</u>

(TV, 3 leaflets). Between the RV and the pulmonary artery (PA) is the pulmonic valve (PV). Between the LA and LV is the mitral valve (MV, 2 leaflets). Between the LV and the aorta is the aortic valve (AV). The PV and AV valves are called semilunar valves--these prevent reflux of blood back into their respective ventricles during diastole. See Fig. 2.15. The TV and MV are attached via chordae tendinae to papillary muscles on their respective ventricles to prevent reflux into the corresponding atria during systole. Improper functioning of the valves is one of the causes of heart murmurs. A schematic of the heart and circulation is:

blood travels from left to right ( ——→ ) in the diagram

SVC = superior vena cava      //// = oxygenated blood
IVC = inferior vena cava

**Fig. 2.15 – Schematic of the Circulatory System**

The heart is made of striated muscle. This differs from skeletal muscle (Section 2.15.1) by: (1) being made of distinct cells, (2) having specializations of cell membranes called intercalated discs to decrease resistance to impulse conduction, (3) being able to initiate beats without the need of a nerve impulse, and (4) being largely involuntary. The microscopic structures are similar (see Section 2.15.1).

Heart beats are divided into systole (contraction) and diastole (relaxation) on the basis of the state of the ventricles. Beats originate in the sinus node which is considered the pacemaker of the heart. Impulses from here activate the atria to contract (diastole), then pass to the atrioventricular (AV) node. From this point, impulses pass down the bundle of His to the left and right branch bundles to the Purkinje fibers which activate the left and right ventricles causing them to contract (systole). Beats can originate in other parts of the heart if the sinus node fails. Also, some of the bundles or fibers may become injured so that they cannot conduct impulses--then the impulses find alternate paths. Sympathetic nerves serve to increase the heart rate and force of contraction. Parasympathetic nerves (e.g., the Vagus nerve) decreases the heart rate. During systole the ventricles are ejecting blood into the large vessels (PA, aorta), and during diastole the ventricles are being filled with blood from the atria. Note that the RV pumps blood to the lungs and the LV pumps blood to the rest of the body.

## 2.9.1.2    The Blood Vessels

Blood Vessels consist of arteries, arterioles, capillaries, and veins.  Vessels are made of (to different degrees), from the inside out, an intima (endothelial cell lining), a media (consisting of muscle and elastic tissue), and an adventitia (connective tissue covering).  Arteries contain a lot of muscle and/or elastic tissue and deliver blood from the heart (not always oxygenated blood).  The contraction of the ventricles in systole imparts energy and pressure to the blood as they enter the arteries.  This causes expansion (elastic nature) of the arteries during systole which stores the energy part.  During diastole the elastic recoil converts the stored energy to pressure and maintains the pressure.  The blood pressure is higher during systole than diastole in the arteries.  But because of the recoil of the arteries and the effect of the arterioles (see below) the diastolic blood pressure remains well above zero in the arteries.  An average blood pressure is 120/80 (systolic/diastolic) measured in mm Hg.  Arterioles connect arteries and capillaries and are the location of the greatest resistance to blood flow.  Blood pressure varies directly as the flow of blood (amount of blood pumped by the heart) and directly as the resistance to flow.

$$\text{blood pressure} \propto (\text{heart output}) \times (\text{resistance}).$$

Resistance to flow varies inversely as the fourth power of the radius (r) of the vessel:    resistance $\propto 1/r^4$

Arterioles can change their radii greatly.  So, arterioles are very important determinators of blood pressure.  Sympathetic nerves can constrict the arterioles, that is, make the radius smaller.  Capillaries contain only endothelial cells which allow transport of substances across them.  Nearly all the transfer of substances between the blood and the tissues occur across the capillaries.  The hydrostatic pressure, generated by the heartbeat, tends to push fluid and molecules (not cells) out of the capillary.  The oncotic pressure, due primarily to the presence of proteins like albumin in the blood, tends to pull fluid and molecules into the capillary.  Hence, the net transfer of fluid depends on the balance of these two.  On the arterial side of the capillary, the hydrostatic pressure dominates and fluid, etc., leaves the capillary and enters the tissue space (not cells directly).  At the venule end of the capillary, the oncotic pressure dominates and this draws fluid, etc. (different substances than exited), back into the capillary (Fig. 2.16).  Not all the fluid and proteins are pulled back in; these are returned to the blood vessels via the lymphatics (Section 2.10.1).

CAPILLARY BED

Arterial side                                              Venous side

fluids,proteins

hydrostatic>oncotic                oncotic>hydrostatic            lymphatic

(pressures are inside the vessel)

net direction of fluid movement

**Fig. 2.16 – Capillary Fluid Exchange**

The veins have less muscle and elastin than arteries, have valves to prevent backward flow of blood away from the heart, and carry blood to the heart. Veins can contain a lot of blood under low pressure, i.e., they have a high capacitance (can act as a reservoir). Veins are assisted by the action of muscle contractions to move blood forward (the heart valves prevent backward movement). Anatomically, the blood vessels consist of three main divisions. (1) The systemic circulation supplies blood to the head, extremities, and trunk. The main artery is the aorta and the main veins are the inferior and superior vena cavas. (2) The pulmonary circulation supplies blood to the lungs. (3) The coronary circulation supplies blood to the heart. The coronary arteries arise at the base of the aorta at the aortic valve. The arteries give rise to the coronary veins which enter the coronary sinus (on the atria) which empties into the RA.


2.9.1.3     The Blood


Blood consists of formed elements: (1) red blood cells (RBC or erythrocytes), (2) white blood cells (WBC), and (3) platelets; and many non-formed elements: proteins, lipids, hormones, dissolved gases, ions, carbohydrates.

RBCs contain hemoglobin (made of four proteins called globin, and heme, which is a porphyrin ring, and iron--II) and are biconcave discs ( ⬭  ◎ ).

The hematocrit is the percentage of whole blood that is RBCs. The plasma is whole blood minus the formed elements. Serum is plasma after clotting has occurred. Hemoglobin (Hb) carries oxygen ($O_2$) attached to iron (Fe). $O_2$ is picked up slowly by Hb at low $O_2$ tension, but this rapidly accelerates as $O_2$ tension increases, and it eventually levels off at high $O_2$ tension (Fig. 2.17). (The tension of a gas is the pressure of the gas).

Fig. 2.17 – Hemoglobin–Oxygen Saturation Curve


This is due to the allosteric nature of the Hb molecule. The first subunit binds $O_2$ slowly, but once bound, the bound $O_2$ causes a conformational change in the second subunit which causes it to pick up the next $O_2$ faster. This is repeated in the third and fourth subunits until the Hb is saturated. Hb releases $O_2$ more readily at low pH than at high pH--the Bohr effect. Hb picks up $O_2$ in the lung and releases it in the tissues. Release and uptake is primarily a function of $O_2$ tension (pressure) gradients, but pH and other factors pay a role. Carbon dioxide is transported from the tissues to the lungs dissolved in blood, as bicarbonate, and bound to Hb and some other proteins.  Its uptake (at tissues) by blood and release (in the lungs) by blood is also a function of $CO_2$ pressure gradients. Gases diffuse from regions of higher pressure to regions of lower pressure.

WBCs are mostly neutrophils (a type of granulocyte) and lymphocytes. Eosinophils, basophils and monocytes are also found in the blood. Neutrophils are involved in inflammatory reactions and are responsible for pus formation.  They can phagocytize bacteria and other foreign substances.  Lymphocytes are the key elements in the immunologic response system.  Platelets are fragments of cells called megakaryocytes (located in the bone marrow).  They play a part in the clotting of blood.  All of the formed elements arise from precursor cells in the bone marrow.

Proteins in the blood are albumin (maintains oncotic pressure and acts as a nonspecific carrier protein) and globulins.  Globulins include the immunoglobulins which are antibodies, carrier proteins, and the coagulation factors (fibrinogen, prothrombin, etc.). Calcium is also required for clotting; agents like EDTA and oxalate complex calcium and may prevent clotting.  Vitamin K is responsible for formation of some of the clotting factors, and, thus, the clotting of blood.

2.9.1.4      Summary

The function of the circulatory system is to maintain tissue oxygenation, supply nutrients and remove wastes.  This function is compromised when the heart, blood vessels, or blood fail to perform as intended.  Also, the lungs are critical in $O_2$ and $CO_2$ homeostasis. Malfunction in these systems can lead to a decreased flow of suitable blood (e.g., enough $O_2$) to tissues and this can lead to their death. Also, a fall in blood pressure or loss of blood volume can have similar effects.

2.9.2      QUESTIONS TO REVIEW THE CIRCULATORY SYSTEM

(1)   Which statement(s) is(are) correct?

      (a)  Veins and arteries carry both oxygenated and deoxygenated
           blood.
      (b)  Veins carry only deoxygenated blood.
      (c)  Arteries carry only oxygenated blood.
      (d)  Both (b) and (c).

(2)   Which of the following is not part of the conduction system of
      the heart?

      (a)  artrioventricular node        (b)  chordae tendinae
      (c)  Bundle of His                 (d)  Purkinje fibers

(3)   Cells in the blood are normally derived from precursor cells
      in the:

      (a)  liver  (b)  spleen  (c)  bone marrow  (d)  connective
                                                      tissue

(4) All are types of white blood cells except:

    (a) megakaryocyte         (b) neutrophil
    (b) eosinophil            (d) lymphocyte

(5) The mitral valve is located between the

    (a) left atrium and left ventricle
    (b) left and right ventricles
    (c) left and right atria
    (d) superior vena cava and the heart

(6) Which agent below chelates calcium and may prevent clotting of blood?

    (a) Vit D    (b) EDTA    (c) Vit K    (d) $NH_3$

(7) All of the following are true about albumin except:

    (a) found in the plasma
    (b) plays a role in immunologic reactions
    (c) made in the liver
    (d) plays a role in maintaining the colloid oncotic pressure of the blood

(8) The beats of the heart are initiated by:

    (a) the brain                 (b) the sympathetic nerves
    (c) the parasympathetic nerves   (d) the sinoatrial node

(9) Chordae tendinae:

    (a) hold muscles to bones
    (b) hold muscles to muscles
    (c) hold bones to bones
    (d) found in the heart

(10) The Bohr Effect on hemoglobin function:

    (a) The electrons in the hemoglobin are easily ionized.
    (b) Hemoglobin can also carry $CO_2$.
    (c) Affinity of hemoglobin for oxygen increases with altitude.
    (d) Hemoglobin releases oxygen more readily at lower pHs.

(11) Hematocrit:

    (a) the number of red blood cells in the blood
    (b) the percentage of blood that is red blood cells
    (c) the amount of hemoglobin
    (d) the total amount of blood in the body

(12) Hemoglobin:

    (a) does not carry carbon dioxide;
    (b) is normally free (not in cells) in the blood;
    (c) is composed of protein, porphyrin, and iron;
    (d) is normally found in the plasma portion.

(13) Which statement is correct concerning the heart?

    (a) Right ventricle pumps blood to the body excluding the lung.
    (b) Right ventricle pumps blood to the lung.
    (c) Left ventricle pumps blood to the lung.
    (d) Left ventricle pumps blood to the body including the lung.

(14) Which is the correct sequence of blood passing through the heart? (R=right, L=left, A=atrium, V=ventricle, SVC=Superior Vena Cava, IVC=Inferior Vena Cava)

    (a) RA to RV to SVC/IVC to LA to LV to Lungs to aorta to RA
    (b) SVC/IVC to LA to LV to lungs to RA to RV to aorta to SVC/IVC
    (c) SVC/IVC to RA to RV to lungs to LA to LV to aorta to SVC/IVC
    (d) RA to RV to LA to LV to lungs to aorta to IVC/SVC to RA

(15) Systole refers to

    (a) the contraction phase of the atria;
    (b) the relaxation phase of the atria;
    (c) the contraction phase of the ventricles;
    (d) the relaxation phase of the ventricles.

(16) Heart muscle differs from skeletal muscle in all the following except:

    (a) having striations
    (b) being made of distinct cells
    (c) having intercalated discs
    (d) having the capacity to originate beats without nervous impulses

(17) Sympathetic impulses

    (a) increase the heart rate;
    (b) decrease the heart rate;
    (c) do not affect the heart rate.

(18) In diastole

    (a) the aortic valve is closed;
    (b) the tricuspid valve is closed;
    (c) the mitral valve is closed;
    (d) the ventricles are contracting.

(19) Layers of blood vessels include all of the following except:

    (a) tendinae  (b) media  (c) adventitia  (d) intima

(20) Arteries

    (a) conduct blood toward the heart;
    (b) help maintain blood pressure due to their elastic recoil properties;
    (c) always carry oxygenated blood;
    (d) contain a large media, a small adventitia, and no intima.

(21) The greatest resistance to blood flow is in the:

    (a) capillaries  (b) veins  (c) arteries  (d) arterioles

(22) All of the following might increase blood pressure except:

    (a)  increase in sympathetic tone of vessels
    (b)  increase in the radius of a vessel
    (c)  increase in blood output by the heart
    (d)  increase in resistance of vessels

(23) Exchange of substances between tissues and the blood occurs in the:

    (a) veins  (b) capillaries  (c) arterioles  (d) arteries

(24) The oncotic pressure of blood:

    (a)  has no effect on the movement of fluid
    (b)  causes fluid to move into the tissues from the blood vessels
    (c)  causes fluid to move into the blood vessels from the tissues

(25) On the venous side of the capillary

    (a)  hydrostatic pressure exceeds oncotic pressure and causes fluid to move into the tissues;
    (b)  oncotic pressure exceeds hydrostatic pressure and causes fluid to move into the tissues;
    (c)  hydrostatic pressure exceeds oncotic pressure and causes fluid to move into the blood vessel;
    (d)  oncotic pressure exceeds hydrostatic pressure and causes fluid to move into the blood vessel.

(26) Regarding the fluid that escapes from the blood on the arterial side of the capillaries:

    (a)  some of the fluid and proteins is carried off by lymphatics;
    (b)  all of the fluid is returned to the blood at the venous end of the capillary;
    (c)  the fluid normally contains red blood cells;
    (d)  none of the above.

(27) The coronary circulation supplies the:

    (a) brain  (b) heart  (c) lungs  (d) trunk

(28) Select the following which is most likely a red blood cell:

61

(29) Hemoglobin

    (a)  binds $O_2$ uniformly at all $O_2$ tensions;
    (b)  binds $O_2$ rapidly at low $O_2$ tensions;
    (c)  binds $O_2$ slowly at low $O_2$ tensions;
    (d)  does not become saturated at high $O_2$ tensions.

(30) Which of the following is involved in the immune response?

    (a) neutrophils  (b) lymphocytes  (c) platelets  (d) basophils

(31) Clotting:

    (a) platelets  (b) neutrophils  (c) lymphocytes  (d) eosinophils


2.9.3      ANSWERS TO QUESTIONS IN SECTION 2.9.2


(1) a  (2) b  (3) c  (4) a  (5) a  (6) b  (7) b  (8) d  (9) d
(10) d  (11) b  (12) c  (13) b  (14) c  (15) c  (16) a  (17) a  (18) a
(19) a  (20) b  (21) d  (22) b  (23) b  (24) c  (25) d  (26) a  (27) b
(28) a  (29) c  (30) b  (31) a


2.9.4      DISCUSSION OF ANSWERS TO QUESTIONS IN SECTION 2.9.2


All are adequately discussed in the Section except the following:


QUESTION #22 (Answer: b) Sympathetic tone means there is a decrease in the radius of the vessels. A decrease in the radius of the vessels means an increase in resistance (resistance $\propto 1/r^4$). This means that the pressure increases (pressure $\propto$ resistance). An increase in radius causes a drop in blood pressure:
    as radius increases, the resistance decreases
    (resistance $\propto 1/r^4$).
    as resistance decreases, the pressure decreases
    (pressure $\propto$ resistance)
Options (c) and (d) are straight from the Section.


2.9.5      VOCABULARY CHECKLIST FOR THE CIRCULATORY SYSTEM


____ atrium               ____ ventricles
____ tricuspid valve      ____ pulmonic valve
____ mitral valve         ____ aortic valve
____ chordae tendinae     ____ papillary muscles
____ intercalated discs    ____ sinus node
____ diastole           ____ atrioventricular node
____ bundle of His       ____ Purkinje fibers
____ systole            ____ vagus nerve
____ intima              ____ media
____ adventitia         ____ artery
____ vein               ____ arteriole

____ capillary      ____ blood pressure
____ resistance      ____ hydrostatic pressure
____ oncotic pressure      ____ red blood cells
____ white blood cells      ____ hemoglobin
____ hematocrit      ____ plasma
____ serum      ____ allosteric
____ Bohr effect      ____ neutrophils
____ eosinophils      ____ basophils
____ lymphocytes      ____ platelets
____ albumin      ____ globulins

## 2.9.6     CONCEPTS, PRINCIPLES, ETC. CHECKLIST FOR THE CIRCULATORY SYSTEM

____ structure-function relations of heart
____ relation of heart muscle and skeletal muscle
____ effects of nerves on heart rate
____ changes in heart during systole and diastole
____ structure of blood vessels in general
____ structure-function of arteries, arterioles, veins, capillaries
____ control of blood pressure
____ fluid and particle transport across the capillary
____ the different circulations in the body
____ structure-function of red blood cells and hemoglobin

## 2.10     Lymphatic System

## 2.10.1     REVIEW OF THE LYMPHATIC SYSTEM

The lymphatic system consists of lymph nodes and lymphatic vessels. Lymph nodes are points of mergence of several different lymphatic vessels. They contain lymphocytes and macrophages. Lymphocytes are involved in the antibody response to antigens (foreign materials). Removing particulate (bacteria, dead cells, etc.) matter by phagocytosis and helping lymphocytes in the immune response are functions of the macrophage which performs a similar function all over the body (especially in the lung, liver and spleen). Lymph nodes often swell and become tender during infection or inflammation due to this function. The location of the swollen gland (e.g., at the angle of the jaw) is important in localizing the infection (e.g., the throat) or even a cancer (i.e., metastasis from the primary cancer) because nodes drain lymphatic vessels from given regions of the body.

Lymphatic vessels are generally one cell thick being made of endothelial cells (like the cells lining blood vessels). These vessels begin as blind pouches in all tissues of the body. They remove fluid, proteins, and particulate matter that arise in tissues directly or by extravasation from the blood vessels. Once in the lymphatics, the lymph (the above materials) is "filtered" at the lymph nodes and eventually re-enters the circulatory system by flowing into the large veins in the thorax (chest cavity) via the thoracic duct. Lymph flow is passive and requires muscle action (acting as a pump) to move lymph along the vessels. If lymph vessels are destroyed, if lymph nodes are blocked, or it there is no muscle action, the lymph does not flow and the fluid remains in the tissues and that tissue swells up (becomes edematous). Note also that gravity would tend to retard the flow of lymph back into the blood vessels. So, the return of fluid and proteins to the circulation from the tissues and protection against foreign materials are the key functions of the lymphatic system. A schematic is:

**Fig. 2.18 - Lymphatics**

2.10.2        <u>QUESTIONS TO REVIEW THE LYMPHATIC SYSTEM</u>

(1)   The lymphatic system

    (a)   returns fluid and proteins to blood vessels;
    (b)   has a direct connection to the heart;
    (c)   consists of vessels only;
    (d)   is not integral to the function of the body.

(2)   Lymph nodes

    (a)   are found in veins;
    (b)   contain lymphocytes only;
    (c)   may contain lymphocytes and macrophages;
    (d)   are not directly important in protecting the body against disease.

(3)   Macrophages

    (a)   are found in lymph nodes only;
    (b)   are phagocytic cells;
    (c)   are the lining cells of lymphatic vessels;
    (d)   all the above.

(4)  An enlarged lymph node may mean:

    (a)  infection
    (b)  inflammation
    (c)  cancer
    (d)  all of the above

(5)  Lymph moves toward the veins due to:

    (a)  tissue pressure
    (b)  muscle action
    (c)  pumping action of heart
    (d)  gravity

2.10.3      ANSWERS TO QUESTIONS IN SECTION 2.10.2

(1) a      (2) c      (3) b      (4) d      (5) b

2.10.4      DISCUSSION OF ANSWERS TO QUESTIONS IN SECTION 2.10.2

All questions are adequately discussed in the Section.

2.10.5      VOCABULARY CHECKLIST FOR THE LYMPHATIC SYSTEM

____ lymph node      ____ lymphocyte          ____ macrophage
____ lymph           ____ lymphatic vessel

2.10.6      CONCEPTS, PRINCIPLES, ETC.  CHECKLIST FOR THE LYMPHATIC
            SYSTEM

____ structure of lymphatic system
____ role of lymphatic system in disease prevention and recognition
____ role of lymphatic system in fluid and protein homeostasis
____ composition of lymph
____ movement of lymph through the vessels

65

**2.11**     **Renal (Kidney, Etc.) System and Body Fluid Composition and Homeostasis**

**2.11.1**     REVIEW OF RENAL SYSTEM AND BODY FLUID COMPOSITION AND HOMEOSTASIS

**2.11.1.1**     Body Fluid Composition

Human body fluids divide conveniently into an intracellular (IC) compartment and an extracellular (EC) compartment. The EC compartment is further divided into an interstitial (I) compartment (outside of cells and outside of the circulation) and a plasma (P) compartment (circulatory component). Each compartment has a particular substance that tends to maintain its volume. Potassium ($K^+$) ion is the main molecule of the IC compartment. Sodium ($Na^+$) ion is the main molecule of the EC compartment. And protein, in addition to $Na^+$, is important in the plasma compartment.

In the plasma there are cations, $Na^+$ and $K^+$ primarily, balanced by anions, chloride ($Cl^-$) and bicarbonate ($HCO_3^-$) primarily. Also, there are many small organic molecules such as glucose, amino acids, etc. Larger organic molecules such as proteins and fat complexes are also present.

The acidity, measured by the pH, is relatively constant at pH $\approx$ 7.40 for the plasma. The major sources of acidity are the $CO_2$ (produced in tissues) and acids from the oxidation of glucose, fats, and amino acids such as pyruvate, lactate, or sulfur (from sulfur containing amino acids). Bicarbonate (basic) is produced by the kidney to balance these acids. The ratio of dissolved $CO_2$ and $HCO_3^-$ is the determinator of the pH. As $CO_2$ increases the pH decreases and as $HCO_3^-$ increases the pH increases:

$$\left( pH \propto \frac{\left[ HCO_3^- \right]}{P_{CO_2}} \right.$$

where $P_{CO_2}$ is the partial pressure of $CO_2$). Remember that $CO_2$ undergoes this reaction with water,

$$CO_2 + H_2O \rightleftharpoons H_2CO_3$$
$$\text{carbonic acid}$$

and carbonic acid dissociates to give $H^+$, $H_2CO_3 \rightleftharpoons H^+ + HCO_3^-$ (remember $H^+$ is measured by the pH).

The plasma also contains waste products of the tissues, one of the most important being urea. Urea,

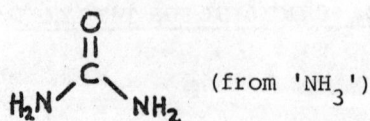

(from 'NH$_3$')

is the result of the breakdown of nitrogen containing organic molecules, especially amino acids. Creatinine is a product of muscle metabolism and is also continuously released into the plasma. Both are excreted by the kidneys.

## 2.11.1.2    The Kidney (Human)

The structure and function of the kidney will be described by following the path of blood through the kidney and the formation of urine by the kidney.

Blood from the renal artery passes to a tuft of capillaries called the glomerulus which sits in a space created by Bowman's Capsule. Filtration of the blood occurs, but larger proteins and formed elements (i.e. cells) are not filtered through the glomerulus. This initial filtrate which contains water, ions, all non-polymeric organic molecules, and small proteins first passes into Bowman's Capsule (BC) and then into the proximal convoluted tubule (PCT) which is continuous with BC. In the PCT, proteins, amino acids, sugars and other nutrients are reabsorbed by active transport by the tubular cells. Sodium, potassium and bicarbonate are reabsorbed as is most of the water. Hydrogen ion and ammonium ions are secreted into the tubular lumen by the PCT cells. Also, toxic substances and waste molecules are secreted into the lumen by the PCT cells. The fluid remaining in the lumen continues into the descending limb of the Loop of Henle (LOH) where $Na^+$ is picked up from the medulla (inside of kidney) interstitium. The filtrate continues around the LOH to the ascending limb of the LOH where $Cl^-$ is being actively extruded into the medulla and $Na^+$ passively follows. A $Cl^-$ pump that requires energy as ATP is responsible for this extrusion against the concentration gradient. This countercurrent multiplier system between the limbs of the LOH maintains a high concentration of $Na^+$ in the medulla. The filtrate (urine) passes on to the distal convoluted tubule (DCT) where $Na^+$ in the lumen is exchanged for $K^+$ (and $H^+$) in the cells stimulated by aldosterone (from the adrenal gland). The filtrate (now urine) continues to the collecting duct (CD) which dips into the medulla with its large $Na^+$ concentration. The $Na^+$ in the medulla draws most of the water out of the CD into the medulla, where the water is picked up by a system of blood vessels called the vasa rectae. ADH (antidiuretic hormone; vasopressin) is synthesized in the hypothalamus and stored in and released from the posterior pituitary. It acts on the CD to increase water resorption and results in a more concentrated urine. The urine now passes to the calyces to the pelvices to the ureter to the bladder to the urethra to the outside (Fig. 2.19). Excretion is the passing of the urine to the outside.

Fig. 2.19 - The Kidney

## 2.11.1.3    Summary of Homeostasis of Body Fluids

The body regulates the composition of its body fluids within fairly narrow limits. This is because too much or too little of most substances is toxic to cells. The kidney is the central regulator. In general, substances taken into the body (by gastrointestinal tract, lungs, skin or directly into vessels) and substances made in the tissues are in balance with substances used by the tissues and excreted by the body (in the lungs, gastrointestinal tract, skin, and kidneys). That is, Input=Output. This results in fairly constant levels of most substances in the blood. Changes in the function or amount of the load imposed on any of the above can destroy homeostasis and cause changes in body fluid composition.

The heart and blood vessels (2.9.1) serve their part by keeping blood flowing to all the organs and tissues. This allows a constant exchange between the tissues and the blood. If cardiovascular function decreases, fluid nutrients can't get to tissues and wastes accumulate in tissues and the blood. Also, if the heart output falls too much the kidney cannot function. The lymphatic vessels (2.10.1) return fluid and protein to the cardiovascular system to help maintain its function. When lymphatic function decreases, fluid accumulates in the tissues, and the heart has less blood to pump which compromises its function. The lungs (2.8.1) remove $CO_2$ from the body and supply the $O_2$ needed. If lung function is affected, the acidity of blood is affected as well as the production of energy (need $O_2$). The skin (2.12.1) plays a role in the passage of water and ions ($Na^+$, $K^+$, $Cl^-$) in the form of sweat. If sweating is excessive, water and ion loss can compromise the circulation. The gastrointestinal tract (2.13.1) is responsible for the intake of nutrients and excretion of certain wastes and ions ($Na^+$, $K^+$, $Cl^-$, $HCO_3^-$) and water. So, malfunctions, as in diarrhea, can lead to body fluid abnormalities.

Finally, the kidney serves the role of fine tuning the body fluids. After the other systems have upset or tried to correct the homeostasis, the kidney, through the mechanisms described in Section 2.11.1.2, can return the body fluids to a new (not necessarily the same) homeostasis. When kidneys malfunction, substances collect in the blood (e.g., urea) and/or are excreted (e.g., sugar, excess $Na^+$) that would ordinarily not be retained or excreted.

## 2.11.2    QUESTIONS TO REVIEW THE RENAL SYSTEM AND BODY FLUID COMPOSITION AND HOMEOSTASIS

(1)    Functions of the kidneys include all except

    (a)    excretion of $NH_3$ from protein oxidation as urea;
    (b)    regulation of fluids and electrolytes;
    (c)    elimination of toxic substances;
    (d)    elimination of carbon dioxide directly.

(2)    All are part of the human kidney except:

    (a)    glomerulus        (b)    loop of Henle
    (c)    Malpighian tubules    (d)    collecting ducts

(3)     Filtration of <u>blood</u> occurs at which structure in the kidney?

    (a)   loop of Henle    (b)   collecting ducts
    (c)   tubules             (d)   glomerulus

(4)     Select the correct statement concerning the antidiuretic hormone (ADH):

    (a)   synthesized in the posterior pituitary gland
    (b)   acts on the collecting duct of the kidney
    (c)   also called aldosterone
    (d)   all of the above are correct

(5)     Select the correct sequence of filtered blood thru the kidney:

    (a)   Bowman's Capsule, glomerulus, tubules, collecting duct
    (b)   glomerulus, Bowman's capsule, collecting ducts, tubules
    (c)   Bowman's capsule, collecting ducts, glomerulus, tubules
    (d)   glomerulus, Bowman's Capsule, tubules, collecting duct

(6)     The volume of fluid in the plasma is maintained by

    (a)   protein   (b)   $Na^+$   (c)   $Na^+$ and protein   (d)   $K^+$

(7)     The cations of $Na^+$ and $K^+$ are balanced in the plasma by

    (a)   $Cl^-$   (b)   $HCO_3^-$   (c)   $Cl^-$ and $HCO_3^-$   (d)   proteins

(8)     The acidity of the plasma is caused by

    (a)   oxidation of glucose and fats;
    (b)   metabolism of sulfur containing amino acids;
    (c)   production of $CO_2$ by the tissues;
    (d)   all of the above.

(9)     Carbon dioxide when dissolved in water

    (a)   has base properties;
    (b)   has acid properties;
    (c)   is neutral.

(10)    Urea

    (a)   is a product of protein metabolism;
    (b)   contains only carbon, hydrogen, and oxygen;
    (c)   is excreted by the lungs;
    (d)   all of the above.

(11)    The _____ is part of the circulatory system.

    (a)   Bowman's Capsule    (b)   loop of Henle
    (c)   medulla           (d)   glomerulus

(12)    All of the following substances are filtered at the glomerulus except:

    (a)   platelets   (b)   proteins   (c)   glucose   (d)   sodium

(13)   Reabsorption of most of the water, glucose, amino acids, sodium and other nutrients occurs at:

(a)   loop of Henle
(b)   collecting duct
(c)   proximal convoluted tubule
(d)   distal convoluted tubule

(14)   The high concentration of sodium in the medulla is maintained by the:

(a)   proximal convoluted tubule
(b)   distal convoluted tubule
(c)   loop of Henle
(d)   collecting duct

(15)   The movement of $Cl^-$ out of the ascending limb of the Loop of Henle occurs by:

(a)   diffusion
(b)   active transport
(c)   osmosis
(d)   facilitated diffusion

(16)   In the distal convoluted tubule

(a)   $K^+$ moves into the lumen;
(b)   $H^+$ moves into the tubular cells;
(c)   $Na^+$ moves into the lumen;
(d)   $Na^+$ is actively extruded into the medulla.

(17)   Malfunction in which of the following systems might result in body fluid disturbances?

(a)   heart     (b)   skin     (c)   lung     (d)   all of them


2.11.3        ANSWERS TO QUESTIONS IN SECTION 2.11.2


( 1)   d   (2)   c   (3)   d   (4)   b   (5)   d   (6)   c   (7)   c   (8)   d
( 9)   b   (10)   a   (11)   d   (12)   a   (13)   c   (14)   c   (15)   b   (16)   a
(17)   d


2.11.4        DISCUSSION OF ANSWERS TO QUESTIONS IN SECTION 2.11.2


All questions adequately discussed in the Section.


2.11.5        VOCABULARY CHECKLIST FOR RENAL SYSTEM AND BODY FLUID COMPOSITION AND HOMEOSTASIS


____   intracellular compartment              ____   aldosterone
____   distal convoluted tubule              ____   collecting duct
____   extracellular compartment             ____   vasa rectae
____   interstitial compartment              ____   ADH
____   plasma compartment                    ____   urea
____   proximal convoluted tubule            ____   calyx
____   descending limb of loop of Henle      ____   pelvis

| | |
|---|---|
| ____ ascending limb of loop of Henle | ____ nephron |
| ____ countercurrent multiplier system | ____ creatinine |
| ____ glomerulus | ____ cortex |
| ____ medulla | ____ filtration |
| ____ reabsorption | ____ secretion |
| ____ excretion | ____ Bowman's capsule |

2.11.6      CONCEPTS, PRINCIPLES, ETC.   CHECKLIST FOR RENAL SYSTEM
            AND BODY FLUID COMPOSITION AND HOMEOSTASIS

____ role of different substances in maintaining volumes of fluid
     compartments
____ balance of cations and anions in fluids
____ origin of acidity in plasma and role of $CO_2$ and $HCO_3^-$
____ structure/function of kidney
____ factors involved in body fluid composition homeostasis
____ systems and their role in body fluid homeostasis

## 2.12      The Skin and Thermoregulation

2.12.1      REVIEW OF THE SKIN AND THERMOREGULATION

2.12.1.1      The Skin

The layers of the skin are the epidermis, dermis, and subcutaneous
tissue.  The epidermis (Fig. 2.20) is a layer comprised of several
types of related cells and melanocytes.  The deepest layer of the
epidermis, the basal layer, contains cells which are dividing.  As
these cells move toward the surface, they lose their nucleus and
produce a protein called keratin (which is stable and water
insoluble).  At the surface, these cells have no nucleus, are dead,
are essentially keratin and are called the stratum corneum which is
the scaly dry surface layer of the skin.  Melanocytes synthesize
melanin (a black to dark-brown pigment) which is responsible for the
color of the skin.  It also responds to ultraviolet light to produce
tanning of the skin.

The dermis is internal to the epidermis and contains most of the
accessory structures of the skin.  Blood vessels end in the dermis.
Sensory endings for pain, temperature and touch are found here and in
the subcutaneous tissue.  Hair follicles and sebaceous glands
(secrete an oily fat substance; if clogged cause acne), and sweat
glands originate here. All of these exit at the epidermis. General
connective tissue cells, fibroblasts, and macrophages among other
cells may be found in the dermis.

The subcutaneous tissue contains primarily fat cells.

Fig. 2.20 - The Skin

Functions of the skin include:

(1)    protection from physical agents (wind, water, etc.)—afforded
       by the stratum corneum and melanocytes (radiation),

(2)    protection from microbial agents especially bacteria—
       afforded by the stratum corneum and some secretions of the
       sebaceous glands,

(3)    thermoregulation (see 2.12.1.2),

(4)    waste removal (e.g., excess water, salts, urea, others)—via
       the sweat glands,

(5)    site of the first activation of vitamin D—by ultraviolet
       light,

(6)    sensation—by the many nerve endings.


2.12.1.2    Thermoregulation

Thermoregulation is the regulation of the internal body temperature
between the narrow limits necessary for life.  Too high or low a
temperature can cause proteins (enzymes especially) to become less
effective or totally inactive (denatured) and cause the protoplasm
to gel (become more solid).

Normally, the body temperature is a balance between heat produced by
metabolism and heat loss by the various means described below.
Processes that increase body metabolism increase body heat, this is
especially true of muscle activity (e.g., shivering).  Regulation of
body temperature is centered in the hypothalamus (in the brain).

Pyrogens released during bacterial infections, among other causes,
can affect the hypothalamus in a way that it allows the body
temperature to rise higher than normal, and fever results.

The mechanisms of heat conservation include those that are always
present and those called upon in emergencies:  ( * = most important)

(A) Mechanisms always present:

    *(1) subcutaneous fat as insulation;
    (2) presence of hair or fur (lower animals).

(B) Mechanisms called upon as needed:

    *(1) shivering--contractions of muscles produce heat;
    *(2) constriction of vessels to skin--prevents heat loss from surface;
    (3) piloerection of hair on skin--traps air against skin that once warmed serves as an insulation;
    (4) increase in metabolic rate.

The mechanisms of heat loss include those that are always present and those called upon in emergencies:

(A) Mechanisms always present:

    (1) loss of heat by radiational cooling;
    (2) low level of evaporation of moisture from skin--for a liquid to evaporate, heat must be supplied; this heat comes from the skin which is cooled.

(B) Mechanisms called upon as needed:

    *(1) sweating and consequent evaporation of water--the sweat itself removes heat from the body and more is lost when this evaporates;
    *(2) dilation of vessels to the skin--increases the amount of radiational cooling.


2.12.2    <u>QUESTIONS TO REVIEW THE SKIN AND THERMOREGULATION</u>


(1) Layers of the skin include all except:

    (a) epidermis          (b) dermis
    (c) lamina propria    (d) subcutaneous tissue

(2) Dead cells are found in the:

    (a) subcutaneous tissue    (b) dermis
    (c) epidermis          (d) no dead cells are in the skin

(3) Melanocytes are found in the:

    (a) dermis            (b) epidermis
    (c) subcutaneous tissue    (d) none of the above

(4) The dermis usually contains all of the following except:

    (a) hair follicles      (b) sweat glands
    (c) fat cells          (d) fibroblasts

(5) All are functions of the skin except:

    (a) exchange of gases      (b) thermoregulation
    (c) activation site of Vitamin D  (d) protection from bacteria

(6) The main effect of extremes of temperature is on the functions of:

    (a) carbohydrates         (b) phosopholipids
    (c) proteins             (d) nucleic acids

(7) Control of body temperature is localized in the:

    (a) skin   (b) heart   (c) cerebrum   (d) hypothalamus

(8) Select the mechanism that is <u>not</u> used to conserve heat:

    (a) shivering          (b) dilation of blood vessels
    (c) piloerection        (d) subcutaneous fat

(9) Select the mechanism that is <u>not</u> used to lose heat:

    (a) sweating          (b) increase in metabolic rate
    (c) radiational cooling    (d) dilation of blood vessels

2.12.3       ANSWERS TO QUESTIONS IN SECTION 2.12.2

(1) c  (2) c  (3) b  (4) c  (5) a  (6) c  (7) d  (8) b  (9) b

2.12.4       DISCUSSION OF ANSWERS TO QUESTIONS IN SECTION 2.12.2

All questions adequately discussed in Section.

2.12.5       VOCABULARY CHECKLIST FOR SKIN AND THERMOREGULATION

| | | | |
|---|---|---|---|
| ____ | epidermis | ____ | hair follicles |
| ____ | Vitamin D | ____ | keratin |
| ____ | sebaceous glands | ____ | hypothalamus |
| ____ | stratum corneum | ____ | sweat glands |
| ____ | pyrogens | ____ | melanocytes |
| ____ | fibroblasts | ____ | shivering |
| ____ | melanin | ____ | subcutaneous tissue |
| ____ | piloerection | ____ | dermis |
| ____ | fat cells | ____ | radiational cooling |

2.12.6       CONCEPTS, PRINCIPLES, ETC. CHECKLIST FOR SKIN AND THERMOREGULATION

____ structure of skin
____ functions of the skin
____ general concept of thermoregulation
____ mechanisms of heat conservation
____ mechanisms of heat loss

**2.13**    **Digestive System**

2.13.1    <u>REVIEW OF THE DIGESTIVE SYSTEM</u>

2.13.1.1    <u>Structure/Function Relationships of the Digestive System</u>

The structure and function of the digestive system will be discussed by following a bolus of food through it.

The <u>teeth</u> and the <u>tongue</u> are responsible for breaking food down into swallowable chunks (called boluses). Adults have 32 teeth, children have 20 (called deciduous teeth). Each quadrant (quarter) contains two <u>incisors</u> (for cutting), one <u>canine</u> (for tearing), two <u>premolars</u> (for crushing), and 3 <u>molars</u> (for grinding). <u>Salivary glands</u> secrete alkaline <u>saliva</u> to moisten food for swallowing, protect against bacteria, and begin digestion of starch. <u>Swallowing</u> is initiated voluntarily but becomes involuntary as food enters the pharynx. The <u>swallowing center</u> is located in the medulla, and the hypoglossal (XII) and glossopharyngeal (IX) nerves are responsible for the esophageal phase after the bolus passes from the pharynx. The bolus enters the <u>stomach</u> from the esophagus where it may be stored for several hours. Grinding and liquefying the food are the main functions of the stomach accomplished by its strong muscles. <u>Hydrochloric acid</u> and <u>intrinsic factor</u> (for absorption of Vit $B_{12}$) are secreted by parietal cells, and <u>pepsin</u> (digests proteins) is secreted by the chief cells of the stomach. <u>Mucus</u> is secreted by goblet cells to protect the stomach from the acid. The acid kills many bacteria and its secretion is controlled by the vagus nerve and <u>gastrin</u>. Food (now <u>chyme</u>) is propelled to the duodenum by <u>peristalsis</u> (propulsive contractions in the gut) through a relaxed <u>pyloric sphincter</u>. Chyme entering the duodenum causes <u>secretin</u> (causes bicarbonate and fluid to be released from the pancreas) and <u>cholecystokinin-pancreozymin</u> (causes primarily enzymes and water to be released from the pancreas and bile to be released by the gall bladder) to be released. The <u>pancreas</u> secretes inactive enzymes called <u>zymogens</u>. <u>Trypsinogen</u> which is converted to <u>trypsin</u> by <u>enterokinase</u>, located in the duodenal mucosa, activates itself and other zymogens. Other enzymes are chymotrypsin, lipases, and amylases. <u>Bile</u> is secreted by the liver and stored in and released from the gall bladder. <u>Bile salts</u> in bile emulsify lipids to make them more available for digestion. The duodenum has an alkaline pH. Chyme passes into the jejunum where the mucosa contains disaccharidases and peptidases for the final breakdown of nutrients before they are absorbed by active transport. The <u>small intestine</u> is composed of the <u>duodenum</u>, <u>jejunum</u> and <u>ileum</u> in that order. The duodenum is important for absorption of $Ca^{+2}$ and $Fe^{+3}$, the jejunum for most sugars, amino acids, fats, etc., and the ileum absorbs Vit $B_{12}$ (complexed to intrinsic factor) and bile salts. In the <u>colon (large intestine)</u> the remaining water from the small intestine is largely absorbed as are most ions--this compacts the chyme into feces. <u>Feces</u> are stored in the <u>sigmoid colon</u> and <u>rectum</u> until they are defecated. The <u>appendix</u> is attached to a part of the colon called the <u>cecum</u>.

The small intestines are thrown into folds called <u>villi</u>. Individual cells have convolutions of the cell membrane called <u>microvilli</u>.

Both of these increase the surface area for absorption of nutrients. Crypts are regions at the base of villi where new cells are generated.

The liver is a vital organ reflected in its numerous functions. The major functions will be listed: (1) synthesis and storage of glycogen to be converted to glucose under the stimulation of epinephrine or glucagon; (2) gluconeogenesis--the synthesis of glucose from amino acids stimulated by glucagon and epinephrine via cAMP; by removal of storage glycogen and gluconeogenesis the liver plays an important role in regulation of blood glucose; (3) proteins--synthesizes coagulation factors, albumin, and various others; (4) synthesizes bile and cholesterol; (5) contains numerous macrophages (called Kupffer cells) for defense against foreign materials (e.g., bacterial); (6) contains a system for detoxification and degradation of toxins, drugs, and normal metabolites; (7) fats--packages fats for transport, oxidizes fatty acids to ketone bodies for use by other tissues; (8) amino acids-- deaminates (removes nitrogen), produces urea; (9) can interconvert fats, carbohydrates, and amino acids, (10) stores substances such as iron and Vit $B_{12}$; and (11) red blood cells--potential site for production of RBCs in the adult, site of destruction of old red blood cells.

## 2.13.1.2    The Digestion of Key Nutrients

The digestive functions will be reviewed by discussing each of the major nutrients in turn.

Carbohydrates (approximately 4 kcal/gm). A small amount of carbohydrate digestion occurs in the mouth (salivary amylase) and the stomach (acid digestion). Pancreatic amylases digest the starch to disaccharides (maltose, isomaltose) and glucose. These disaccharides and sucrose (cane sugar, sugar beets) and lactose (from milk) are broken down, respectively, by maltases, sucrases, and lactases located on the outer surface of mucosal cells. The resulting monosaccharides then enter by active transport (glucose and galactose) or facilitated transport (the above and fructose, mannose, xylose, arabinose). The active transport mechanisms involve a coupling with $Na^+$ via a Na-K-ATPase and a specific carrier for glucose both located in the mucosal cell. Carbohydrates are not essential (for life) to the diet. But, they normally provide (in the US) 50+% of calories. Cellulose cannot be digested by humans.

Lipids. Triglycerides are hydrolyzed by lipase from the pancreas. Bile salts aid this by emulsifying and solubilizing the fat. Fatty acids, monoglycerides, diglycerides, and glycerol are the products of lipases. These products can diffuse across the mucosa. Glycerol and short chain fatty acids go directly to the liver via the venous portal system. Long chain fatty acids, and the mono- and diglycerides are resynthesized into triglycerides and packaged with proteins as chylomicrons which are absorbed into lymphatics and then go to the liver. In the liver, the lipids are reorganized into lipoproteins (lipid plus special proteins) and shipped to adipose cells primarily. Linolenic and linoleic acids are essential fatty acids (cannot be synthesized by humans). Fats are the long term energy storage compounds (approximately 9 kcal/gm). The molecules discussed above are in Figure 2.21, on the following page.

ester linkage

$R-\overset{O}{\overset{\|}{C}}-OH$

$R= CH_3(CH_2)_n-$

n= even number
usually 12,
14,16,18

FATTY ACID

$H-\overset{H}{\underset{}{C}}-OH$
$H-\overset{}{\underset{}{C}}-OH$
$H-\overset{}{\underset{H}{C}}-OH$

GLYCEROL

$H-\overset{H}{\underset{}{C}}-O-\overset{O}{\overset{\|}{C}}-R_1$
$H-\overset{}{\underset{}{C}}-O-\overset{O}{\overset{\|}{C}}-R_2$
$H-\overset{}{\underset{H}{C}}-O-\overset{O}{\overset{\|}{C}}-R_3$

TRIGLYCERIDE

$H-\overset{H}{\underset{}{C}}-O-\overset{O}{\overset{\|}{C}}-R_1$
$H-\overset{}{\underset{}{C}}-O-\overset{O}{\overset{\|}{C}}-R_2$
$H-\overset{}{\underset{H}{C}}-OH$

DIGLYCERIDE

$H-\overset{H}{\underset{}{C}}-O-\overset{O}{\overset{\|}{C}}-R$
$H-\overset{}{\underset{}{C}}-OH$
$H-\overset{}{\underset{H}{C}}-OH$

MONOGLYCERIDE

**Fig. 2.21 - Lipids**

Proteins. Some protein digestion occurs in the stomach by pepsin (secreted as inactive pepsinogen which is activated by stomach acid or other pepsins). Enterokinase (intestinal enzyme) converts trypsinogen to trypsin which then converts trypsinogen and chymotrypsinogen (both from the pancreas) and all other pancreatic zymogens to active forms. The result of these digestions are oligopeptides and dipeptides which are cleaved by mucosal enzymes, e.g., carboxypeptidases. Several intestinal active transport systems exist. Absorbed amino acids go to the liver via the venous portal system. There are about 8-10 essential amino acids which have to be supplied in the diet (some are isoleucine, leucine, phenylalanine, histidine). Protein provides about 4 kcals/gm.

2.13.2     QUESTIONS TO REVIEW THE DIGESTIVE SYSTEM

(1)    Which type of tooth, in the normal adult with a full set of teeth, has the incorrect maximum number in parenthesis?

   (a)  incisors (4)              (b)  canines (4)
   (c)  premolars (8)            (d)  molars (12)

(2)    All are functions of saliva except:

   (a)  digestion of starch       (b)  digestion of protein
   (c)  lubrication of food       (d)  protection against
                                        bacteria

(3)    Select the incorrect association:

   (a)  stomach--grinds and liquefies food
   (b)  pancreas--digestive enzymes
   (c)  small intestine--absorption of fluid and food
   (d)  colon (large intestine)--absorption of food

(4)    Select the incorrect association:

   (a)  chymotrypsin--protein      (b)  trypsin--carbohydrates
   (c)  amylase--carbohydrates     (d)  lipases--fats

77

(5)   The correct sequence of structures in the gut is

      (a)  stomach, esophagus, small intestine, large intestine;
      (b)  esophagus, stomach, large intestine, small intestine;
      (c)  esophagus, stomach, small intestine, large intestine;
      (d)  esophagus, small intestine, stomach, large intestine.

(6)   Which of the following is not a function of the liver?

      (a)  synthesis of insulin
      (b)  synthesis of carbohydrates, proteins, fats
      (c)  detoxifies drugs
      (d)  synthesis of bile

(7)   Most nutrients are absorbed in the:

      (a)  esophagus              (b)  stomach
      (c)  small intestine        (d)  large intestine

(8)   Digestion of carbohydrates occurs mostly by enzymes from the:

      (a)  pancreas  (b)  liver  (c)  stomach  (d)  salivary glands

(9)   All of the following carbohydrates can be digested by humans
      except:

      (a)  starch  (b)  sucrose  (c)  cellulose  (d)  maltose

(10)  Monosaccharides cross the intestinal wall mainly by:

      (a)  active transport        (b)  diffusion
      (c)  facilitated transport   (d)  both (a) and (c)

(11)  Select the incorrect statement concerning bile salts:

      (a)  break down (digest) lipids
      (b)  emulsify and solubilize lipids
      (c)  synthesized in the liver
      (d)  stored in the gall bladder

(12)  The products of triglyceride hydrolysis by lipases in the
      intestine may include:

      (a)  fatty acids            (b)  monoglycerides
      (c)  diglycerides           (d)  all of these

(13)  Which is the main long—term energy storage substance in
      animals?

      (a)  carbohydrates          (b)  fats
      (c)  proteins               (d)  nucleic acids

(14)  All of the following enzymes are important in the digestion of
      proteins except:

      (a)  amylase  (b)  pepsin  (c)  trypsin  (d)  chymotrypsin

(15)  The enzyme reponsible for the activation of trypsinogen in the
      intestine is:

      (a)  pepsin                 (b)  enterokinase
      (c)  chymotrypsin           (d)  carboxypeptidase

(16)   Swallowing is:

(a)  voluntary     (b)  involuntary     (c)  both

(17)   Secretion of bicarbonate and fluid from the pancreas is
       stimulated by:

(a)  secretin                    (b)  cholecystokinin
(c)  enterokinase                (d)  gastrin

(18)   Acid secretion from the stomach may be stimulated by:

(a)  gastrin  (b)  vagus nerve  (c)  neither  (d)  both

(19)   Select the enzyme not made in the pancreas:

(a)  trypsin  (b)  lipase  (c)  amylase  (d)  pepsin

(20)   Vitamin $B_{12}$ is absorbed in the:

(a)  ileum     (b)  jejunum  (c)  duodenum  (d)  stomach

(21)   Iron is absorbed in the:

(a)  stomach   (b)  jejunum  (c)  ileum  (d)  duodenum

(22)   The absorptive area of the small intestine is increased by
       structures called:

(a)  crypts                      (b)  villi
(c)  microvilli                  (d)  both (b) and (c)

(23)   The liver does not play a role in the metabolism of:

(a)  fats
(b)  carbohydrates
(c)  proteins
(d)  it plays a role in the metabolism of all of these

(24)   The digestion of starch by amylase produces:

(a)  galactose                   (b)  glucose
(c)  maltose                     (d)  both (b) and (c)

(25)   The digestion of small peptides and disaccharides occurs

(a)  in the stomach lumen;
(b)  in the lumen of the bowel;
(c)  on the mucosal cell surface;
(d)  inside the mucosal cell.

(26)   Certain lipids, in contrast to other nutrients, leaving the
       intestine enter the:

(a)  portal system               (b)  lymphatics
(c)  arteries                    (d)  no different from
                                      other nutrients

(27)   Chylomicrons primarily contain:

(a)  carbohydrates               (b)  lipids
(c)  proteins                    (d)  nucleic acids

**2.13.3** ANSWERS TO QUESTIONS IN SECTION 2.13.2

( 1)  a    (2)  b    (3)  d    (4)  b    (5)  c    (6)  a    (7)  c
( 8)  a    (9)  c   (10)  d   (11)  a   (12)  d   (13)  b   (14)  a
(15)  b   (16)  c   (17)  a   (18)  d   (19)  d   (20)  a   (21)  d
(22)  d   (23)  d   (24)  d   (25)  c   (26)  b   (27)  b


**2.13.4** DISCUSSION OF ANSWERS TO QUESTIONS IN SECTION 2.13.2

All answers are adequately discussed in the Section.


**2.13.5** VOCABULARY CHECKLIST FOR THE DIGESTIVE SYSTEM

| | |
|---|---|
| ____ incisor | ____ peristalsis |
| ____ small intestine | ____ canine |
| ____ pyloric sphincter | ____ jejunum |
| ____ premolar | ____ secretin |
| ____ feces | ____ molar |
| ____ cholecystokinin-pancreozymin | ____ sigmoid colon |
| ____ stomach | ____ rectum |
| ____ large intestine (colon) | ____ pancreas |
| ____ zymogens | ____ saliva |
| ____ trypsin | ____ pepsin |
| ____ mucus | ____ appendix |
| ____ cecum | ____ enterokinase |
| ____ bile | ____ gastrin |
| ____ chyme | ____ villi |
| ____ microvilli | ____ bile salts |
| ____ ileum | ____ duodenum |
| ____ liver | ____ crypts |
| ____ sucrase | ____ mucosal cells |
| ____ amylase | ____ gluconeogenesis |
| ____ starch | ____ maltase |
| ____ chylomicrons | ____ lactase |
| ____ chymotrypsin | ____ triglycerides |
| | ____ salivary gland |


**2.13.6** CONCEPTS, PRINCIPLES, ETC.  CHECKLIST FOR THE DIGESTIVE SYSTEM

____ types and purposes of teeth
____ process of swallowing
____ role of stomach, intestines  in digestion and absorption
____ role of pancreas in digestion
____ functions of the liver
____ location of absorption of the key nutrients
____ digestion of key nutrients
____ digestive enzymes

2.14.1    REVIEW OF THE SKELETAL SYSTEM

Bone is composed of a crystal part (mostly hydroxyapatite which is a complex of $Ca^{+2}$ and $PO_4^{-3}$, but also $Na^+$, $K^+$, $Mg^{+2}$ and other anions) and an organic part (mostly the fibrous protein, collagen). Collagen, whose fibrils are arranged end to end, serves as the focus for the deposition of the crystals. This is the basic composition of all types of bone.

Bone can be formed without a cartilaginous model (intramembranous bones such as skull bones) or can be formed from a cartilaginous model (endochondral bone formation, such as long bones). The cartilage is first removed and then the bone is laid down in its place. Bone does not come from the cartilage. Osteoblasts make the inorganic matrix which crystallizes around the collagen. Osteoblasts become osteocytes (mature bone cells) when bone formation is complete. Bone is in a dynamic state with bone formation (osteoblasts) and bone destruction (osteoclasts) occurring simultaneously and continuously. Haversian systems (Fig. 2.22) are present in mature bone. They consist of central nutrient blood vessels and nerves which connect by canaliculi to osteocytes located in lacunae arranged circumferentially around the central canal.

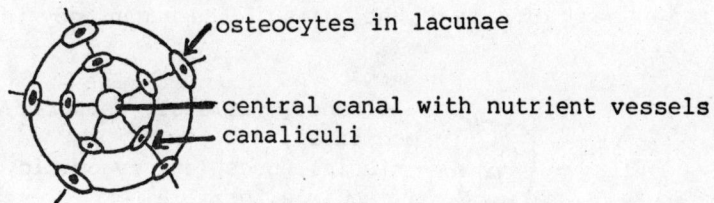

osteocytes in lacunae

central canal with nutrient vessels

canaliculi

Fig. 2.22 – Haversian Canal System

When bone is laid down it may be spongy or compact. Spongy bone (Fig. 2.23) has many air pockets, like a sponge, with the bone present as spicules. Compact bone (Fig. 2.24) is densely packed bone with no air spaces. It is very strong bone and is found where great strength is required as in the cortex of long bones:

spicules of bone

air pockets (or marrow)

Fig. 2.23 – Spongy Bone

Haversian Canal Systems

dense bone between canals

Fig. 2.24 – Compact Bone

Bones in the human are of two types, flat bones and long bones. Flat bones (Fig. 2.25) include the skull bones, ribs and vertebrae, contain red marrow (much blood cell production), are found where little movement is required, and perform protective functions in general.  Long bones (Fig. 2.26) include the bones of the hands, feet, arms and legs, contain yellow marrow, are involved in locomotion and motion primarily.

Fig. 2.25 - Flat Bone

Fig. 2.26 - Long Bone

Joints allow for motion between bones.  The contacting and mobile surfaces between bones are covered by cartilage.  Ligaments help hold bones together at the joint--that is, they are attached bone to bone.  Tendons connect muscles to bones--they also help hold bones together at joints.

Parathyroid hormone (PTH) causes $Ca^{+2}$ (and phosphate) to be removed from the bony matrix, thus causing demineralization of bone.  The $Ca^{+2}$ appears in the serum.  The bone matrix serves as a storage depot for many cations ($Ca^{+2}$, $K^+$, $Mg^{+2}$, $Na^+$) and serves to buffer (help control the levels of) these in the blood (as well as an $H^+$ buffer).  PTH is stimulated by low serum calcium.  Calcitonin is secreted from special cells in the thyroid gland.  It is stimulated by high serum calcium and causes $Ca^{+2}$, etc., to be deposited in bone.  A schematized drawing of some of the bones of the human body is in Fig. 2.27.

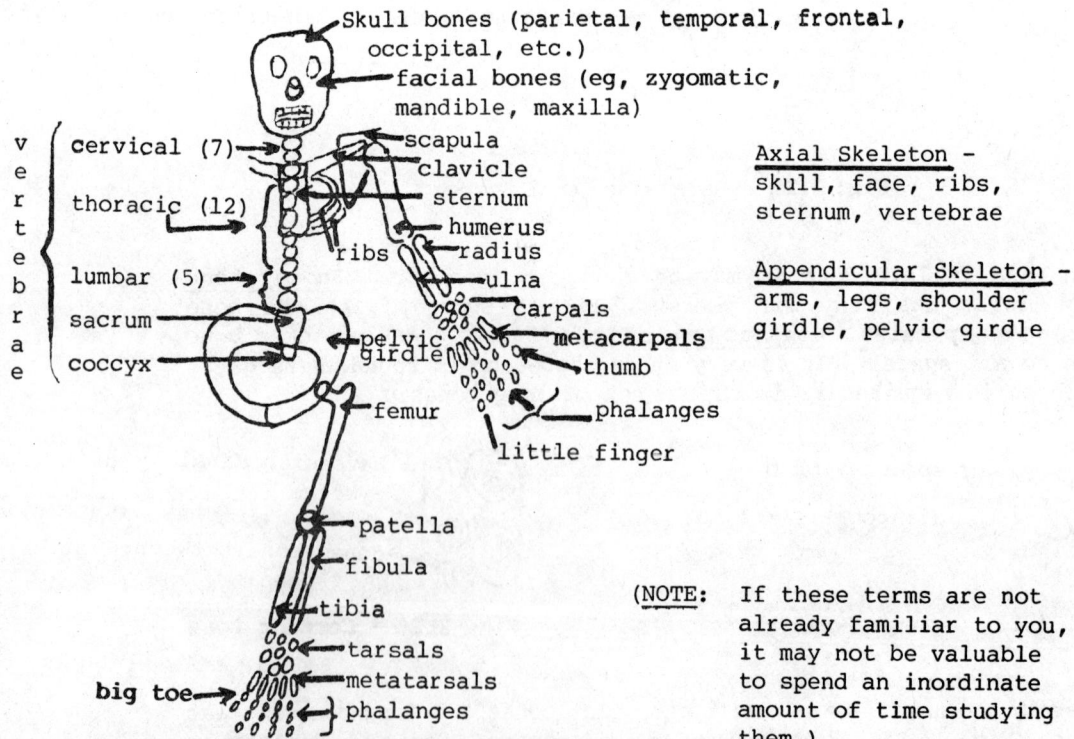

Axial Skeleton - skull, face, ribs, sternum, vertebrae

Appendicular Skeleton - arms, legs, shoulder girdle, pelvic girdle

(NOTE:  If these terms are not already familiar to you, it may not be valuable to spend an inordinate amount of time studying them.)

Fig. 2.27 - Human Skeleton

(1)     All bone is formed

    (a)   from a cartilage model;
    (b)   without a cartilage model;
    (c)   either (a) or (b);
    (d)   neither (a) nor (b).

(2)     Parathyroid Hormone:

    (a)   demineralization of bone
    (b)   mineralization of bone
    (c)   increases basal metabolic rate
    (d)   Graves' disease results when in excess

(3)     Which cell makes bone?

    (a)   osteoblast        (b)   osteocyte
    (c)   osteoclast       (d)   all of these

(4)     Haversian Canals:

    (a)   markings seen on Mars
    (b)   nutrient systems of bone
    (c)   found in the inner ear
    (d)   communication between the left and right cerebral
        hemispheres

(5)     Components of a <u>mature</u> Haversian canal system would include
all except:

    (a)   osteoblasts      (b)   lacunae
    (c)   canaliculi       (d)   blood vessels

(6)     Components of the human axial skeleton include all except:

    (a)   sternum   (b)   vertebral column   (c)   hips   (d)   skull

(7)     Components of the appendicular human skeleton include all
except:

    (a)   shoulder girdle    (b)   arm bones
    (c)   ribs            (d)   leg bones

(8)     The humerus, radius and ulna are found in the:

    (a)   vertebral column    (b)   shoulder girdle
    (c)   arm            (d)   leg

(9)     All are parts of the vertebral column except:

    (a)   cervical   (b)   thoracic   (c)   caudal   (d)   lumbar

(10)    The parietal and occipital bones are found in the:

    (a)   vertebral column    (b)   skull
    (c)   hip girdle       (d)   foot

(11) The bones of the wrist are called:

    (a) carpals             (b) metacarpals
    (c) tarsals              (d) metatarsals

(12) The hip bone connects the _____ to the _____.

    (a) femur, sternum        (b) humerus, sacrum
    (c) femur, sacrum         (d) humerus, sternum

(13) Phalanges are found in the:

    (a) fingers  (b) toes  (c) both  (d) neither

(14) Bone is composed of _____ and _____.

    (a) calcium; phosphate    (b) globular proteins; ions
    (c) collagen; hydroxyapatite  (d) none of the above

(15) _____ serves as the focus of the deposition of the crystal matrix.

    (a) collagen           (b) osteocytes
    (c) hydroxyapatite     (d) cartilage

(16) The hormone that mobilizes $Ca^{+2}$ from bone:

    (a) thyroxin           (b) parathyroid hormone
    (c) calcitonin         (d) Vit D


## 2.14.3    ANSWERS TO QUESTIONS IN SECTION 2.14.2

( 1) c  (2) a  (3) a  (4) b  (5) a  (6) c  (7) c
( 8) c  (9) c  (10) b  (11) a  (12) c  (13) c  (14) c
(15) a  (16) b


## 2.14.4    DISCUSSION OF ANSWERS TO QUESTIONS IN SECTION 2.14.2

All questions are adequately discussed in the Section.


## 2.14.5    VOCABULARY CHECKLIST FOR THE SKELETAL SYSTEM

____ hydroxyapatite        ____ collagen
____ intramembranous    ____ endochondral
____ osteoblasts          ____ osteocytes
____ osteoclasts          ____ Haversian systems
____ canaliculi           ____ lacunae
____ spongy bone        ____ compact bone
____ flat bones          ____ long bones
____ parathyroid hormone  ____ calcitonin

**2.14.6** <u>CONCEPTS, PRINCIPLES, ETC.  CHECKLIST FOR THE SKELETAL</u>
<u>SYSTEM</u>

____ composition of bone
____ formation of bone
____ types of bone (histologically, grossly)

**2.15      Muscles (Esp. Skeletal)**

**2.15.1     <u>REVIEW OF MUSCLES</u>**

The three types of muscles are smooth, striated (skeletal), and
cardiac.  <u>Smooth muscle</u> is composed of distinct spindle shaped cells
with central nuclei and no visible markings.  They are innervated by
the autonomic nervous system and are largely involuntary.  Smooth
muscles can contract slowly and maintain contractions for long
periods of time.  This feature is useful for their function in organs
where they are found.  These include the gut (for peristalsis and
churning of food), in blood vessels (for regulation of blood
pressure), and in many ducts (e.g., the ureter for peristalsis).

<u>Cardiac muscle</u> is composed of distinct cells separated by condensed
cell membranes called intercalated discs.  Heart cells are connected
by gap junctions (specialized cell membrane regions) to speed
impulse conduction.  Cardiac muscle appears striated.  The muscle
fibers are highly branched--this probably adds to their strength.
Innervation is by the autonomic nervous system but beats are
originated by specialized muscle cells (see section 2.9.1.1).

<u>Skeletal muscle</u> are a <u>syncytium</u> (many cells fused together with loss
of intervening membranes and retention of nuclei) and appear
striated.  Skeletal muscles are innervated by the somatic nervous
system and are voluntary.  The control of voluntary movements
originates in a portion of the <u>cerebral cortex</u> (surface of cerebrum)
and are coordinated by impulses from the <u>cerebellum</u>.  Skeletal
muscles contract rapidly but tire easily.  A simple <u>twitch</u> of a
muscle involves the following steps:   (1) impulse from a nerve
stimulates the muscle, (2) a brief latent period, (3) then the phase
of contraction, and (4) a phase of relaxation.  If the muscle is
stimulated during the relaxation phase it can be made to contract
again.  If these stimuli are in rapid succession the contractions can
be made to <u>summate</u> to a sustained contraction called <u>tetanus</u> (Fig.
2.28(a, b).

**Fig. 2.28(a) - Phases of Contraction**

tetanus

Rapid sequence of stimuli (↑) cause muscle to contract continuously until it reaches a maximal state of contraction (tetanus).

**Fig. 2.28(b) - Tetanus**

Muscle <u>tone</u> differs from tetanus in that groups of muscle fibers of a muscle alternatingly contract and relax. This allows form and position (at rest) to be maintained.

Skeletal muscle uses $O_2$ (oxygen) in aerobic metabolism (Sec. 2.2.1) when it is available. In the absence of $O_2$, the production of energy requires that there be a final electron acceptor. This electron acceptor becomes pyruvate which is converted to lactate (Fig. 2.29).

pyruvate                lactate

e.g., NADH could transfer an $H:^-$ and $H^+$ is picked up from solution.

**Fig. 2.29 - Formation of Lactate**

The amount of lactate formed becomes a measure of the lack of $O_2$ (the usual electron acceptor). This is then the <u>oxygen debt</u> that muscles incur during exercise when their rate of $O_2$ demand exceeds that supplied. After exercise, the lactate is converted back to pyruvate, and the electrons are passed to $O_2$ as $O_2$ is supplied to the muscles and the oxygen debt is repaid. <u>In summary</u>, during exercise the energy metabolism of muscle switches from aerobic to anaerobic and an oxygen debt is incurred which is repaid when the exercise ends.

The skeletal muscles act across joints to move body parts. Each muscle has an <u>origin</u> and an <u>insertion</u>. In general, the origin is stationary, and when the muscle contracts, the insertion (and the bone it is attached to) moves toward the origin (Fig. 2.30).

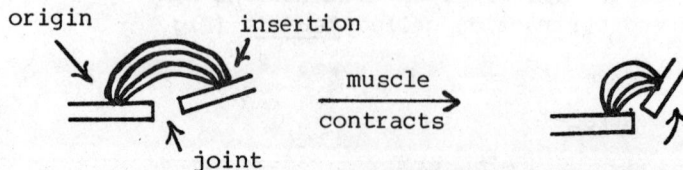

origin          insertion

muscle
contracts

joint

**Fig. 2.30 - Attachments of a Muscle**

Muscles work in pairs (or in more complex arrangements). For a muscle that moves a joint in one direction there is an <u>antagonistic</u> <u>muscle</u> that will move the joint in the opposite direction (i.e., undo that motion).  There are also synergistic muscles that aid in the motion caused by a given muscle.  At the elbow, the triceps (extension) and biceps (flexion) are examples of antagonistic muscles.  At the shoulder, the deltoid (raises arm) and supraspinatous (raises arm) are examples of synergistic muscles. Complex neural pathways insure coordination of the muscle groups.  A flexor decreases the angle of a joint.  An extensor increases the angle of a joint.  An abductor moves a limb away from the midline. An adductor moves a limb toward the midline.

The functioning unit of the muscle is the myofibril (muscle fibers are composed of myofibrils).  Myofibrils are composed of linearly arranged sarcomeres.  A sarcomere is limited by regions that anchor the actin (thin filaments) called the Z-lines.  Myosin (thick filaments) alternate with the actin and are not anchored.  Bands are labeled as shown in Fig. 2.31.

Fig. 2.31 - Components of a Sarcomere

When the muscle contracts, the Z-lines move together, the I and H bands decrease in size, and the A-band remains the same size.  The actin complex is composed of actin, tropomyosin and troponin.  Actin has sites which bind to heavy meromyosin when contraction occurs. Tropomyosin is an $\alpha$-helical protein wound around the actin (which is two intertwined $\alpha$-helical chains) and blocks the myosin binding site.  Troponin is a regulator protein bound to tropomyosin and has a site for binding $Ca^{+2}$ and a site that inhibits myosin's binding to actin.  When there is no $Ca^{+2}$ present, the troponin and tropomyosin prevent myosin binding and, hence, contraction.  When $Ca^{+2}$ is present, the $Ca^{+2}$ binds to troponin causing a conformational change which in turn causes tropomyosin to shift, uncovering the actin binding region for myosin, and contraction proceeds.  Myosin is composed of light meromyosin (the tail) and heavy meromyosin (the head).  The head binds to actin and contains an ATPase to break the bonds to actin.  Contraction is caused by the heads of myosin alternatingly binding and releasing actin in a rachet-like fashion. The sarcolemma (cell membrane of muscle) sends a system of membranes (T-tubules) into the muscle.  When an impulse from a nerve reaches the sarcolemma, this is transmitted down the T-tubules which release $Ca^{+2}$ into the sarcoplasm (muscle cell interior) for contraction. The sarcoplasmic reticulum (specialized smooth endoplasmic reticulum) abuts upon the T-tubules; its role is to remove the $Ca^{+2}$ from the sarcoplasm.


2.15.2        QUESTIONS TO REVIEW MUSCLES


(1)   All of the following are muscle proteins except:

      (a)  actin  (b)  myosin  (c)  fibrinogen  (d)  troponin

87

(2)   One of the histologic muscle types has striated fibers and is
      involuntary.  It is:

      (a)   smooth muscle          (b)   skeletal muscle
      (c)   cardiac muscle         (d)   none

(3)   Select the muscle type composed of distinct cells:

      (a)   smooth                 (b)   skeletal
      (c)   cardiac                (d)   both (a) and (c)

(4)   Intercalated discs are found in which type of muscle?

      (a)   skeletal  (b)  cardiac  (c)  smooth  (d)  all

(5)   Which type of muscle is a syncytium?

      (a)   skeletal  (b)  cardiac  (c)  smooth  (d)  all

(6)   All are true concerning smooth muscle except:

      (a)   composed of distinct spindle cells
      (b)   largely involuntary
      (c)   have intercalated discs
      (d)   found in the gut

(7)   All are true concerning cardiac muscle except:

      (a)   it is a syncytium
      (b)   it is striated
      (c)   it is involuntary
      (d)   gap junctions speed conduction

(8)   All are true concerning skeletal muscle except:

      (a)   they are a syncytium
      (b)   they are involuntary
      (c)   they are responsible for locomotion
      (d)   they contract rapidly but tire readily

(9)   Select the incorrect statement concerning muscles:

      (a)   ligaments attach bone to bone
      (b)   flexors decrease the angle at a joint
      (c)   adductors move a limb away from the midline
      (d)   tendons attach muscle to bone

(10)  The A-band of striated muscle represents:

      (a)   myosin only            (b)   actin only
      (c)   both (a) and (b)       (d)   neither (a) nor (b)

(11)  The Z-line as seen in striated muscle anchors:

      (a)   both actin and myosin  (b)   neither actin nor myosin
      (c)   actin                  (d)   myosin

(12)  During muscle contraction, all of the following occur except:

      (a)   Z-lines move together  (b)   A-band decreases in size
      (c)   I-band decreases in size (d)   H-band decreases in size

(13) Which of the following ions is of most importance in the mechanical contraction of muscle?

    (a) $Na^{+1}$  (b) $Ca^{+2}$  (c) $K^{+1}$  (d) $Cl^{-1}$

(14) Muscle tone depends upon

    (a) continual low level contraction of all fibers in the muscles;
    (b) summation of twitches to a plateau;
    (c) presence of short fibers that constantly appear contracted;
    (d) alternating contractions of different fiber groups in a muscle.

(15) During exercise

    (a) muscles depend on the Kreb's Cycle for energy;
    (b) $O_2$ becomes the electron acceptor;
    (c) lactate levels decrease;
    (d) energy metabolism changes from aerobic to anaerobic.

(16) Troponin

    (a) binds $Ca^{+2}$;
    (b) binds to tropomyosin;
    (c) inhibits myosin's binding to actin;
    (d) all of the above.

(17) The phase of contraction of a muscle occurs when

    (a) tropomyosin binds and releases actin;
    (b) myosin alternately binds and releases actin;
    (c) actin alternately binds and releases myosin;
    (d) none of the above.


2.15.3    ANSWERS TO QUESTIONS IN SECTION 2.15.2

( 1)  c  (2)  c  (3)  d  (4)  b  (5)  a  (6)  c  (7)  a
( 8)  b  (9)  c  (10)  c  (11)  c  (12)  b  (13)  b  (14)  d
(15)  d  (16)  d  (17)  b


2.15.4    DISCUSSION OF ANSWERS TO QUESTIONS IN SECTION 2.15.2


QUESTION #10  (Answer:  c)  Technically, the band is visible as such because of the myosin, but within the limits of the band actin is also present.


2.15.5    VOCABULARY CHECKLIST FOR MUSCLES


____ smooth muscle      ____ origin
____ cardiac muscle      ____ insertion

| ____ sarcomere | ____ skeletal muscle |
|---|---|
| ____ synergistic | ____ actin |
| ____ tetanus | ____ antagonistic |
| ____ myosin | ____ muscle tone |
| ____ flexor | ____ tropomyosin |
| ____ pyruvate | ____ extensor |
| ____ troponin | ____ lactate |
| ____ abductor | ____ sarcolemma |
| ____ adductor | ____ sarcoplasmic reticulum |
| ____ myofibril | ____ T-Tubules |

## 2.15.6   CONCEPTS, PRINCIPLES, ETC.  CHECKLIST FOR MUSCLES

____ types of muscle and differences between them
____ locus of control of voluntary muscles
____ difference between tone and tetanus
____ concept of oxygen debt
____ muscles as movers of bones
____ antagonistic and synergistic muscles
____ molecular mechanism of muscle contraction

## 2.16   Nervous System

## 2.16.1   REVIEW OF THE NERVOUS SYSTEM

## 2.16.1.1   The Central and Peripheral Nervous Systems; Nerve Conduction

Histologically, the nervous system is composed of neurons and glial cells.  Neurons conduct impulses, and glial cells provide some sort of supportive function.  There are many kinds of neurons and glial cells--only a typical neuron will be discussed.  A neuron has a cell body or soma that is characterized by having Nissl bodies (ribosomes), one or more short branched projections off the body called dendrites, and, usually, one long projection called an axon. Although impulses can travel in either direction in a dendrite or an axon, dendrites usually convey impulses toward the soma, and axons usually convey impulses away from the soma.  This directionality is achieved by the presence of synapses between adjacent neurons or a neuron and an effector (muscle or gland).  Synapses typically include an axon ending with transmitter substance, a synaptic cleft, and a dendrite or muscle or gland with receptors for the transmitter substance (Fig. 2.32).

Fig. 2.32 - Neuron

An impulse causes the axon to release the chemical transmitter; this diffuses across the cleft to the receptors and induces an impulse there which is then transmitted. An impulse or action potential is set up in a neuron when the potential difference (voltage) across its membrane reaches a threshold potential. The resting potential of a neuron is determined by the balance of $Na^+$ (most outside) and $K^+$ (most inside) on each side of the cell membrane--the outside is positive relative to the inside. An impulse or transmitter substance can disturb the ionic balance in such a way that $Na^+$ moves inside and $K^+$ moves outside (only $Na^+$ moves in the early phase of the action potential). This causes the cell potential to move toward the threshold potential. Once the threshold potential is reached, the action potential is initiated and this moves down the neuron to the axon end, releases transmitter and the process continues as such.

A Na-K ATPase maintains the concentration across the nerve membrane by active transport of the ions. Myelin sheaths (condensed cell membranes) around axons increase the speed of conduction (saltatory conduction). Details in Fig. 2.33.

Fig. 2.33 - Various Potentials of a Nerve

The refractory period is that time during which the nerve cannot respond to a stimulus.

Anatomically, the nervous system is divided into the central nervous system (CNS), consisting of the brain and spinal cord, and the peripheral nervous system (PNS), consisting of the cranial nerves (CN) and peripheral nerves (PN). The PNS may be divided into the autonomic nervous system (ANS) and the somatic nervous system (SNS). The ANS and SNS also have components in the CNS. The ANS is divided into the sympathetic and parasympathetic branches. The SNS contains the sensory (afferent--toward the CNS) and motor (efferent--away from the CNS) nerves.

Hindbrain (rhombencephalon), midbrain (mesencephalon), and forebrain (prosencephalon) are the gross divisions of the brain. The hindbrain consists of the myelencephalon (medulla) and metencephalon (pons). The midbrain is not further divided. The forebrain consists of the diencephalon (hypothalamus and thalamus) and the telencephalon (the cerebral hemispheres). The cerebellum is a derivative of the metencephalon. Respiratory and circulatory regulation, coughing, and vomiting reflexes, are functions of the medulla. Note that these are functions basic to life. The cerebellum is concerned with muscle coordination. No general functions are localized in the midbrain or pons; they serve important relay functions. The hypothalamus is the important regulator of the internal environment (controls hormones of the pituitary via releasing factors, thirst and hunger centers, water balance, temperature regulation) and also behavior (sexual, aggressive). The thalamus is the relay center for nearly all sensory input. The cerebrum (especially the cerebral cortex, i.e., surface) is the integrating and interpretation center for all sensory input and voluntary motor activity. In addition, memory, learning, emotions, etc., are also located here (Fig. 2.34).

The spinal cord (SC) has an interior of gray matter (neuron cell bodies) surrounded by white matter (myelinated axons). Serving as a path between the brain and the periphery (senses and muscles or glands) is the primary function of the SC. Descending tracts (from the brain to the SC) and ascending tracts (from SC to brain) are in the white matter. Sensory nerves enter dorsally and motor nerves exit ventrally. Several reflexes are at the SC level, e.g., the knee jerk (Fig. 2.35).

The sympathetic system (SS) peripherally consists of a chain of ganglia (neuron cell bodies outside the CNS) called the sympathetic chain which is parallel to and adjacent to the spinal cord. From these, nerves travel to many organs and tissues and may affect them all simultaneously (i.e., in a diffuse manner). In general, the SS moves the organism away from homeostasis as in the "fight or flight" phenomenon. Sympathetic discharges, e.g., cause the heart rate to increase, digestive process to stop, circulation to the skin to decrease, and blood flow to the heart and muscles to increase. The ganglia of the parasympathetic system (PS) are located near the end-organ, and it can exert specific effects directed at one organ or tissue. The PS tends to maintain homeostasis and, in general, opposes actions of the SS. Actions of the PS include slowing of the heart rate and increasing the digestive processes. The Vagus nerve (cranial nerve X) is a very important parasympathetic nerve to the heart and abdominal viscera. Acetylcholine is the postganglionic (after the synapses in the ganglia discussed above) transmitter in the PS. Norepinephrine is the postganglionic transmitter for the SS. The PS originates from the cranio-sacral CNS, and the SS originates from the thoraco-lumbar CNS.

There are 31 spinal nerves (SN). They are classified according to the level of their connection with the spinal cord--8 cervical, 12 thoracic, 5 lumbar, 5 sacral, 1 coccygeal. Each nerve contains motor and sensory components.

There are 12 cranial nerves (CN). Olfactory (I) for smell. Ocular (II) for vision. Oculomotor (III), Trochlear (IV) and Abducens (VI) for eye movements. Trigeminal (V) for sensory perception (pain, temperature, touch, pressure) over the face and head and for mastication (chewing). The Facial (VII) for taste and facial expression. The Vestibulocochlear (VIII) for balance and hearing. The Glossopharyngeal (IX) for taste and swallowing. The Vagus (X) for voice, swallowing, digestive functions (secretions, peristalsis), and slowing heart rate. The Spinal Accessory (XI) helps rotate head and move shoulders. The Hypoglossal (XII) for tongue movement.

The brain and spinal cord are covered by meninges. These are, from the outside in: the dura mater (tough fibrous layer), the arachnoid (vascular and nutrient layer), and the pia mater (fragile layer directly attached to nervous tissue).

Summary of the above information is in Fig. 2.36.

Lateral View of the Brain

**Fig. 2.34 -- The Cerebral Cortex**

**Fig. 2.35 -- The Spinal Cord**

Divisions of the Nervous System

| Nervous System | | | | | | | | |
|---|---|---|---|---|---|---|---|---|
| CNS | | | | | | | PNS | |
| Brain | | | | | | SC | ANS | SNS |
| Hindbrain | | Mid-Brain | Forebrain | | | | PS | SS |
| Myelen-cephalon | Meten-cephalon | " | Dien-cephalon | | Telen-cephalon | | | |
| Medulla | Pons | Cere-bellum | " | Thal-amus | Hypo-thalamus | Cerebral Hemispheres | | |

**Fig. 2.36 - Summary of CNS Organization**

The simplest functional organization of the nervous system is into
reflex arcs. The basic structure consists of a sensory neuron which
detects a stimulus and transmits it to the spinal cord where a motor
neuron is stimulated which transmits the impulse to an effector
(gland or muscle) and which causes the organism to respond (Fig.
2.37).

**Fig. 2.37 - Reflex Arc**

Not all neurons stimulate other neurons. Some inhibit other neurons. This adds another level of functional complexity. In the example above the afferent neuron could have also stimulated an interneuron (in the spinal cord) which could have inhibited the motor neuron of the antagonist of the muscle that contracted:

Stimulus—>

sensory
interneuron—
motor

muscle #2
antagonist to #1 relaxes

motor +

muscle #1
contracts

+ = stimulates

- = inhibits

This can be magnified many times thereby affording numerous possibilities for antagonistic or synergistic actions in the nervous system.

## 2.16.1.2    The Human Ear

The human ear is divided into an external ear (pinna and auditory canal), the middle ear (the tympanic membrane and the three bones—malleus or hammer, incus or anvil, and stapes or stirrup), and the internal ear (the cochlea, the semicircular canals, and the origin of the vestibulocochlear nerve). The tympanic membrane (eardrum) is attached to the malleus which attaches to the incus which attaches to the stapes which attaches to the oval window of the cochlea. The outer and middle ear function to match the impedance of the air outside and the fluid of the cochlea inside. This mechanism results in more efficient transmission of sound. Sound waves are transmitted from the stapes via the oval window to the fluid in the cochlea. This fluid sets up vibrations in the basilar membrane which causes special hair cells to send impulses to the auditory part of the vestibulocochlear (VIII) nerve which transmits them to the auditory cortex in the temporal lobe of the cerebrum. The basilar membrane, tectoral membrane, and hair cells run the full length of the cochlea and together constitute the organ of Corti. The distance from the oval window that the vibration of the basilar membrane is a maximum determines the frequency (pitch) of the sound—highest frequencies are closest to the oval window. The round window, at the other end of the cochlea, serves as a release of pressure imparted to the cochlear fluid by the stapes (Fig. 2.38).

The vestibular system is continuous anatomically but not functionally with the cochlea. The system is filled with fluid (endolymph) and contains the sacculus, the utricle and three perpendicular semicircular canals. Each semicircular canal has an ampulla region which contains hair cells sensitive to changes in angular acceleration. The utricle and sacculus contain a special sensory region called the macula which has crystals of calcium carbonate on it. These regions are sensitive to changes in gravity (position) and linear acceleration. Impulses travel from these special regions via the vestibular portions of the vestibulocochlear nerve (VIII) to the CNS. The vestibular system helps maintain posture, balance, spatial orientation, and stabilization of eye movements.

Ear

CROSS SECTION OF COCHLEA          ORGAN OF CORTI

**Fig. 2.38 - The Ear**

### 2.16.1.3   The Human Eye (Fig. 2.39)

Anatomically, the eye is separated by the lens into an anterior
region filled by the aqueous humor and a posterior region filled by
the vitreous humor. There are three layers in the eye. The sclera
(dense connective tissue) is the outermost. It is covered
anteriorly by the conjunctiva (whites of the eyes). It is continuous
with the clear portion called the cornea which is important in
focusing light. Inside the sclera is the choroid which contains the
blood vessels and black pigment to prevent light scattering.
Continous with the choroid in front are the iris (which gives the eye
its color and opens and shuts to let light in through the pupil) and
the ciliary muscle (which controls the shape of the lens and helps to
focus or accommodate the eye to distance). The innermost layer is
the retina which is the light sensitive layer containing rods and
cones. Rods are located peripherally in the eye, are concerned with
vision in dim light and peripheral vision, and contain rhodopsin
(retinal from Vit A and a protein called opsin). Light converts
retinal from a cis to a trans form which causes rhodopsin to fall
apart and somehow sets up an impulse which is eventually transmitted
to the optic nerve (Cranial Nerve II). Cones are located more
centrally, are concerned with bright light and color vision, contain
iodopsin (light sensitive substance) and are maximally concentrated

at the <u>fovea</u> (or macula area) which has the highest visual acuity (ability to see clearly points that are close together).

<u>Light passes</u> through the cornea where it is refracted (bent). It then passes through the aqueous humor and then through the pupil. The pupil size is regulated by the iris which is regulated by the parasympathetic (causes pupil to get smaller) and the sympathetic (causes pupil to get larger) systems. Next, the light passes through the lens where it is refracted further and focused upon the retina (after it passes through the vitreous). The lens is flat for objects far away (ciliary muscle relaxed), and it is rounded for objects nearby (ciliary muscle contracted--parasympathetic). Light then stimulates the cones and rods of the retina. From here nerve impulses are transmitted via the Ocular nerve (II) to the visual center in the occipital cortex of the cerebrum.

<u>Emmetropia</u> means that light is focused on the retina (by the cornea-lens system) when objects are near or far. <u>Myopia</u> (near-sightedness) means light is focused on the retina only when objects are near but not when objects are far away. A cause may be an eyeball that is too long and correction is by diverging (concave) glasses (i.e., lens). <u>Hypermetropia</u> (far-sightedness) means light is focused on the retina when objects are far away and not when they are near. A cause may be an eyeball that is too short and correction is by converging (convex) glasses. To <u>summarize</u> (Fig. 2.40) the problem in myopia is a cornea-lens system that refracts light relatively (for the eyeball length) too strong and focuses light in front of the retina when the object is far away. In hypermetropia, the problem is a cornea-lens system that refracts light relatively too weak and focuses light behind the retina when objects are near.

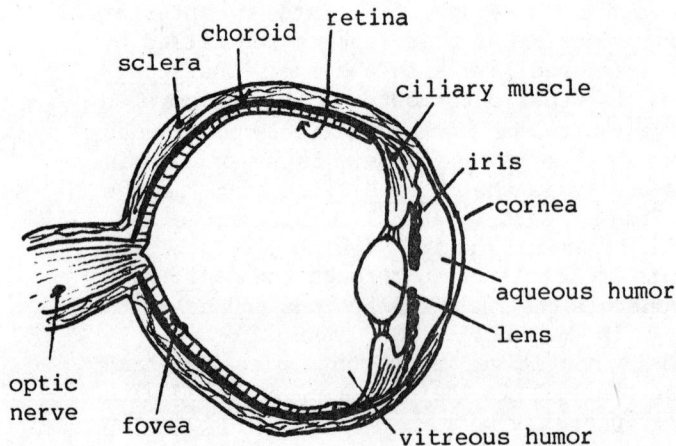

**Fig. 2.39 - The Eye**

object close      object far away      correction with diverging lens

(a) MYOPIA

object close      object far away      correction with converging lens

(b) HYPERMETROPIA

**Fig. 2.40 – Myopia (a) and Hypermetropia (b)**

2.16.2      QUESTIONS TO REVIEW THE NERVOUS SYSTEM

(1) Select the incorrect statement concerning the spinal cord:

     (a) gray matter is central
     (b) white matter is peripheral
     (c) sensory nerves enter ventrally
     (d) motor nerves exit ventrally

(2) Which is(are) not part of the central nervous system?

     (a) thalamus            (b) hypothalamus
     (c) spinal cord          (d) cranial nerves

(3) Glial cells are found in the:

     (a) muscular system        (b) endocrine system
     (c) nervous system         (d) skeletal system

(4) All are specifically associated with a neuron except:

     (a) lack of a nucleus       (b) Nissl bodies
     (c) dendrite             (d) axon

(5) What entity of neurons allow for one-way conduction of impulses in the nervous system?

     (a) axons    (b) dendrites    (c) synapses    (d) somas

(6) Which of the following can conduct impulses away from the neuron cell body or toward it?

     (a) axon    (b) dendrite    (c) both    (d) neither

(7)  When the potential difference across a nerve membrane equals
     the threshold, what results?

     (a)  an action potential
     (b)  synthesis of transmitter substances
     (c)  destruction of transmitter substances
     (d)  nothing until the resting potential is exceeded

(8)  What ion(s) determine the resting potential of a nerve cell?

     (a)  sodium                      (b)  potassium
     (c)  calcium                     (d)  both (a) and (b)

(9)  The concentrations of ions across the cell membrane is
     maintained by:

     (a)  diffusion                   (b)  active transport
     (c)  osmosis                     (d)  facilitated transport

(10) Myelin sheaths are found:

     (a)  surrounding tendons         (b)  covering the brain
     (c)  covering muscles            (d)  around axons of
                                           neurons

(11) During the early phase of the action potential

     (a)  only $Na^+$ moves;
     (b)  only $K^+$ moves;
     (c)  $Na^+$ moves into the cell and $K^+$ moves out;
     (d)  $Na^+$ moves out of the cell and $K^+$ moves in.

(12) The refractory period occurs

     (a)  before threshold is exceeded;
     (b)  before the action potential;
     (c)  after the action potential;
     (d)  roughly during the action potential.

(13) The peripheral nervous system includes:

     (a)  spinal nerves              (b)  cranial nerves
     (c)  spinal cord                (d)  both (a) and (b)

(14) The autonomic nervous system includes:

     (a)  sympathetic system    (b)  parasympathetic system
     (c)  somatic nervous system (d)  both (a) and (b)

(15) The hindbrain contains:

     (a)  thalamus  (b)  medulla  (c)  cerebrum  (d)  spinal cord

(16) All are associated with the forebrain except:

     (a)  diencephalon               (b)  telencephalon
     (c)  myelencephalon             (d)  hypothalamus

(17) All are functions of the medulla except:

     (a)  voluntary movements        (b)  respiratory regulation
     (c)  circulatory regulation     (d)  cough reflex

(18)   The cerebellum:

    (a)   regulates respiration    (b)   is the site of memory
    (c)   coordinates motor activity    (d)   is the site of behavior

(19)   Select the incorrect statement concerning the sympathetic nervous system:

    (a)   sympathetic ganglia are near the spinal cord
    (b)   causes the heart rate to incresae
    (c)   increases blood flow in certain tissues
    (d)   moves the organism toward homeostasis

(20)   Select the incorrect statement concerning the parasympathetic system:

    (a)   ganglia are located near the end-organ
    (b)   increases the heart rate
    (c)   maintains homeostasis
    (d)   increases digestive actions

(21)   Vagus Nerve:

    (a)   parasympathetic    (b)   supplies gut and the heart
    (c)   a cranial nerve    (d)   all are correct

(22)   Select the correct sequence of the meninges from outside inward:  (A=arachnoid, D=dura, P=pia)

    (a)   A,D,P    (b)   D,P,A    (c)   P,A,D    (d)   D,A,P

(23)   Frequency (pitch) is determined in the ear by the:

    (a)   oval window    (b)   basilar membrane
    (c)   tympanic membrane    (d)   medial geniculate body

(24)   Which structure is not found in the middle ear of humans?

    (a)   cochlea    (b)   tympanic membrane    (c)   anvil    (d)   incus

(25)   Organ of Corti:

    (a)   brain    (b)   eye    (c)   ear    (d)   bone

(26)   Hearing is localized in which lobe of the cerebral cortex?

    (a)   frontal    (b)   parietal    (c)   temporal    (d)   occipital

(27)   All are components of the vestibular system except:

    (a)   semicircular canals    (b)   sacculus
    (c)   organ of Corti    (d)   utricle

(28)   Semicircular canals are sensitive to:

    (a)   linear acceleration    (b)   angular acceleration
    (c)   gravity    (d)   all of the above

(29)   The vestibular system is important for all except:

    (a)   balance    (b)   posture
    (c)   spatial orientation    (d)   voluntary movement

(30)  A reflex arc usually consists of

   (a)  sensory neuron, motor neuron, and their synapse in the
        spinal cord;
   (b)  sensory and motor neurons only;
   (c)  as in (a) and always an interneuron;
   (d)  none of the above.

(31)  Which structure is anterior to the lens in the human eye?

   (a)  aqueous humor          (b)  vitreous humor
   (c)  retina                 (d)  choroid

(32)  From the outside in, the sequence of layers of the eye is:
      (C=choroid, R=retina, S=sclera)

   (a)  S,C,R     (b)  C,R,S     (c)  R,S,C     (d)  S,R,C

(33)  Select the incorrect association of structure and function in
      the eye:

   (a)  cornea--scatters light
   (b)  choroid--prevents light scattering
   (c)  iris--regulates amount of light that enters eye
   (d)  ciliary muscle--controls shape of the lens

(34)  Select the _incorrect_ statement concerning rods and cones of
      the eye:

   (a)  rods are for vision in dim light
   (b)  rods are located peripherally in the eye
   (c)  cones are for color vision
   (d)  cones contain rhodopsin

(35)  All are function or properties of cones of the eye except:

   (a)  provide for high visual acuity
   (b)  peripheral vision
   (c)  color vision
   (d)  vision in bright lights

(36)  Select the correct path of light through the eye (anterior to
      posterior):

   (a)  cornea, aqueous humor, lens, vitreous humor, retina
   (b)  lens, aqueous humor, cornea, vitreous humor, retina
   (c)  cornea, vitreous humor, lens, aqueous humor, retina
   (d)  retina, cornea, aqueous humor, lens, vitreous humor

(37)  Select incorrect statement:

   (a)  converging lenses will correct for myopic eyes
   (b)  light is focused in front of the retina when objects are
        distant in myopic eyes
   (c)  light is focused behind the retina when objects are near
        in hypermetropic eyes
   (d)  convex lens will correct hypermetropic eyes

## 2.16.3     ANSWERS TO QUESTIONS IN SECTION 2.16.2

( 1)  c    (2)  d    (3)  c    (4)  a    (5)  c    (6)  c    (7)  a
( 8)  d    (9)  b   (10)  d   (11)  a   (12)  d   (13)  d   (14)  d
(15)  b   (16)  c   (17)  a   (18)  c   (19)  d   (20)  b   (21)  d
(22)  d   (23)  b   (24)  a   (25)  c   (26)  c   (27)  c   (28)  b
(29)  d   (30)  a   (31)  a   (32)  a   (33)  a   (34)  d   (35)  b
(36)  a   (37)  a


## 2.16.4     DISCUSSION OF ANSWERS IN SECTION 2.16.2

All questions are adequately discussed in the Section.


## 2.16.5     VOCABULARY CHECKLIST FOR THE NERVOUS SYSTEM

| | |
|---|---|
| _____ glial cell | _____ afferent |
| _____ sympathetics | _____ neuron |
| _____ efferent | _____ parasympathetics |
| _____ Nissl body | _____ sensory nerves |
| _____ vagus nerve (X) | _____ axon |
| _____ motor nerves | _____ acetylcholine |
| _____ dendrite | _____ hindbrain |
| _____ norepinephrine | _____ soma |
| _____ myelencephalon | _____ spinal nerves |
| _____ synapse | _____ medulla |
| _____ cranial nerves | _____ transmitters |
| _____ metencephalon | _____ olfactory (I) |
| _____ action potential | _____ pons |
| _____ Ocular (II) | _____ threshold potential |
| _____ diencephalon | _____ Oculomotor (III) |
| _____ resting potential | _____ thalamus |
| _____ trochlear (IV) | _____ Na-K ATPase |
| _____ hypothalamus | _____ trigeminal (V) |
| _____ myelin sheath | _____ telencephalon |
| _____ abducens (VI) | _____ refractory period |
| _____ cerebral hemispheres | _____ Facial (VII) |
| _____ central nervous system | _____ spinal cord |
| _____ vestibulocochlear (VIII) | _____ peripheral nervous system |
| _____ brain | _____ glossopharyngeal (IX) |
| _____ autonomic nervous system | _____ white matter |
| _____ Spinal Accessory (XI) | _____ somatic nervous system |
| _____ gray matter | _____ Hypoglossal (XII) |
| _____ dura mater | _____ arachnoid |
| _____ pia mater | _____ meninges |
| _____ reflex arc | _____ interneuron |
| _____ middle ear | _____ inner ear |
| _____ outer ear | _____ semicircular canals |
| _____ tympanic membrane | _____ malleus |
| _____ incus | _____ stapes |
| _____ oval window | _____ cochlea |
| _____ hair cells | _____ basilar membrane |
| _____ tectoral membrane | _____ organ of Corti |
| _____ frequency (pitch) | _____ round window |

| | |
|---|---|
| ____ vestibular system | ____ endolymph |
| ____ ampulla | ____ utricle |
| ____ sacculus | ____ macula |
| ____ aqueous humor | ____ vitreous humor |
| ____ sclera | ____ cornea |
| ____ choroid | ____ iris |
| ____ pupil | ____ lens |
| ____ ciliary muscle | ____ retina |
| ____ rods | ____ rhodopsin |
| ____ retinal | ____ opsin |
| ____ cones | ____ iodopsin |
| ____ fovea | ____ emmetropia |
| ____ hypermetropia | ____ myopia |

## 2.16.6  CONCEPTS, PRINCIPLES, ETC. CHECKLIST FOR THE NERVOUS SYSTEM

____ structure of nerve cell
____ structure and function of synapse
____ origin and propagation of the action potential
____ organization and functions of the central nervous system
____ organization and functions of the peripheral nervous system
____ structure and function of the sympathetic system
____ structure and function of the parasympathetic system
____ coverings of the brain
____ structure of a reflex arc
____ basic idea of antagonism/synergism in the nervous system
____ structure and function of the ear
____ structure and function of the eye
____ structure and function of the semicircular canals

## 2.17  Endocrine System

### 2.17.1  REVIEW OF THE ENDOCRINE SYSTEM

Hormones are substances released from special secretory tissues, called endocrine glands, into the blood. From there they circulate to their target tissue, combine with the target receptor and exert their effect. Hormones are regulators, not catalysts (as enzymes are), of organism homeostasis. The major glands are the hypothalamus, pituitary, thyroid, parathyroid, adrenal, pancreas, gut, ovaries, testis, liver, kidney, pineal gland, thymus gland, skin and placenta. Gut hormones (gastrin, secretin, cholecystokinin-pancreozymin) are discussed in Section 2.13.1. Ovarian, placental and testicular hormones and FSH, LH and prolactin are discussed in section 2.18.1.

The hypothalamus synthesizes releasing factors (RF), inhibiting factors (IF), vasopressin (antidiuretic hormone--ADH) and oxytocin.

Vasopressin causes the kidney to retain water. Oxytocin causes contraction of certain smooth muscles and plays a role in uterine contractions of labor and milk ejection in lactation. Oxytocin and vasopressin are stored in the posterior pituitary until released. RFs and IFs act upon the anterior pituitary (AP). RFs cause the corresponding hormones of the AP to be synthesized and released from it. IFs inhibit release of the corresponding hormones. All of the hormones of the hypothalamus are peptides or proteins. Examples are TRF (TSH Releasing Factor) and PIF (Prolactin Inhibiting Factor).

The anterior pituitary (AP) synthesizes and releases several trophic (growth stimulating and supporting) hormones among others. Hormones secreted are thyroid stimulating hormone (TSH), adrenal cortex stimulating hormone (ACTH), follicle stimulating hormone (FSH), and luteinizing hormone (LH) which are all trophic hormones to the glands indicated by their names. The AP also secretes growth hormone (GH) and prolactin (also called lactogenic hormone). GH functions via somatomedin (produced in the liver) to stimulate the growth of many tissues in the body. Oversecretion of GH results in Giantism (if before adolescence) or acromegaly (if as an adult). All of the AP hormones are proteins or glycoproteins. MSH (melanocyte stimulating hormone) is secreted by the intermediate lobe of the pituitary gland.

The thyroid gland produces thyroxin and calcitonin. Thyroxin, which is a modified tyrosine with iodine attached, works by increasing the rate of metabolism. Calcitonin decreases the calcium in the blood by causing it to move into the bones.

The adrenal gland is composed of a cortex and medulla. The cortex is stimulated by ACTH to synthesize glucocorticoids (the primary one being cortisol) which perform many functions incuding regulation of blood sugar (increases it) and fighting stress (e.g., infections). Mineralocorticoids (primary one is aldosterone) are also synthesized by the cortex but usually as a result of stimulation by angiotensin II (see below). Aldosterone causes the kidney to retain sodium (and hence water) and secrete potassium. The medulla synthesizes epinephrine which is a sympathetic stimulant (see Section 2.15.1.1). The cortical hormones are steroids. The medullary hormones are modified tyrosines.

Parathyroid glands (located on the thyroid gland, but not part of it) secrete parathyroid hormone (PTH, a protein) which regulates calcium and phosphorus metabolism. Calcium and phosphate are resorbed from bone under the infuence of PTH.

The pancreas secretes insulin (from $\beta$-cells) and glucagon (from $\alpha$-cells) among other hormones and substances. Insulin acts to lower blood glucose by causing cells to take up glucose, it also causes amino acid and fatty acid uptake. Glucagon works to increase blood glucose by stimulating glycogenolysis (glycogen breakdown) and gluconeogenesis (synthesis of glucose from amino acids) by the liver. Insulin and glucagon are both proteins. Diabetes mellitus is due to a deficiency of insulin.

Vitamin D is taken in as a nutrient, then goes through a series of activation steps. First, it is activated by ultraviolet light in the skin, then it is hydroxylated successively in the liver and kidney. Its main role is to increase absorption of calcium by the gut through the stimulation of the synthesis of a calcium binding protein. Vit D is a steroid.

The kidney secretes renin, erythropoietin, and helps in the synthesis of active Vit D (above). Renin is an enzyme molecule that splits a small peptide called angiotensin I off the renin substrate (produced in the liver). Angiotensin I is further split by enzymes in the lung or blood to yield angiotensin II which is a potent constrictor of blood vessels and also stimulates synthesis and release of aldosterone from the adrenal. Erythropoietin is a protein hormone which stimulates the bone marrow to synthesize more red blood cells.

The pineal gland probably produces a host of hormones, but the best known is melatonin which is a modified tryptophan. The pineal gland suppresses pituitary, gonadal (ovary and testis), adrenal and thyroid function. These effects may be mediated via the hypothalamus.

Thymosin is produced by the thymus gland and plays a role in the immunologic system.

Hormones regulate themselves by means of a process called feedback inhibition. A gland produces a hormone and this hormone, or a product, feeds back at some level to shut off its synthesis. This is illustrated in Fig. 2.41. Note the following points:

(1) Long Loop - the specific hormone feeds back on the hypothalamus to inhibit release of the RF. This then prevents release of the trophic hormone which prevents the synthesis of the specific hormone. As this decreases, its inhibition on the hypothalamus decreases and more of the RF is released which causes more trophic hormone to be released, etc. This cycle can continue as such or be modified positively or negatively by factors outside of the axis (hypothalamus-pituitary-gland) shown.

(2) & (3) Short Loops - Mechanisms as above, but the hormones feed back on the gland that stimulated their synthesis (i.e., the pituitary) instead of a point farther removed (i.e., the hypothalamus).

For a given hormone all combinations of the above may exist.

(-) ≡ inhibition of that gland

(+) ≡ stimulation of that gland

Fig. 2.41 - Feedback Loops

Hormones exert their actions in many ways (some still unknown). Some protein hormones seem to act via cAMP by combining with specific receptors on the target cell membrane. Some steroids exert their effect by combining with receptors in the target cell cytoplasm (they diffuse through the lipid cell membrane). They then move into the nucleus to interact with DNA to cause synthesis of mRNA, which makes specific proteins (usually enzymes).

## 2.17.2    QUESTIONS TO REVIEW THE ENDOCRINE SYSTEM

(1)    Insulin:

    (a)    secreted by the pancreas
    (b)    a protein
    (c)    involved in the metabolism of glucose, amino acids, fats
    (d)    all of the above

(2)    Vitamin D:

    (a)    is actually a hormone after modification in the body
    (b)    increases absorption of calcium from the gut
    (c)    requires metabolic changes in the skin, liver, and kidney to function
    (d)    all of the above

(3)    Select the incorrectly paired hormone and disease or deranged process associated with an excess/deficiency of it:

    (a)    growth hormone--acromegaly
    (b)    insulin--diabetes mellitus
    (c)    cortisol--abnormal calcium/phosphate metabolism
    (d)    thyroxin--altered metabolic rate

(4)    All of the following hormones are correctly paired with one of its major functions except:

    (a)    thyroxin--increases metabolic rate
    (b)    glucocorticoids--increases blood sugar levels
    (c)    aldosterone--role in "fight or flight" sympathetic response
    (d)    parathyroid hormone--regulation of calcium/phosphorus metabolism

(5)    Select the endocrine gland that is incorrectly paired with its hormone product:

    (a)    adrenal cortex--cortisol
    (b)    adrenal medulla--aldosterone
    (c)    adrenal medulla--epinephrine
    (d)    adrenal cortex--mineralocorticoids

(6)    Select the hormone incorrectly paired with its target tissue:

    (a)    TSH--thyroid gland    (b)    ACTH--anterior pituitary
    (c)    LH--ovary or testis    (d)    MSH--melanocytes

(7)    Which hormones are synthesized by the hypothalamus?

    (a)    releasing factors    (b)    vasopressin
    (c)    oxytocin    (d)    all of the above

(8) Hormones synthesized and released by the anterior pituitary is(are)

(a) Thyroid Stimulating Hormone (TSH);
(b) Folicle Stimulating Hormone (FSH);
(c) Growth Hormone;
(d) all of the above.

(9) Which of the following tissues secrete hormones?

(a) pancreas                  (b) ovaries
(c) gastrointestinal tract    (d) all of the above

(10) All of the following are general characteristics of hormones except

(a) hormones are secreted into the blood;
(b) hormones are regulators not initiators of homeostatic processes;
(c) hormones are all proteins;
(d) hormones do not function like enzymes.

(11) All of the following are general characteristics of hormones except

(a) hormones regulate themselves by feedback inhibition;
(b) hormones may be proteins, peptides, steroids, or modified amino acids;
(c) some protein hormones act via cAMP;
(d) most steroid hormones act via cAMP.

(12) Melatonin is produced by the:

(a) pineal gland              (b) skin
(c) liver                     (d) pituitary gland

(13) Thymosin is concerned with:

(a) metabolic rate           (b) immunologic competence
(c) calcium/phosphate        (d) none of the above

(14) Calcitonin:

(a) decreases serum calcium
(b) has no effect on serum calcium
(c) is made in the parathyroid gland
(d) is a steroid

(15) All of the following are true about glucagon except:

(a) causes glycogenolysis
(b) is a steroid
(c) causes gluconeogenesis
(d) made in the pancreas

106

(16)   In the hypothalamic-pituitary-adrenal axis, if the long feedback loop holds then

   (a)   ACTH inhibits the production of ACTH-RF by the hypothalamus;
   (b)   cortisol inhibits the production of ACTH by the pituitary;
   (c)   cortisol inhibits the ACTH-RF produced by the hypothalamus;
   (d)   none of the above.


## 2.17.3   ANSWERS TO QUESTIONS IN SECTION 2.17.2

( 1)  d   (2)  d   (3)  c   (4)  c   (5)  b   (6)  b   (7)  d
( 8)  d   (9)  d  (10)  c  (11)  d  (12)  a  (13)  b  (14)  a
(15)  b  (16)  c


## 2.17.4   DISCUSSION OF ANSWERS IN SECTION 2.17.2

All questions of adequately discussed in the Section except:

QUESTION #16   (Answer:  c)  In the long feedback loop, the specific hormone (cortisol) of the gland (adrenal) feeds back past the pituitary to the hypothalamus.


## 2.17.5   VOCABULARY CHECKLIST FOR THE ENDOCRINE SYSTEM

| | |
|---|---|
| ____ hormone | ____ ACTH |
| ____ thyroid gland | ____ mineralocorticoids |
| ____ hypothalamus | ____ FSH |
| ____ thyroxin | ____ aldosterone |
| ____ releasing factors | ____ LH |
| ____ calcitonin | ____ epinephrine |
| ____ inhibiting factors | ____ growth hormone |
| ____ adrenal gland | ____ parathyroid gland |
| ____ vasopressin | ____ prolactin |
| ____ adrenal cortex | ____ PTH |
| ____ oxytocin | ____ giantism |
| ____ adrenal medulla | ____ pancreas |
| ____ pituitary | ____ acromegaly |
| ____ glucocorticoids | ____ insulin |
| ____ TSH | ____ MSH |
| ____ cortisol | ____ glucagon |
| ____ gluconeogenesis | ____ glycogenolysis |
| ____ Vitamin D | ____ kidney |
| ____ renin | ____ renin substrate |
| ____ angiotensin I | ____ angiotensin II |
| ____ erythropoietin | ____ pineal gland |
| ____ melatonin | ____ thymus gland |
| ____ thymosin | ____ long loop |
| ____ short loop | ____ trophic hormone |
| ____ feedback inhibition | |

2.17.6    CONCEPTS, PRINCIPLES, ETC.   CHECKLIST FOR THE ENDOCRINE
          SYSTEM


____  characteristics of hormones
____  the different endocrine glands and hormones
____  role of the hypothalamus and pituitary gland
____  concept of feedback inhibition
____  general mechanisms of action of hormones



## 2.18    Reproductive System



## 2.18.1    REVIEW OF THE REPRODUCTIVE SYSTEM



### 2.18.1.1    Male and Female Anatomy


Male anatomy    The testicles are located outside the body because
spermatogenesis requires a temperature lower than body temperature.
The scrotum is the sack that contains the testicles.  Sperm travels
from the testis to the epididymis (where sperm maturation is
completed) to the vas deferens to the ejaculatory duct to the penile
urethra to the exterior.   The seminal vesicles and prostate gland
contribute fluid to the ejaculate (which averages 1-2cc).  The penis
consists of a glans penis (very sensitive) and a shaft (consisting of
cavernous tissue for blood engorgement).   Penile erection (mostly
parasympathetic stimulation) results from veins of the penis
clamping down and, hence, holding blood in the penis.  Ejaculation is
a reflex mediated by the sympathetic nervous system.  Males continue
to produce sperm from puberty onwards.

Female anatomy    The labia are composed of the major folds or labia
majora (analogous to the scrotum), and the minor folds or labia
minora (analogous to the penile shaft).   The clitoris (located
between the minor folds ventrally) is analogous to the glans penis
and is also very sensitive. The vagina, the passage from the
external genital opening, terminates in the cervix (part of the
uterus), which has an os (opening) to the uterine cavity (where the
fertilized egg implants). The placenta derives from the uterus and
the developing embryo. Connected to the uterus are the Fallopian
tubes that lead to the ovaries (but are not connected to them).



### 2.18.1.2    Meiosis and Gametogenesis


Meiosis   (Fig. 2.42) Meiosis has two phases.   The first, a
reductional division is different from mitosis (Section 2.5.1.3).
Prophase I - the DNA coils to become the chromosome, and there is
exact pairing (synapsis) of the pairs of homologous chromosomes
allowing crossing-over to occur.    The nuclear membrane
disintegrates, and the centrioles migrate to opposite poles of the
nucleus.  Metaphase I - the two members of the homologous pair align

along the equatorial plane. The disposition of the maternal and paternal members of the pair toward either pole is random. The spindle fibers attach to the centromere of only one member of each homologous pair. Anaphase I - chromosomes of each homologous pair separate and move toward opposite poles, the centromeres do not divide. Telophase I - cytokinesis occurs. In spermatocytes the distribution of the cytoplasm is equitable giving two cells of equal size. In oocytes, the division is unequal giving one secondary oocyte and one polar body. Interphase I - a short period in which chromosomes may uncoil somewhat and the nuclear membrane may be partially reconstituted. The daughter cells now contain the haploid number of chromosomes each composed of two daughter chromatids. Prophase II, metaphase II and anaphase II are all like the corresponding mitosis phases. Telophase II is like mitosis but has haploid cells.

Gametogenesis in Males (Fig. 2.43) The first step is a differentiation of spermatogonia (2n) into primary spermatocytes (2n) into secondary spermatocytes (1n) into spermatids (1n) by meiosis. The second step is called spermiogenesis in which spermatids (1n) are transformed into sperm (1n). A sperm consists of a head, a middle part and a tail. The head contains an acrosome (contains digestive enzymes to penetrate egg, probably derived from the Golgi apparatus) and nuclear material (DNA) surrounded by very little cytoplasm. The midpiece contains mitochondria for power. The tail has the structure of a centriole and provides locomotion. Leydig cells (produce testosterone) and Sertoli cells (support sperm development) are also in the testis. Sperm deposited in the vagina by the penis reach the cervix within 90 seconds and migrate up the Fallopian tubes to fertilize the ovum there.

Gametogenesis in Females (Fig. 2.44) The ovary consists of oogonia (2n) which divide and differentiate (before birth) into primary (1⁰) oocytes (2n) which become surrounded by follicular cells (from the mesenchymal stroma), and together constitute the primordial follicle. The primary oocytes are arrested in the prophase of the first meiotic division, and they may remain as such from birth to menopause. There are about 5 million oogonia, but only 1 million primary oocytes at birth and about 40,000 at puberty--the remainder degenerate (become atretic follicles). Beginning at puberty, a group of primordial follicles begin differentiation to Graffian follicles, and the 1⁰ oocyte (2n) becomes the secondary (2⁰) oocyte (1n). The 2⁰ oocyte is surrounded by the zona pellucida (a gel-like substance), this is surrounded by follicular cells, and these are surrounded by thecal cells (which secrete estrogens). Next, ovulation occurs by expelling the secondary oocyte and zona pellucida plus some follicular cells (corona radiata together) into the Fallopian tubes. If fertilization occurs in the Fallopian tubes (the usual location), the secondary oocyte completes meiosis to become an ovum (1n) and fuses with the sperm--if it is not fertilized, it degenerates. The follicular and thecal cells left behind become the corpus luteum which is the main source of progesterone which maintains pregnancy. The other follicles that began to develop degenerate because only one follicle completes development and is ovulated from one ovary during each cycle. Polar bodies result from the division of the primary oocyte, the secondary oocyte, and possibly the first polar body. Polar bodies have nuclear material but no cytoplasm. Hence, each primary oocyte (2n) produces only one gamete.

## 2.18.1.3    The Menstrual Period (Not Specifically Requested in The MCAT Student Manual)

The female period is typically 28 days and consists of a menstrual flow (menses), a follicular phase (ovary)/proliferative phase (uterus), ovulation, and a luteal phase (ovary)/secretory phase (uterus) in that order. The first day of menses is conveniently taken as the first day of the cycle. Shedding of the uterine lining occurs during the menstrual flow. Development of the follicle under the stimulation of FSH (Follicle Stimulating Hormone) and proliferation of the cells of the uterine lining under the stimulation of estrogen (from the ovary) occurs in the follicular/proliferative phase. A rapid increase of estrogen triggers a surge of LH (Luteinizing Hormone) at midcycle which causes ovulation to occur (at about 14 days prior to the first day of menses). Just before ovulation, there is a slight dip in body temperature which then rises with ovulation--the progesterone is responsible for the temperature rise. During the luteal/secretive phase, the corpus luteum secretes progesterone, which, with estrogen, causes the uterus to secrete different substances. If fertilization and implantation occur, the corpus luteum continues to secrete progesterone under the stimulation of HCG (Human Chorionic Gonadotropin) from the placenta. If implantation does not occur, the corpus luteum degenerates and there is no progesterone to support the uterus, and menses (shedding of the uterine lining) occurs. Then the cycle repeats itself as FSH and estrogen concentrations rise. Menstrual cycles occur until nearly all the oocytes are depleted--this results in menopause.

**Fig. 2.42 - Meiosis**

**Fig. 2.43 - Gametogenesis in Males**

follicle cells
thecal cells
follicle cells
1° oocyte (2n)
Meiosis I
2° oocyte (1n)
polar body
Meiosis II
+ O + O + O

oogonium (2n)   primordial follicle   Graffian follicle   ovum (1n)   polar bodies

**Fig. 2.44 – Gametogenesis in Females**

2.18.2    QUESTIONS TO REVIEW THE REPRODUCTIVE SYSTEM

(1)    The testicles are located outside the body because

   (a)    that is the normal embryologic location;
   (b)    there is direct connection from the epididymis to the penile urethra;
   (c)    there is a need for autonomic peripheral nerves;
   (d)    spermatogenesis requires a temperature lower than body temperature.

(2)    Sperm travels through all of the following structures except:

   (a)    ureter             (b)    urethra
   (c)    vas deferens     (d)    epididymis

(3)    What structure is directly attached to the ovary?

   (a)    vagina           (b)    uterus
   (c)    Fallopian tubes   (d)    none of the above

(4)    The placenta of humans is composed of tissue derived from the

   (a)    uterus and developing embryo;
   (b)    uterus only;
   (c)    developing embryo only;
   (d)    none of the above.

(5)    The menstrual period (total cycle) is typically closest to:

   (a)    2 weeks        (b)    4 weeks
   (c)    2 months      (d)    1 year

(6)    The sequence of stages of the menstrual cycle (in reference to the ovary) following the menstral flow is:    (F=follicular phase, L=luteal phase, O=ovulation)

   (a)    F,O,L   (b)    L,O,F   (c)    O,F,L   (d)    F,L,O

(7)    Ovulation usually occurs

   (a)    1-3 days after menses (blood flow);
   (b)    14 days before menses;
   (c)    1-3 days before menses;
   (d)    during menses.

(8)   The corpus luteum secretes:

      (a)  progesterone  (b)  LH  (c)  FSH  (d)  HCG

(9)   The organ in the female analogous to the glans penis in the
      male is the:

      (a)  vagina                    (b)  labia minora
      (c)  labia majora              (d)  clitoris

(10)  Which hormone below is found primarily during the first half
      (follicular/proliferative phase) of the menstrual cycle?

      (a)  FSH  (b)  progesterone  (c)  prolactin  (d)  HCG

(11)  Synapsis and crossing over of chromosomes occur in which phase
      of meiosis?

      (a)  Interphase I             (b)  Prophase I
      (c)  Prophase II              (d)  Metaphase I

(12)  When do the centromeres divide in meiosis?

      (a)  Anaphase I               (b)  Anaphase II
      (c)  Telophase I              (d)  Telophase II

(13)  Which substance is not secreted by the ovary or uterus in a
      pregnant female?

      (a)  FSH                      (b)  HCG
      (c)  progesterone            (d)  estrogen

(14)  In males, gametes are formed in the:

      (a)  vas deferens             (b)  Leydig cells
      (c)  epididymis               (d)  seminiferous tubules

(15)  Polar bodies:

      (a)  the poles of magnets
      (b)  result from gametogenesis in the male
      (c)  result from gametogenesis in the female
      (d)  dipoles

(16)  Fertilization of the ovum by the sperm usually occurs in the:

      (a)  ovary  (b)  Fallopian tubes  (c)  uterus  (d)  vagina

(17)  Select the incorrect association:

      (a)  oogonia--1n              (b)  primary oocyte--2n
      (c)  secondary oocyte--1n     (d)  ova--1n

(18)  Corpus luteum:

      (a)  mature ovum              (b)  no hormones
      (c)  before ovulation         (d)  after ovulation

(19)  Tissue/cells not found in the testis:

      (a)  seminiferous tubules     (b)  Leydig cells
      (c)  spermatogonia            (d)  seminal vesicles

(20)   The primary oocyte remains arrested in what phase of meiosis from birth to puberty:

(a)   Prophase I              (b)   Prophase II
(c)   Metaphase I             (d)   Metaphase II

(21)   Which of the following contains no developing ovum?

(a)   Graffian follicle       (b)   primordial follicle
(c)   corpus luteum           (d)   none of the above

(22)   Select the incorrect association:

(a)   spermatogonia--2n       (b)   primary spermatocytes--2n
(c)   secondary spermatocytes--1n  (d)   spermatozoa--2n

(23)   Which is not associated with the male reproductive system?

(a)   Epididymis              (b)   Leydig cells
(c)   Thecal cells            (d)   Sertoli cells

(24)   The number of mature gametes resulting from meiosis of the primary oocyte in the female:

(a)  1      (b)  2      (c)  3      (d)  4

(25)   The number of mature gametes resulting from meiosis in the male:  \

(a)  1      (b)  2      (c)  3      (d)  4

(26)   The key difference(s) in Anaphase I of meiosis and anaphase of mitosis is:

(a)   crossing over occurs in Anaphase I of meiosis
(b)   centromeres divide in Anaphase I of meiosis
(c)   homologous chromosomes move to opposite poles in Anaphase I of meiosis
(d)   all of the above

2.18.3      ANSWERS TO QUESTIONS IN SECTION 2.18.2

( 1)  d   (2)  a   (3)  d   (4)  a   (5)  b   (6)  a   (7)  b
( 8)  a   (9)  d   (10)  a   (11)  b   (12)  b   (13)  a   (14)  d
(15)  c   (16)  b   (17)  a   (18)  d   (19)  d   (20)  a   (21)  c
(22)  d   (23)  c   (24)  a   (25)  d   (26)  c

2.18.4      DISCUSSION OF ANSWERS TO QUESTIONS IN SECTION 2.18.2

All questions adequately discussed in the Section.

## 2.18.5 VOCABULARY CHECKLIST FOR THE REPRODUCTIVE SYSTEM

_____ scrotum
_____ spermatogonia
_____ testicles
_____ secondary spermatocytes
_____ epididymis
_____ vas deferens
_____ spermiogenesis
_____ penile urethra
_____ spermatids
_____ seminal vesicles
_____ sperm
_____ prostate gland
_____ acrosome
_____ penis
_____ menses
_____ Sertoli cells
_____ ejaculation
_____ oogonia
_____ labia minora
_____ primary oocytes
_____ Anaphase I
_____ ovulation
_____ Telophase I
_____ secretory phase
_____ Interphase I
_____ FSH
_____ Telophase II
_____ estrogens
_____ luteal phase

_____ vagina
_____ cervix
_____ zona pellucida
_____ os
_____ thecal cells
_____ placenta
_____ ovary
_____ ovulation
_____ Fallopian tubes
_____ corona radiata
_____ meiosis
_____ corpus luteum
_____ reductional division
_____ polar bodies
_____ Leydig cells
_____ glans penis
_____ follicular phase
_____ Prophase I
_____ proliferative phase
_____ Metaphase I
_____ labia majora
_____ follicular cells
_____ clitoris
_____ primordial follicle
_____ LH
_____ atretic follicle
_____ progesterone
_____ Graffian follicle
_____ HCG
_____ penile erection

## 2.18.6 CONCEPTS, PRINCIPLES, ETC. CHECKLIST FOR THE REPRODUCTIVE SYSTEM

_____ male anatomy, female anatomy; relationships and differences between them
_____ meiosis and how it differs from mitosis and differences in males and females
_____ gametogenesis in males
_____ gametogenesis in females
_____ the menstrual period

## 2.19 Behavior

## 2.19.1 REVIEW OF BEHAVIOR

General behavioral responses, the effect of neurological changes upon behavior, and behavioral relationships in populations will be discussed. Motivation is considered to be the driving force of all behavior, innate and learned. It is believed that the internal state of the animal determines this motivation. A simple example being hunger causing the animal to search out food. The hypothalamus is probably a major control center. Much needs to be learned concerning motivation.


## 2.19.1.1    Basic Behavioral Responses


Behavioral responses may be divided broadly into those considered innate versus those considered learned. Innate implies a predominant inherited component that is only slightly modifiable by external factors. Learned implies a behavior that is largely modifiable by external factors, but it still depends, to some extent, upon inherited characteristics. Note that inheritance tends to set the limits of possible behavior, and the environment (external) determines the realization of behavior within those limits. In general, the limits set by inheritance increase as the evolutionary scale is ascended, and this implies that environmental factors may also play a greater role within those widened limits.

Innate types of behavior are reflexes, taxis, instincts, and biorhythms. Reflexes may be considered as the basic unit of behavior, even though they may be difficult to discern or not be present in advanced behaviors. The simplest reflex involves a stimulus perceived by a sensor, and the conduction of the stimulus to an effector which gives the response, e.g., the knee jerk reflex. There are more complex reflexes. Reflexes are, in general, rigid and automatic and essentially not modifiable by external factors. Taxis is a simple orienting movement usually in some relation to a stimulus, but not necessarily so. It may involve one or more reflexes. An example is the preference of a paramecium to be in a region of higher acidity (but not very high) than one of lower acidity. Instinct is generally considered to be rigid and stereotyped behavior little affected by learning. There is a strong inherited component, but the correct environmental opportunity must be present for it to express itself. For example, bird songs may be considered instinctive, but if a baby bird is not exposed to the song of its species during a given time period, it may not be able to sing. The inherited component allows the capacity for a specific type of song, but the correct environmental situation must be present. Note there is little room for "learning" because other species of birds cannot "teach" the baby birds their songs. Biorhythms exist not only for behaviors but for physiological functions as well. They tend to depend upon, or at least correlate with, environmental cycles such as day length (or night length), precipitation, and temperature. Daily cycles (24 hrs ) are called Circadian Rhythms. Many hormones are secreted in Circadian cycles, i.e., a peak secretion followed by a minimum secretion within a 24-hour period. Mating patterns of many animals follow seasonal cycles. The mechanisms of these cycles are not known, but the internal metabolism of the animal is suspected to play a role. Also, most of these cycles can be modified by environmental factors. For example, a 24-hour cycle can be changed to a 22-hour cycle.

Learning is the process whereby behavior is changed in an enduring (not necessarily permanent) manner by experiences and the environment. Changes in behavior due to learning must be distinguished from behavioral changes due to maturation (e.g., babies cannot physically walk until a certain age). Also the ability to learn can vary with a setting, may depend on a critical period during which "teaching" must occur, and may be delayed from the time of the "teaching." Note that all forms of learning are dependent upon adequate motivation. Types of learning include habituation, conditioning, trial and error, imprinting, and insight learning or reasoning as its ultimate extension.

Habituation is the gradual decline in the responses to insignificant stimuli due to the lack of positive reinforcement. Conditioning may be viewed as the establishment of active reflex neural pathways (by facilitation) which were present but not used. Conditioning is more complex than the usual reflex. Pavlov conditioning is the classic example of conditioning. If there exists a natural stimulus (called the unconditioned stimulus—US) which elicits a natural response (R), then if an artificial stimulus (called the conditioned stimulus—CS) is paired with the US, eventually the CS alone will elicit the R. This is because the animal comes to interpret the CS and US as interchangeable in eliciting the given R. But if the CS is continually given without the US, the CS will eventually cease to elicit the R—this is called extinction. To summarize:

$$
\begin{array}{ll}
\text{already existing} & \text{US} \longrightarrow \text{R} \\
\text{experimentally add} & \text{CS, US} \longrightarrow \text{R} \\
\text{eventually} & \text{CS} \longrightarrow \text{R}
\end{array}
$$

The intensity, duration, character, and timing relative to US of the CS are all important in eliciting the R. Trial and error learning is just what the words imply, and it is a very common method of learning. Similar to trial and error learning (some consider them to be the same) is operant conditioning. In this there is a response (R) for which there is no clear preceding stimulus. But following the response there is a reinforcement (RI). A positive reinforcement (PRI), also called a reward (such as food), increases the likelihood of future similar responses. A negative reinforcement (NRI), also called punishment (such as electric shock), decreases the likelihood of future responses. Note that the termination of NRI increases the likelihood of future responses. To summarize for operant conditioning:

present                                      future

Response (R) leads to      then       if more rewards (PRI),
   Reinforcement (RI)                      then more responses (R)     [↑PRI → ↑R]
                                        if less rewards (PRI),
   [R ⟶ RI]                                then less responses (R)     [↓PRI → ↓R]
                                        if more punishment (NRI),
                                           then less responses (R)     [↑NRI → ↓R]
                                        if less punishment (NRI),
                                           then more responses (R)     [↓NRI → ↑R]

Imprinting is a form of learning that occurs within a very short critical period, is difficult to reverse, and is not affected by reward or punishment. An example is baby geese who learn that the first object they see is the parent and follow it. Insight learning merges with reasoning and will be considered together. This involves the application of prior learning and knowledge to totally new situations. This is different from generalization from a learning experience in which similar but not identical stimuli may lead to the same response.

An evolutionary scheme of potential behavior patterns and the evolutionary scale is shown in Fig. 2.45.

Relative Dominance

Reflexes

Taxis

Instinct

Reasoning

Learning

protozoa    birds    mammals    man

Invertebrates              Vertebrates

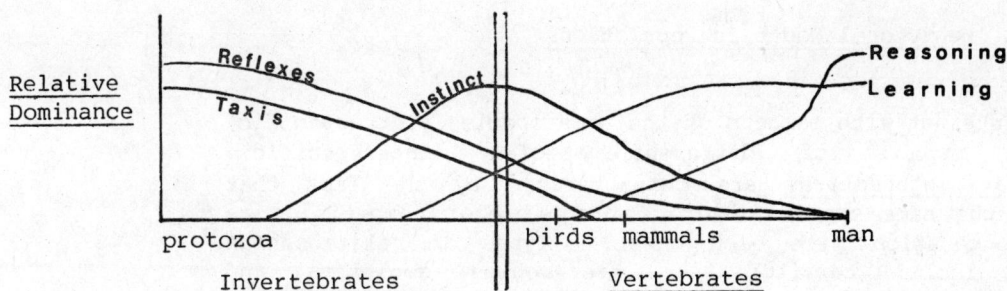

**Fig. 2.45 – Behavior Patterns in Evolution**

2.19.1.2    Effect of Evolution of Neurological Structures Upon Behavior

Irritability, the ability to respond to stimuli, is a universal property of protoplasm. Conduction of the stimulus and response to it exist as well. These are the basic units of the neurological mechanism of behavior. As evolution progressed, specific cells called neurons became specialized for receiving stimuli (in special sense organs), conducting stimuli as nerve impulses, coordination and integration of stimuli (as in the CNS--see Section 2.16.1), and in conducting impulses to effectors to cause responses. The general changes in the nervous system as evolution progressed are: (1) increased centralization into a CNS, (2) an increase in the complexity for pathways within the CNS, (3) an increase in segregation within the CNS of cells performing different functions, (4) an increase in the concentration of integration and coordinating functions in the brain, (5) an increase in one-way conduction paths such as sensory and motor nerves (see Section 2.16.1), and (6) an increase in the number and complexity of sense organs. All of these changes allowed for the reception of an increased variety, complexity and number of stimuli, an increase in the interpretation of these, and an increase in the number of possible responses. All of these added up to more complex behaviors.

The brain proceded to evolve from the three basic divisions-- hindbrain, midbrain, forebrain--to the complex structure found in humans (see Section 2.16.1). The medulla of the hindbrain became a control center for autonomic and some somatic functions. The cerebellum of the hindbrain developed rapidly to coordinate muscular movements. Initially, the optic lobes of the midbrain were the dominant control center, but this eventually gave way to the thalamus which gave way to the cerebrum. Through fishes, the cerebrum was primarily an olfactory (smell) center. But in amphibians a neocortex (gray matter of neuron bodies) began to grow over the surface of the cerebrum. Two paths emerged in the reptiles. One group with a continued growth of the neocortex led to mammals. The other group with no neocortex, but a dominance of the internal part of the cerebrum, led to birds. Initially, the neocortex of mammals was concerned with sensory and motor functions. But in humans, these covered less of the neocortex, and associational areas came to dominate. The neocortex and especially the associational areas of man led to more complex behaviors characterized by more complex types of learning and reasoning, while in birds, where there was no neocortex (or very little), more innate behaviors (e.g., instinct) and simpler learning modes (e.g., imprinting) remained dominant.

## 2.19.1.3    Behavioral Modes in Populations

Organisms interact with members of the same species (intraspecific)
and with members of different species (interspecific).
Intraspecific interactions are characterized by the fact that
members of the same species exhibit antagonism or competition as
well as cooperation with each other.    Types of relationships
established include territoriality, hierarchies, societies, and
competition. Territoriality is the establishment of a specific area
by each member, usually the male of a species, for its own use.
Members tend to avoid each others' territories. Areas are delimited
in various ways such as behavioral demonstrations, fecal droppings,
scents, etc.    These territories serve the purposes of spacing
members of a species, decreasing competition and antagonism,
increasing social stability, and controlling the size of the
breeding population. Dominant members of a species usually get the
better territories, and, hence, usually survive better because they
have access to better food, mates, and living conditions. If members
of a species are organized into a group, dominance patterns become
apparent in the form of hierarchies.    Hierarchies are established
usually during the first encounter between members of a species.
This occurs by behavioral demonstrations of aggression usually, and,
if necessary, by outright fighting.    Various types of hierarchies
exist such as despotism (one individual dominant over others without
ranking of other members), straight chains (each individual is
dominant over those below it in a sequential manner), closed loops
(where no one individual is dominant over all other individuals),
and other more complex patterns. Societies are highly structured
groups where there are clearly defined social roles and divisions of
labor.    In general, insect societies are dominated by a single
female, a division of labor based on biological differences, and
behavioral patterns tend to be instinctive with little room for
modification.    In general, human societies consist of an aggregation
of individuals and family groups, the division of labor is not based
upon biological differences or castes, there is a considerable
choice of roles, and behavioral patterns are based on learning and
are highly modifiable. Competition between members of a species can
be intense because they require the same types of resources.    Wide
fluctuations in numbers occur when imbalances between numbers of a
species and resources exist.

Interspecific interactions include symbiosis (commensualism,
mutualism, and parasitism), predation, and competition. Symbiosis
means the living together of different organisms. Commensualism is
when one species benefits and the other is not affected by the
relationship.    Mutualism is when both species benefit from the
relationship. Parasitism is when one species benefits and the other
is harmed by the relationship. Parasitism merges with commensualism
on one end and predation on the other.    It differs from predation
because the parasite is usually tied to its host, whereas a predator
lives independently of its prey.    Also, a parasite is specific for
its host and is specialized (which usually means loss of all
unnecessary organs and functions).    The best adapted parasites do
not kill their hosts. Predators are free-living from their prey,
have less specificity for prey (i.e., they can prey on a variety of
organisms), and can greatly affect the numbers of their prey.    The
prey usually increase and the predators then increase after a lag
period.    As the predators increase, the number of prey decrease and
fewer predators are supported and they decrease. This allows prey to
increase   and   the   cycle   recurs.    Predators   are,   in   general,

beneficial to prey species because prey are prevented from outgrowing and, hence, ruining their needed resources. Interspecific competition is considered in the context of niches which include every factor (food, physical environment, other species, etc.) that affects the life of an organism. The habitat is just the physical environment. The guiding concept is the Competitive Exclusion Principle which states that two different species canot occupy the same niche for long. One of several options must occur because resources become limited: (1) extinction of one of the species, (2) the range of one or both of the species is restricted, and (3) evolution of one or both species which results in greater differentiation.

2.19.1.4    Communication Between Individuals

Communication is the process of affecting behavior of individuals to assure survival and/or reproduction of the species through a variety of signals transmitted between its members. Communicative signals also permit structural complexity within groups of organisms, and may affect the development of species outside the usual mechanisms of evolution. Signals received by the senses (smell, taste, vision, and hearing), individually or in combination, are the basis of communication.

Pheromones are chemicals produced by cells and transmitted via air, water, objects, etc., to a second individual. They may be effective over long distances. They are extremely potent in small amounts. Pheromone communication is the most common type and is found from single organisms to mammals, including plants. A releasor pheromone causes a behavioral response in the receiving organism. It plays a role in reproduction, territorial determinations, recognition of individuals, trail marking, etc. A primer pheromone causes a physiological change (often via hormonal changes) in the receiving organism that may be permanent. An example is the suppression of additional queens in a variety of insects.

Visual communication involves colors, shapes, visual cues, etc. Humans, birds, butterflies, e.g., utilize this method heavily. It is more restricted than pheromones. It is also used for territory delineations and especially sexual/reproductive functions. Auditory communication is valuable in situations in which vision is restricted (night, water, dense foliage, etc.). It is fairly common and effective. Its uses are similar to visual communication.

2.19.2    QUESTIONS TO REVIEW BEHAVIOR

(1)    Motivation

    (a)  is not dependent upon the internal physiological state;
    (b)  is not required for innate behavior;
    (c)  is required for learned behavior;
    (d)  all of the above.

(2)    Which region of the brain is thought to be most associated with motivation?

    (a)  hypothalamus          (b)  thalamus
    (c)  cerebrum              (d)  medulla

119

(3)   Innate behavior differs from learned behavior by the former being

   (a)   highly modifiable by external factors;
   (b)   slightly modifiable by external factors;
   (c)   totally unaffected by external factors.

(4)   Select the correct statement:

   (a)   innate behavior depends on inherited factors only
   (b)   learned behavior depends on environmental factors only
   (c)   both types of behavior depend on both inherited and environmental factors
   (d)   both (a) and (b)

(5)   The wider the behavioral limits set by inherited factors

   (a)   the greater the role exerted by environmental factors;
   (b)   the lesser the role exerted by environmental factors;
   (c)   has no effect on the role exerted by environmental factors.

(6)   All are innate types of behavior except:

   (a)   reflexes                (b)   taxis
   (c)   instincts               (d)   imprinting

(7)   The most basic of the following units is the:

   (a)   reflex                  (b)   taxis
   (c)   instinct                (d)   imprinting

(8)   An instinct:

   (a)   is little affected by learning
   (b)   always is expressed as a behavior
   (c)   has a strong inherited component that requires no environmental opportunity
   (d)   all of the above

(9)   A Circadian Rhythm

   (a)   has a cycle of about 4 months as the seasons;
   (b)   exists only for behavioral cycles;
   (c)   is not affected by environmental factors;
   (d)   none of the above.

(10)  All of the following are types of learning except:

   (a)   habituation             (b)   maturation
   (c)   conditioning            (d)   imprinting

(11)  Facilitation may be involved in

   (a)   habituation             (b)   conditioning
   (c)   imprinting              (d)   reflexes

(12)  In Pavlovian conditioning,

   (a)   the unconditioned stimulus cannot elicit the response until it has been paired with the conditioned stimulus;
   (b)   the response is created by experiment;

(c) the conditioned stimulus is a natural (already existing in nature) stimulus;

(d) extinction may occur if the conditioned stimulus is continually given without the unconditioned stimulus.

(13) Operant conditioning is similar to:

(a) trial and error learning     (b) Pavlovian conditioning
(c) imprinting     (d) habituation

(14) In operant conditioning,

(a) a decrease in negative reinforcement increases the likelihood of future responses;
(b) positive reinforcement precedes the response;
(c) a stimulus precedes the response;
(d) all of the above.

(15) All of the following are correct about imprinting except:

(a) it is a form of learning
(b) rewards can increase its likelihood of occurrence
(c) must occur within a very short critical period
(d) it is not the same as instinct

(16) All of the following are correct about reasoning except:

(a) it is similar to generalization
(b) it is similar to insight learning
(c) it requires application of prior experiences to totally new situations
(d) it is unrelated to motivation

(17) All of the following modes of behavior are dominant among invertebrates except:

(a) learning     (b) instinct
(c) reflexes     (d) taxis

(18) Modes of behavior dominant in humans include all except:

(a) reasoning     (b) learning
(c) reflexes     (d) all of these are dominant

(19) All of the following occurred in the evolution of the nervous system except:

(a) increased centralization into a central nervous system
(b) increased complexity of pathways in the central nervous system
(c) increased segregation in the periphery of neurons performing specific functions
(d) increased number and complexity of sense organs

(20) The earliest control center in the brain was probably the:

(a) cerebellum     (b) midbrain
(c) thalamus     (d) cerebrum

(21) In early vertebrates (fishes, amphibians) the cerebrum was primarily concerned with:

(a) smell                              (b) vision
(c) all sensory modalities             (d) integration of
                                           information

(22) The development of what structure was important in separating behavioral potentials of birds and mammals?

(a) midbrain                           (b) thalmus
(c) neocortex                          (d) cerebellum

(23) The neocortex of man differs from that of other mammals by having a dominance of which area(s)?

(a) sensory                            (b) association
(c) autonomic                          (d) motor

(24) Types of intraspecific competition include all except:

(a) territoriality                     (b) mutualism
(c) hierarchies                        (d) societies

(25) Function(s) of territoriality are(is):

(a) spacing members of a species
(b) decreasing competition among members of a species
(c) increasing social stability of a species
(d) all of the above

(26) In hierarchies

(a) there is always one dominant individual;
(b) social stability is usually decreased;
(c) dominance by an individual is usually established in the first encounter;
(d) all of the above.

(27) Human societies are characterized by all except

(a) aggregation of individuals and families;
(b) roles based on biological differences;
(c) behavioral patterns are greatly modifiable by learning;
(d) all of the above are correct.

(28) Insect societies are characterized by all except

(a) domination by a single female;
(b) division of labor based on biological differences or castes;
(c) behavioral patterns based upon instincts;
(d) all of the above are correct.

(29) Types of interspecific interactions include all except:

(a) hierarchies                        (b) parasitism
(c) mutualism                          (d) predation

(30) "One species benefits and the other not affected" is called:

    (a) mutualism           (b) predation
    (c) commensualism     (d) parasitism

(31) "Both species benefitting from a relationship" is called:

    (a) mutualism           (b) predation
    (c) commensualism     (d) parasitism

(32) "One species benefitting and the other being harmed in a relationship" is called:

    (a) mutualism           (b) commensualism
    (c) parasitism         (d) none of these

(33) Parasitism, at its extremes, is similar to:

    (a) commensualism     (b) predation
    (c) neither (a) nor (b)   (d) both (a) and (b)

(34) A parasite differs from a predator by

    (a) being specific for its host;
    (b) being tied (versus living free) to its host;
    (c) both (a) and (b);
    (d) neither (a) nor (b).

(35) Predators in general

    (a) increase the number of prey in an area;
    (b) decrease the number of prey in an area;
    (c) have no effect on the number of prey.

(36) "Two different species cannot occupy the same niche for long" is a statement of the:

    (a) Hardy-Weinberg Law
    (b) Darwin's Natural Selection Theory
    (c) Competitive Exclusion Principle
    (d) none of the above

(37) Which of the following may occur if two different species occupy the same niche?

    (a) extinction of one of the species
    (b) range restriction of one of the species
    (c) evolution of one of the species
    (d) all of the above may occur

(38) If a bright light is placed near a planarian, it will move toward the light. This will occur repeatedly as the light is moved. This is an example of:

    (a) taxis           (b) reflex
    (c) habituation       (d) conditioning

(39) A sound is produced that startles a pigeon. The sound is repeated a second time but has less of an effect on the pigeon. By the tenth time the pigeon is not affected by the sound. This

process is best characterized as:

(a) Pavlov Conditioning   (b) habituation
(c) Operant Conditioning   (d) insight learning

## For Questions 40, 41, and 42

Ducklings will run and hide if a hawk flies overhead. Actually, it is the pattern of the hawk's shape and motion that is detected by the ducklings. This effect can be created in a lab setting by a moving hawk-shaped cardboard. A bell is rung when the cardboard is presented to the ducklings who continue to seek shelter. Eventually, the bell is rung but without the cardboard hawk, and the ducklings still seek shelter.

(40) This is an example of:

(a) trial and error learning   (b) imprinting
(c) Pavlovian conditioning   (d) operant conditioning

(41) The bell is called the:

(a) conditioned stimulus   (b) unconditioned stimulus
(c) positive reinforcement   (d) negative reinforcement

(42) If the bell continues to be rung without the presence of the cardboard hawk, a process called _____ will occur:

(a) forgetting   (b) insight learning
(c) extinction   (d) facilitation

(43) Some citizens decided that the wolf population in a fairly isolated but fertile valley had grown too large and was destroying too many deer. To save the deer, they decided to destroy all the wolves, the only natural predators of the deer in the valley. They succeeded in removing all of the wolves. Over a representative period of time, which graph probably shows the growth of the deer? (a) = initial level of deer before wolf eradication; ↑ = elimination of all wolves.

(44)

species #1 ≡ ————
species #2 ≡ - - - - - - -

The above graph probably represents what type of relationship

124

between these species?

(a) commensualism     (b) mutualism
(c) parasitism        (d) predation

(45) Cows do not have digestive enzymes to digest cellulose. Cellulose is a very important component of a cow's diet. The cellulose is digested by bacteria in the cow's stomach. These bacteria can use some of the cellulose products for their own purposes. This relationship is called:

(a) commensualism     (b) mutualism
(c) parasitism        (d) competition

(46) Bacterial species #1 and bacterial species #2 are very similar in their requirements for life. The "diet" of both consists primarily of small organic molecules. The following experiments are done as shown in the graphs below:

The bacteria alone or in combination are placed in identical culture media.

This experiment may be considered to be an example of:

(a) commensualism
(b) the Competitive Exclusion Principle
(c) parasitism
(d) predation

2.19.3     ANSWERS TO QUESTIONS IN SECTION 2.19.2

| ( 1) c | (2) a | (3) b | (4) c | (5) a | (6) d | (7) a |
| ( 8) a | (9) d | (10) b | (11) b | (12) d | (13) a | (14) a |
| (15) b | (16) a | (17) a | (18) c | (19) c | (20) b | (21) a |
| (22) c | (23) b | (24) b | (25) d | (26) c | (27) b | (28) d |
| (29) a | (30) c | (31) a | (32) c | (33) d | (34) c | (35) b |
| (36) c | (37) d | (38) a | (39) b | (40) c | (41) a | (42) c |
| (43) c | (44) d | (45) b | (46) b | | | |

2.19.4     DISCUSSION OF ANSWERS TO QUESTIONS IN SECTION 2.19.2

QUESTIONS #1 - #37  Adequately discussed in Section.

QUESTION #38 (Answer: a) The motion is an orienting motion and simply a rigid stereotyped response (as a reflex). There is no evidence of habituation (decreased response to the stimulus) nor that the organism was conditioned. Taxis is the best of the possible answers.

QUESTION #39 (Answer: b) The response of the pigeon decreases with repeated application of the sound which was presented without reinforcement--this is the meaning of habituation. There is no evidence in the question for the other answer options.

QUESTION #40 (Answer: c) All the criteria are present for Pavlovian conditioning. The hiding is a natural response found in ducklings elicited by the natural stimulus of the hawk (or its stand-in). The bell is the conditioned stimulus which eventually can elicit the response after being paired with the unconditioned stimulus (the hawk). But upon repeated presentations of the bell without the hawk the response is elicited less and less--this is the extinction phenomenon.

QUESTIONS #41, #42  See discussion of #40 above.

QUESTIONS #43  (Answer: c)  As soon as the wolves are removed the deer population will begin to increase because the wolves were the major limiting factor of the deer.  So the deer population will increase.  But the resources of the valley are limited and the deer population will reach a brief plateau as the carrying capacity of the valley is reached.  Then, because the valley is relatively isolated and the deer can't move on, they will tend to destroy foliage faster than it can be replenished and the carrying capacity will decrease; hence, the deer population will decrease.  This is as in graph (c).

QUESTION #44  (Answer: d)  Species #2 tends to lag behind species #1 as to peaks and valleys.  Also, as species #2 increases, species #1 decreases; as #1 increases, #2 increases.  And, species #2 is always less abundant than species #1.  Of the relationships given, the predator(#2)/prey(#1) relationship would best explain the graph.  As the prey (#1) increase, more predators can be supported and they increase.  But when the predator:prey ratio reaches a critical point, more prey are destroyed than are created so they decrease.  The decrease in prey causes the predators to decrease because fewer can be supported.  Thus the numbers fluctuate.

QUESTION #45  (Answer: b)  The cow benefits by having the cellulose digested for it.  The bacteria benefit by being provided with an abundant supply of cellulose.  This is the definition of mutualism.

QUESTION #46  (Answer: b)  These two species occupy the same niche as alluded to in the question; they are, therefore, in competition with each other.  The experiments show that, when put with #2, species #1 is decreased in number (goes toward extinction) as is predicted by the Competitive Exclusion Principle.  Parasitism, predation and commensualism are most likely all excluded by the fact that both organisms survive well when grown alone.  Also, it is noted that the diet of both is small organic molecules.

2.19.5      VOCABULARY CHECKLIST FOR BEHAVIOR

| | |
|---|---|
| ____ motivation | ____ reflexes |
| ____ instinct | ____ biorhythms |
| ____ maturation | ____ habituation |
| ____ extinction | ____ reward |
| ____ punishment | ____ imprinting |
| ____ generalization | ____ neocortex |
| ____ territoriality | ____ hierarchies |
| ____ societies | ____ symbiosis |
| ____ commensualism | ____ mutualism |
| ____ parasitism | ____ predation |
| ____ competition | ____ niche |
| ____ insight learning | ____ taxis |
| ____ Circadian Rhythms | ____ conditioning |
| ____ Pavlov conditioning | ____ reasoning |
| ____ conditioned stimulus | ____ operant conditioning |
| ____ unconditioned stimulus | ____ habitat |

____ trial and error learning     ____ positive
____ negative reinforcement          reinforcement
____ Competitive Exclusion Principle    ____ pheromones


2.19.6      CONCEPTS, PRINCIPLES, ETC.    CHECKLIST FOR BEHAVIOR


____ innate behavioral responses
____ learned behavioral responses
____ distinction between innate and learned behavior
____ evolution of innate and learned behaviors
____ evolution of the nervous system
____ behavioral consequences of evolution of the nervous system
____ intraspecific interactions
____ interspecific interactions
____ visual communication
____ auditory communication


## 2.20      Genetics


2.20.1      REVIEW OF GENETICS


Each organism has a set of chromosomes. Chromosomes of eucaryotes are a complex of DNA, histone (basic protein), and non-histone protein. The normal complement of chromosomes is called diploid (2n) as occurs in somatic cells. Gametes (male and female) are haploid (1n). Gametes combine to form the diploid cell. The complement of chromosomes may be divided into autosomes and sex chromosomes (having to do with sex determination). Humans have 22 pairs of autosomes and 1 pair of sex chromosomes (X,Y) for a total of 46. The female is XX, and the male is XY. Either the whole set of chromosomes can be in some multiple of n which is called polyploidy, e.g., 4n = tetraploidy, or one or more chromosomes may be missing or in excess, which is called aneuploidy, e.g., monosomy (only one of a chromosome type is present) or trisomy (three of chromosome type is present). Down's Syndrome (Mongolism) is caused by trisomy 21 (i.e., there are three of the chromosomes numbered 21 instead of two).

On each chromosome there is a sequence of genes. For this Section, a gene is a specific trait. Hence, each locus (or position) on a chromosome is for a specific trait. In the diploid (2n) cell, there is a pair of homologous chromosomes (which pair in meiosis). Homologous chromosomes are similar by having the same sequence of trait loci (except the pair X and Y, see below); hence they are the same size. For any given general trait (e.g., eye color), there are many alternative genes (e.g., blue, brown) for its determination. The alternative genes for a general trait constitute a set of alleles for that trait. Since there is only one locus (usually) for a simple trait on a chromosome, there can be only one allele of that trait per homologous chromosome. Then, for any given trait, there is a maximum of two alleles per diploid cell (one on each homologous chromosome). But the total number of different alleles for a given trait can be greater than two (e.g., there are many different alleles for types of hemoglobin--normal adult, fetal, sickle, hemoglobin C, hemoglobin Milwaukee, etc.). For an individual, the specific alleles present is called the genotype. If the alleles for a given trait on each homologous chromosome are identical, the genotype is called homozygous. If the alleles for a given trait on each homologous chromosome are different, the genotype is called heterozygous. The term genotype can refer to the alleles of a specific trait or the total genetic makeup (all of the alleles) of an individual. Each of the alleles (genes) of a given trait will attempt to express itself via its protein product. If one allele of a pair expresses itself over another (e.g., eye color with brown over blue), that allele is said to be dominant and the other recessive. (Note that these terms go together like oxidation-reduction in chemistry.) If both alleles express themselves, they are called codominant. The expression (what is seen as the trait of the individual) of the genotype is called the phenotype. Note that different genotypes can give rise to the same phenotype, but a given genotype will not usually give rise to different phenotypes.

Gametes (haploid) are formed during meiosis by the separation of homologous chromosomes (diploid state). This results in the separation of each of the alleles into a different gamete. This is Mendel's First Law of Segregation (of alleles of the same trait). Different traits (i.e., loci) may be on the same chromosome or on different chromosomes. If the traits are on different chromosomes, the alleles of these different traits should separate independently of each other into gametes. This is Mendel's Second Law of Independent Assortment (of alleles of different traits). But if different traits are on the same chromosome, they may be far apart or close together. Traits far apart on the same chromosome separate into gametes as if they were on separate chromosomes. This is possible because of crossing-over (reciprocal exchange of parts of homologous chromosomes) during synapsis in the first meiotic prophase. The farther apart two different traits are on a chromosome, the easier it is for cross-over to occur. Alleles of traits which are close together do not separate frequently by the mechanism of crossing-over into different gametes because they tend to remain on the same chromosome. So they cannot independently (of each other) assort, do not follow Mendel's Second Law, and are called linked traits (or genes). (Fig. 2.46). Recombination is the process of separating alleles of linked traits into different gametes, i.e., onto different homologous chromosomes. Linkage (recombination) studies and cytogenetics (study of markings, e.g., bands on chromosomes) are used to map chromosomes as to the loci of traits. Another of Mendel's great contributions to genetics was his recognition that genes are particulate (i.e., not indivisible or blendable). Mendel's mechanisms of assortment and segregation and the later discovered ideas of recombination illustrate mechanisms of genetic variability which can be viewed as the passage to offspring, via gametes, of different combinations of alleles than existed in the parent. Another set of mechanisms responsible for genetic variability is mutations. A mutation may be considered a stable heritable change in genetic material (DNA). Mutations that may occur at the level of the chromosome (see Fig. 2.47) are:

(1)   inversion - sequence of genes on the chromosomes is reversed
(2)   translocations - a part of one chromosome attaches to another
(3)   deletion - a part of the chromosome is missing
(4)   duplication - part of the chromosome is repeated.

| Diploid (2n) cell showing a pair of homologous chromosomes with loci for three different traits with alleles A,a and B,b and D,d. Traits A,a and B,b are linked. Traits A,a and D,d and traits B,b and D,d are not linked. | Mendel's 1st Law, each allele of a given trait (A vs a, B vs b, and D vs d) segregate independently of each other. | Mendel's 2nd Law, consider A,a vs D,d. These alleles of different traits assort independently of each other (also for B,b vs D,d). Not true for A,a vs B,b because these are linked. | Recombination of the linked genes A,a vs B,b. A,a and B,b do not assort independently of each other because they are so close together. One would normally expect A & B or a & b to be together in gametes. But by crossing over, Ab and aB also are possible but at frequencies less than expected. |

Fig. 2.46 - **Mendel's Law; Crossing-over; Recombination; Gamete Formation**

Fig. 2.47 - **Chromosomal Mutations**

In the sex chromosomes, the X is larger than the Y (i.e., has more loci for traits), and hence, traits on the X may not appear on the Y. Traits of this type are called sex-linked traits. Examples in humans are hemophilia, color blindness, and glucose-6-phosphate dehydrogenase deficiency. The X and Y chromosomes are homologous because they can pair (synapse) in meiosis. Sex-linked traits are unique in their inheritance because the male (with only one X chromosome) can express (phenotypes) recessive alleles because there is only one allele present. The female requires both recessive alleles to be present for expression of the recessive trait. Also note that transmission to the male occurs usually only from the mother. Whereas if the daughter is diseased, both mother and father must have passed on the allele. In passing, Barr bodies are inactivated "excess" X chromosomes (only one X remains active). This phenomenon is referred to as the Lyon or Lyon-Russel hypothesis. The above concepts are illustrated in Fig. 2.48.

Given a trait with alleles A=dominant, a=recessive and phenotypes $\underline{A}$ and $\underline{a}$.

| If on autosomes | If on sex chromosomes |
|---|---|

Genotype:   A $\Vert$ A      A $\Vert$ a      a $\Vert$ a          A $\mid$ $\mid$          a $\mid$ $\mid$
                                                           X Y          X Y

Phenotype:   $\underline{A}$          $\underline{A}$          $\underline{a}$              $\underline{A}$          $\underline{a}$

Note that the a allele can only be expressed when it is present on both chromosomes (i.e., it is homozygous).

Note that a (the allele) is alone and is expressed.

**Fig. 2.48 – Autosomal and Sex Chromosomes:  Phenotype Expressions**

Cytoplasmic inheritance is the determination of genetic traits by constituents of the cytoplasm rather than the nucleus.  This inheritance does not follow Mendelian Laws.  The mother (most of the cytoplasm of the zygote comes from the ovum) plays the major role in this type of inheritance.  Chloroplasts (contain DNA), mitochondria (contain DNA), centrioles, and basal bodies of flagella and cilia are examples of structures that replicate without input from the nucleus.

Pedigrees are convenient diagrams for showing the phenotypic appearance of traits in a family.  The basic nomenclature is given in Fig. 2.49.

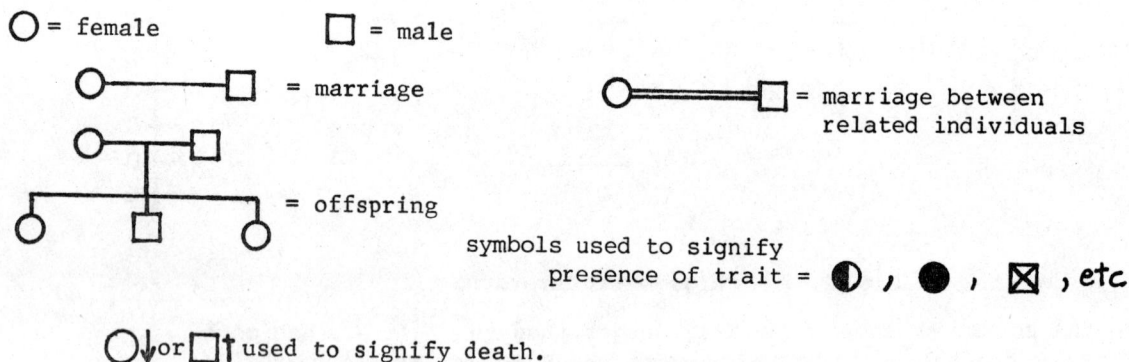

○ = female          □ = male

○——□ = marriage          ○═══□ = marriage between related individuals

= offspring

symbols used to signify presence of trait = ◖ , ● , ⊠ , etc

○↓ or □↑ used to signify death.

**Fig. 2.49 – Pedigree Terminology**

A dominant autosomal or sex-linked trait, with complete penetrance (i.e., the trait appears in all with the allele), will have a pedigree that shows both sexes affected, many individuals affected, passage of trait from affected parent to children even if heterozygous (Fig. 2.50).

*A†*†*a* = homologous chromosomes
with alleles shown on
each

■, ● ≡ *A*†*†a* or *A*†*†A*

Case (1) is probably heterozygous for the trait because
if homozygous then all offspring would be affected.

**Fig. 2.50 - Dominant Pedigree**

An autosomal recessive trait will also show both sexes affected, but
fewer individuals will be affected and passage may be from an
unaffected parent (because heterozygous) to an affected offspring
(Fig. 2.51).

†^? ≡ ? = B or b without
affecting phenotype

(assume BB because
no offspring with
the trait; she could
be Bb)

Both parents are heterozygous for the recessive allele.

**Fig. 2.51 - Recessive Pedigree**

A sex-linked recessive trait usually shows only males affected  and
passage of the trait from an unaffected mother to a son.  A daughter
can get the trait only if the father has it and the mother is, at
least, heterozygous. (Fig. 2.52).

*D*†*|* and *D*†*†d*
X Y        X X

trait loci not found on Y

**Fig. 2.52 - Sex-Linked Pedigree**

<u>Punnet squares</u> are useful ways of determining the genotypes possible
from the mating of two individuals with known genotypes. First  the
possible gametes are determined (Fig. 2.53), then these are combined
in  all  possible  ways.   Then  by  knowing  dominant-recessive
relationships, the frequency of phenotypes can be ascertained.  The

131

Punnet square gives expected ratios only.  Fig. 2.54 and Fig. 2.55 are examples.

♀    ♂

Aa   x   Aa      and A is dominant to a.

possible gametes: ♀ —A,a; ♂ —A,a

GENOTYPE (Diploid): (1) AaBb      (2) AaBB   (3) AABbDd      (4) AaBbDd

POSSIBLE GAMETES:
(Haploid)

AB,Ab,aB,ab    AB,aB    ABD,ABd,AbD,Abd    ABD,ABd,AbD
Abd,aBD,aBd,
abD,abd

**Fig. 2.53 – Gamete Formation by Example**

Punnet square:     Genotype frequency:     Phenotype frequency:

AA = 1      AA same as Aa = 3
Aa = 2            aa = 1
aa = 1

**Fig. 2.54 – Punnet Square With One Trait**

♀     ♂
AaBb   x   AaBb       A dominant to a
                       B dominant to b

possible gametes: ♀ —AB, aB, Ab, ab
               ♂ —AB, aB, Ab, ab

Punnet Square:

**Genotype Frequency**

AABB = 1    aaBb = 2
AABb = 2    AAbb = 1
AaBb = 4    aaBB = 1
AaBB = 2    aabb = 1
Aabb = 2

**Phenotypes Frequency**

A-B- (AABB,AABb,AaBb,AaBB) =
              1+2+4+2=9
aaB- (aaBb,aaBB) = 2+1=3
A-bb (Aabb,AAbb) = 2+1=3
aabb (aabb) = 1

**Fig. 2.55 – Punnet Square With Two Traits**

Simple gene mapping is done utilizing recombinant techniques. This is done with viral and bacterial DNAs. The map is a linear, one-dimensional structure. The map units indirectly represent the percent recombination between various traits (genetic loci). The traits must be measurable in some manner (e.g., nutrient utilization, products produced, temperature dependence, etc.). The combination of traits in the offspring, as compared with the parents, helps determine the recombinant frequencies (percentages) that help determine the gene map. An example of a two-factor (trait) cross:

Parents       Offspring

$$
\begin{array}{c}
a \\
b^+
\end{array} \times
\begin{array}{c}
a^+ \\
b
\end{array} \longrightarrow
$$

$$
\left.\begin{array}{l} a \\ b^+ \end{array}\right\} - 35\% \\
\left.\begin{array}{l} a^+ \\ b \end{array}\right\} - 35\%
$$
   } original genotypes

- the original genotypes are in the highest frequency.

$$
\left.\begin{array}{l} a \\ b \end{array}\right\} - 15\% \\
\left.\begin{array}{l} a^+ \\ b^+ \end{array}\right\} - 15\%
$$
   } recombinant genotypes

- the larger percentage of recombinants, the farther apart the traits are on the map and the less tightly linked the traits are.
- the trait loci (a <u>or</u> $a^+$ and b <u>or</u> $b^+$) are linked (see below).

A series of two-factor crosses may be used to sequence the gene loci. The maximal possible frequency of any recombinant is 50%. If the frequency of recombination between the loci is near 50%, then there is no linkage. The smaller the recombination frequency between two loci, the stronger the linkage (i.e., the closer together the traits. Triple factor (i.e., three traits at three loci) are used to order gene loci. The (original) parental genotypes will appear in the highest frequency, single recombinants next, and double recombinants in the lowest frequency. The probability of the central locus recombining with both outside loci (double recombination) is equal to the products of the probability of it combining with each individually (single recombination).

Example:   Parents

$$
\begin{array}{cc}
x & x^+ \\
y & y^+ \\
z & z^+
\end{array}
$$

| Offspring (8 genotypic classes result) | Genotype Frequency | Recombination Frequency | Recombination Status |
|---|---|---|---|
| x / y / z | 30% | | |
| | | 60% | No recombination |
| $x^+$ / $y^+$ / $z^+$ | 30% | | |
| $x^+$ / $y^+$ / z | 10% | | Recombination between central locus <u>and</u> z. Single recombination. |
| | | 20% | |
| x / y / $z^+$ | 10% | | |
| $x^+$ / y / z | 7% | | Recombination between central locus <u>and</u> x. Single recombination. |
| | | 14% | |
| x / $y^+$ / $z^+$ | 7% | | |
| $x^+$ / y / $z^+$ | 3% | | y is now identified as central locus. This is lowest frequency cross and the y factors are out of place with the others. Double recombination. |
| | | 6% | |
| x / $y^+$ / z | 3% | | |

Note that y is closer to x than to z (lower recombination frequency for x than for z above).

133

There are factors that modify the percentage distributions of the offspring and may affect the analysis. Besides the probability factor (i.e., each cross will not lead to exact ratios just as in Mendelian crosses), conditional lethal mutations may occur and cause some genotypes not to survive and, therefore, not to be counted.

2.20.2    QUESTIONS TO REVIEW GENETICS

(1)    Which of the following is correct for gene mapping?

(a)    only three-factor crosses may be used to sequence gene loci
(b)    the recombination frequencies are always representative of the recombination rates of the gene loci
(c)    the recombination frequency is equal to the map units
(d)    viral DNAs are used for gene mapping

(2)    Cytoplasmic inheritance:

(a)    does not follow Mendelian Laws
(b)    the maternal cytoplasm plays the dominant role
(c)    replication of mitochondria is an example
(d)    all of the above

(3)    Homozygous refers to

(a)    similar types of chromosomes
(b)    having similar functions on an evolutionary basis
(c)    particles in a solution not being separable microscopically
(d)    identical alleles for a given trait

(4)    Which statement is incorrect concerning X and Y chromosomes?

(a)    X is larger than Y
(b)    they are not homologous
(c)    XY is a genotypic male
(d)    traits appearing on X but not on Y are called sex-linked traits

(5)    Select the incorrect statement:

(a)    genotype is the two alleles for a given trait in an individual
(b)    phenotype is the expression of the genotype
(c)    a given genotype will give rise to different phenotypes
(d)    different genotypes may give rise to the same phenotype

(6)    Crossing-over of chromosomes

(a)    involves reciprocal exchanges of homologous chromosomes;
(b)    occurs in metaphase I of meiosis;
(c)    is more frequent between traits located close together;
(d)    prevents independent assortment of traits on the same chromosome.

(7)    Genetic recombination

(a)    occurs by exchange of chromosomes between gametes;
(b)    is the exchange of similar alleles between gametes;
(c)    is the mixing of alleles of different traits on homologous chromosomes by crossing-over;
(d)    is not used to make chromosome maps.

(8) An allele for a trait:

  (a) is a gene
  (b) can be different on homologous chromosomes in a given cell
  (c) both (a) and (b)
  (d) neither (a) nor (b)

(9) Barr bodies:

  (a) the densities associated with desmosomes
  (b) crystals of enzymes seen in lysosomes
  (c) inactivated X-chromosomes seen in certain cells
  (d) synonym for polar bodies resulting during oogenesis

(10) Which of the following is an example of aneuploidy?

  (a) 4n                          (b) trisomy 21
  (c) XO (no Y chromosome)        (d) both (b) and (c)

(11) Select the incorrect statement about the number and type of chromosomes in the normal human male:

  (a) there are 44 autosomal chromosomes
  (b) there are 46 chromosomes total
  (c) there are two X chromosomes
  (d) there is one Y chromosome

(12) In the typical somatic cell, the number of chromosomes is symbolized as:

  (a) 1n    (b) 2n    (c) 3n    (d) 4n

(13) Chromosomes (eucaryotes) are composed of all except:

  (a) histones                    (b) non-histone protein
  (c) DNA                         (d) RNA

(14) Select the incorrect statement:

  (a) a recessive allele is only expressed when it is homozygous
  (b) a dominant allele can be expressed when heterozygous
  (c) a codominant allele may express itself completely or partially when homozygous or heterozygous, respectively
  (d) dominant alleles may not be expressed

(15) Mendel's First Law:

  (a) alleles of the same trait segregate (separate on homologous chromosomes) in the formation of gametes
  (b) alleles of different traits separate independently of each other in the formation of gametes
  (c) genes are particulate in nature
  (d) genes are indivisible (i.e., cannot be subdivided and yet produce a given trait)

(16) Select the incorrect statement regarding homologous chromosomes:

  (a) except for X and Y, they are the same size
  (b) they have identical sequences of genes
  (c) they synapse in meiosis
  (d) except for X and Y, they have the same sequence of loci as traits

135

(17)  Sex-linked traits:

    (a)  are found more in females than in males
    (b)  are found on the Y and X chromosomes
    (c)  allow recessive alleles to be expressed when one such
         allele is present in the male
    (d)  males have a 50% chance of receiving sex-linked alleles
         from the father

(18)  If the genotype for a trait is Aa (A dominant to a), possible
gametes are:

    (a)  Aa only  (b)  AA and aa  (c)  A,a  (d)  Aa,A, and a

(19)  Given the following pedigree, select the correct explanation
assuming that the pedigree is representative of the
inheritance patterns (blackened symbols mean trait is
present):

    (a)  autosomal dominant       (b)  autosomal recessive
    (c)  sex-linked dominant      (d)  sex-linked recessive

(20)  Given the following representative pedigree, select the most
likely pattern of inheritance (blackened symbols mean the
trait is present):

    (a)  autosomal dominant       (b)  autosomal recessive
    (c)  sex-linked dominant      (d)  sex-linked recessive

(21)  Given the following representative pedigree, what is the most
likely pattern of inheritance (blackened symbols mean trait is
present)?

    (a)  autosomal dominant       (b)  autosomal recessive
    (c)  sex-linked recessive     (d)  mutation

(22) If brown eyes (B) is dominant to blue eyes (b), the parents have what genotype for eye color (open symbol: brown eyes; blackened symbol: blue eyes)?

(a) father Bb, mother BB
(b) father BB, mother Bb
(c) father Bb, mother Bb
(d) cannot be determined from information given

(23) Suppose gray (G) is dominant to white (g) coat color for rats. Given the following representative pedigree, what are the most likely genotypes of the parents (open symbol: white; blackened symbol: gray)?

(a) father GG, mother gg
(b) father Gg, mother Gg
(c) father gg, mother Gg
(d) cannot be determined from the information given

(24) Suppose round peas (R) are dominant to wrinkled peas (r) and green peas (G) are dominant to yellow peas (g). The following cross is made:

$$RrGg \times RrGg$$

What are the expected phenotypes and their frequencies in the offspring (assume the traits are not linked)?

(a) 3 round, green: 1 wrinkled, yellow
(b) 2 round, green: 1 round, yellow: 1 wrinked, green
(c) 9 round, green: 3 wrinkled, green:
    3 round, yellow: 1 wrinkled, yellow
(d) all round, green

(25) If red (R) is dominant to white (r) and parents with genotypes RR(male) and rr(female) are crossed, what are the colors and their expected frequencies in the offspring?

(a) 1 red: 3 white        (b) 1 red: 1 white
(c) 3 red: 1 white        (d) all red

(26) If the offspring from Question #25 are crossed with each other, what are the colors and their frequencies in the offspring from this second cross?

(a) 1 red: 2 pink: 1 white     (b) 3 red: 1 white
(c) 1 red: 1 white             (d) all red

137

(27) If the genotype for two traits is AaBB, the possible gametes
are:

(a) Aa,BB                    (b) AB,aB
(d) A,a,B,B                  (d) Ab,ab,AB,aB

(28) Mendel's Second Law:

(a) alleles of the same trait segregate (separate on
homologous chromosomes) in the formation of gametes
(b) alleles of different traits separate independently of
each other in the formation of gametes
(c) genes are particulate in nature
(d) genes are indivisible

(29) Suppose the only alleles that determine blood type are A and
B, and that they are codominant.  If parents, both with Type
AB, have children, what are the ratios of the childrens'
expected blood types?  Type A = AA, Type B = BB, Type AB = AB
(genotypes of each type).

(a) 1 Type A:  2 Type AB:  1 Type B
(b) 1 Type A:  1 Type B
(c) 3 Type AB;  1 Type A:  1 Type B
(d) all Type AB

(30) The following three-factor cross is done.  Which answer* is
correct?

Parent Genotypes:

| r | r$^+$ | Offspring Genotypes | Percentage of Total |
|---|---|---|---|
| s$^+$ | s | r | |
| t | t$^+$ | s$^+$ | 26% |
| | | t | |
| | | r$^+$ | |
| | | s | 26% |
| | | t$^+$ | |
| | | r | |
| | | s$^+$ | 16% |
| | | t$^+$ | |
| | | r$^+$ | |
| | | s | 16% |
| | | t | |
| | | r$^+$ | |
| | | s$^+$ | 6% |
| | | t | |
| | | r | |
| | | s | 6% |
| | | t | |
| | | r$^+$ | |
| | | s$^+$ | 2% |
| | | t | |
| | | r | |
| | | s | 2% |
| | | t$^+$ | |

*Answer choices for Question #30
are on page 139 (across).

138

Question 30 Answer Choices:

(a) the genotypes representing the double recombination are
    r s t and r$^+$ s$^+$ t$^+$
(b) the s locus is farthest from the central locus
(c) the map distance between the three loci is 16 units
(d) the t locus is the central locus


## 2.20.3  ANSWERS TO QUESTIONS IN SECTION 2.20.2

( 1)  d   (2)  d   (3)  d   (4)  b   (5)  c   (6)  a   (7)  c
( 8)  c   (9)  c  (10)  d  (11)  c  (12)  b  (13)  d  (14)  a
(15)  a  (16)  b  (17)  c  (18)  c  (19)  d  (20)  a  (21)  b
(22)  c  (23)  c  (24)  c  (25)  d  (26)  b  (27)  b  (28)  b
(29)  a  (30)  c


## 2.20.4  DISCUSSION OF ANSWERS TO QUESTIONS IN SECTION 2.20.2

QUESTIONS #1 - #9, #15, #28 - Adequately discussed in Section.

QUESTION #10  (Answer: d)  Aneuploidy is the deletion (Y is lost in XO) or addition (an extra #21 is added in trisomy 21) of one or more individual chromosomes.  Polyploidy means a multiplication of the whole set of chromosomes as in 4n.

QUESTION #11  (Answer: c)  The normal male has 44 autosomes, one X and one Y chromosome.  The normal female has 44 autosomes and two X chromosomes.

QUESTION #12  (Answer: b)  2n=diploid.  Gametes are haploid (1n).  Occasionally, somatic cells will be triploid (3n) or tetraploid (4n).

QUESTION #13  (Answer: d)  RNA is made using the DNA of chromosomes as a template; it is not an integral part of a chromosome.

QUESTION #14  (Answer: a) Recessive alleles may be expressed when sex-linked. Dominant alleles may not have penetrance.

QUESTION #16  (Answer: b) A gene is a specific sequence of nucleotides which codes for a specific protein which may be expressed as a phenotypic variation (blue, brown) of a given trait (eye color).  Homologous chromosomes do not usually have an identical sequence of genes; they do have a set sequence of loci for the alleles (contrasting genes) for a given trait.

QUESTION #17  (Answer: c)  This is possible because only the X chromosome carries the trait and the Y is the homologous chromosome in the male.  Hence: a

X Y

The allele, a, will express itself because it is the only allele present for the trait.

QUESTION #18  (Answer: c)  The genotype Aa produces the gametes with A and a separately by Mendel's First Law of Segregation of alleles of the same trait.  Note that A and a are on different but homologous chromosomes.

QUESTION #19  (Answer:  d) Note that the trait appears only in males, can be carried by females, and the males apparently inherit it only from their mothers.

QUESTION #20  (Answer:  a) There is no sex preference and no skipped generations.  It (the trait) is only passed from those parents expressing the disease, and many individuals are affected.  All of this is characteristic of a highly penetrated autosomal dominant allele.  The initial mother (1) is heterozygous for the allele; because if she were homozygous, every one of her children would have the trait.

QUESTION #21  (Answer:  b) There is no sex preference, and since the initial father did not have the disease, it would be improbable that his daughters would have it if it was sex-linked recessive.  A mutuation is unlikely (but possible) because three offspring have the trait, few people are affected, and the trait is not passed by affected individuals.  Autosomal recessive is the most likely, and the initial parents must have been heterozygous for the recessive allele.

QUESTION #22  (Answer:  c) Since both parents have brown eyes, their genotype must be at least B- for each.  Since one child has blue eyes (bb), one b allele must have come from each parent. Therefore, each parent must be Bb.

QUESTION #23  (Answer:  c) The father must be gg because he is white.  The mother is gray and she is, at least, G-.  Since the pedigree is representative, white offspring do appear.  Since each white offspring must get one g from the father, they must also get a g from the mother--otherwise there would be no white offspring. Therefore, the mother must be Gg.

QUESTIONS #24  (Answer:  c) Use the Punnet square to get genotypic frequencies (gametes are RG, Rg, rG, rg for each parent):

|      | RG   | Rg   | rG   | rg   |
|------|------|------|------|------|
| RG   | RRGG | RRGg | RrGG | RrGg |
| Rg   | RRGg | RRgg | RrGg | Rrgg |
| rG   | RrGG | RrGg | rrGG | rrGg |
| rg   | RrGg | Rrgg | rrGg | rrgg |

Then, based on the dominance-recessive relationships given, the phenotypes and their ratios are:

        all R-G- are round, green (RRGG-1, RRGg-2, RrGG-2, RrGg-4) = 9
        all rrG- are wrinkled, green (rrGG-1, rrGg-2) = 3
        all R-gg are wrinkled, yellow (RRgg-1, Rrgg-2) = 3
        rrgg is wrinkled, yellow (rrgg-1) = 1

QUESTION #25  (Answer:  d) Since the gametes will be r and R only, all offspring will be Rr or red.

140

QUESTION #26 (Answer: b) Using the genotype Rr derived in Question #25, determine the genotypes of the new offspring by using a new Punnet Square (gametes are R,r for both parents):

Rr = red

for #25        for #26

Then using the dominance-recessive relationship given, the phenotypes and their ratios are determined:

R- is red (RR-1, Rr-2) = 3

rr is white (rr) = 1.

QUESTION #27 (Answer: b) Each gamete will contain one allele of each trait in all possible combinations with each other. Then each gamete can have an A or a, and it must have a B. This gives AB, aB.

QUESTION #29 (Answer: a) Use the Punnet Square to determine the genotypes (gametes of each parent are A,B):

Using the information relating phenotypes to genotypes given in the question:

        Type A    (AA=1)   = 1
        Type B    (BB=1)   = 1
        Type AB   (AB=2)   = 2

QUESTION #30 (Answer: c) The lowest frequency recombinant is r+ s+ t and r s t+. The locus out of line with the parents is the r locus. Then, r must be the central locus. The t is farther from r (32% recombination frequency) than the s (12% recombination frequency). Map units are not recombination frequency units.

2.20.5        VOCABULARY CHECKLIST FOR GENETICS

____ chromosome          ____ histone             ____ linked traits
____ diploid             ____ autosomes           ____ mutation
____ polyploidy          ____ translocation       ____ sex chromosomes
____ tetraploidy         ____ aneuploidy          ____ duplication
____ monosomy            ____ pedigrees           ____ Barr bodies
____ heterozygous        ____ homozygous          ____ recombination
____ penetrance          ____ genes               ____ Punnet square
____ alleles             ____ homologous          ____ inversion
____ cytoplasmic         ____ chromosomes         ____ deletion
____ inheritance         ____ codominant          ____ phenotype
____ dominant            ____ recessive           ____ genotype
____ crossing-over       ____ sex-linked          ____ Lyon Hypothesis
____ trisomy

141

____ chemical composition of chromosomes
____ the set of human chromosomes and variations
____ organization of chromosomes (genes, alleles, etc.)
____ Mendel's Laws
____ mechanisms of genetic variability
____ sex-linked traits
____ cytoplasmic inheritance
____ use of pedigrees
____ use of Punnet squares
____ two-factor cross
____ three-factor cross
____ recombination frequency
____ map units
____ linkage
____ ordering of gene loci

## 2.21     Evolution and Comparative Anatomy

### 2.21.1     REVIEW OF EVOLUTION AND COMPARATIVE ANATOMY

#### 2.21.1.1     The Mechanism of Evolution

Evolution is the study of the changes that occur in organisms, how
the changes occur, and the results of the changes.  These changes may
be minor and lead to better adaptation to an environment, or they may
be major and lead to a totally different species. Changes come about
when organisms are "selected" on the basis of phenotypic differences
to survive.   These phenotypic differences must be based upon
underlying genetic differences, as found in the germ cells, to lead
to evolutionary change.  The survival of selected organisms leads to
changes in the gene frequencies and gene combinations in the
population,  which  in  turn  leads  to  changes in phenotypic
characteristics and, hence, evolution.

Mutations (see Section 2.20.1) are the ultimate source of all new
genes in the population, and as such, they are the raw material for
all evolutionary changes.  Genes mutate forward to new genes and
backward to the old gene. The mutation pressure is the net change of
these two processes.  Genes arising by mutation tend to be
recessive,  and since they are rarely homozygous, they tend to be
carried silently, i.e. not expressed, in the population for long
periods of time.  Stable alleles are those with low mutation rates
and they tend to increase in frequency. This contrasts with unstable
alleles which have high mutation rates and tend to decrease in
frequency.  This process results in a slow shift in gene frequencies
in the population.  It seems reasonable that mutation alone could
cause evolutionary change.  The major reason that mutation per se
does not cause evolutionary change is that mutation is random and,
consequently,  usually is in a direction away from the organism's

evolutionary trend. So mutation alone has a slow and non-directional effect on evolution with the exception of polyploidy (Section 2.20.1). Polyploidy is the doubling (e.g., 2n→4n), of the set of chromosomes usually by nondisjunction during meiosis. What results is an organism with a larger set of chromosomes which result in phenotypic differences in them. Also, note that mutations in somatic cells have no effect on evolution because they are not passed on to the offspring.

Mutations produce a small but important change in the gene frequencies of the gene pool (Section 2.20.1) of a population. These gene frequencies determine the genotypic ratios which determine the distribution of phenotypes in the population. Genotypic ratios (i.e., numbers and types of genotypes) can be determined from the gene frequencies and the Punnet square method as shown in Fig. 2.56.

allele B = 0.8, allele b = 0.2 as frequencies in the population

Punnet Square to determine genotypes:

|  | B(0.8) | b(0.2) |
|---|---|---|
| B(0.8) | BB (0.64) | Bb (0.16) |
| b(0.2) | Bb (0.16) | bb (0.04) |

genotypic frequencies   BB = 0.64,   Bb = 2(0.16) = 0.32, bb = 0.04.

**Fig. 2.56 – Genotypic Frequencies**

The Hardy-Weinberg Law states that under certain conditions the above gene frequencies and genotypic frequencies remain constant from generation to generation in sexually reproducing populations. This means no evolution would occur under these conditions which are: (1) large populations, (2) no mutations or the existence of mutational equilibrium, (3) no immigration or emigration of the population, and (4) random reproduction. The reason large populations (#1) are required is that gene frequencies undergo random fluctuations called genetic drift. In a small population, these random changes may cause an increase of certain alleles which leads to homozygosity. This effect is small in large populations (e.g., greater than 10,000 breeding individuals). As noted above, mutations always occur so #2 does not hold. Immigration or emigration leads to loss or gain of certain alleles which change gene frequencies. Reproduction includes all the steps from mate selection thru mating and development of the embryo to growth of the young to reproductive maturity. All of these steps, and all in between, must be random for gene frequencies to remain constant (#4). But in all populations, non-random reproduction exists, and this non-random reproduction is called natural selection as first set forth by Darwin. The reason reproduction is non-random is because phenotypes vary, and different phenotypes result in differences in reproductive capabilities. Natural selection does change gene frequencies by causing new combinations of genes which result in new phenotypes. Additionally, recombination and gene mutation, if left alone, can destroy favorable gene combinations and substitute unfavorable combinations for them. Natural selection also serves a conservative function by eliminating these unfavorable combinations. Note that natural selection can act on gene frequencies only when the genetic variation is expressed as phenotypic variation, and that phenotypic variation can lead to changes in gene frequencies only when it reflects underlying genetic variation.

Phenotypic differences are in a distribution in any population. The distribution is often an approximation of the bell shaped curve.

An example is the distribution of height in humans. Environmental factors (meteorologic, geographic, physical, or biologic) also vary greatly. It is a small step to infer that certain characteristics are better suited for certain environments. Or, to look at it differently, environments may select organisms with certain phenotypic characteristics that are most likely to survive in them. As above, if these phenotypic characteristics reflect genetic differences then a change in gene frequencies and evolution can occur. Evironmental factors and reproductive factors (i.e., natural selection) interact with each other.


In summary, mutations provide the raw material for evolution. But it is the selection pressure for certain phenotypes exerted by natural selection and environmental factors that determines the course of evolution.


2.21.1.2    Consequences of Evolution


The consequences of evolution are seen in the changes that may occur in a given species. These changes can be minor and reflected as clines. Clines are gradual variations in a species due to geographic (environmental) variations such as altitude or latitude. Subspecies (races) result when an abrupt environmental change is associated with an abrupt change in characteristics. Finally, the evolutionary changes may be so great as to result in a totally new species--a process called speciation.

A species is viewed as a set of genetically distinct organisms that share a common gene pool (i.e., gene flow is possible between them) and are reproductively isolated from all other such groups. The first step in speciation is usually geographic isolation of two populations of the same species. A barrier (e.g., rivers, oceans, canyons, mountains, etc.) prevent the populations from coming together to mate. The two separate populations will tend to differ because: (1) gene frequencies usually differ, (2) each population experiences different mutations, (3) the different environments will exert different selection pressures, and (4) if small, genetic drift can cause differences. The second factor in speciation then comes into play; it is reproductive isolation. The two populations will begin to differ such that gene flow between them is no longer possible even if they are brought together. This is brought about by intrinsic reproductive isolating mechanisms which act at all the steps of reproduction discussed earlier. These are: (1) ecogeographic isolation (organisms can no longer survive in each other's environment), (2) habitat isolation (organisms may occupy only certain, but different, habitats within the same range), (3) seasonal isolation (the breeding periods may be at different times of the year), (4) behavioral isolation (mating rituals differ), (5) mechanical isolation (nonfitting of genitals), (6) gametic isolation (fertilization cannot occur), (7) hybrid unviability (the offspring cannot reproduce), and (9) developmental isolation (fertilization can occur, but the embryo dies). So, by geographic isolation followed by reproductive isolation, the mechanisms of evolution lead to new species.

General patterns of evolution are divergent (moving from one species to different species, the usual pattern), convergent (moving from separate to common species), or parallel (two species resulting from one but evolving in a parallel fashion). Adaptive radiation is the gradual divergent differentiation of a species, usually as a response to environmental variations. Homologous structures are those that arose from a common structure even though functions may be different. Analogous structures have common functions but arose from different structures.

2.21.1.3      Taxonomy

A hierarchical classification that exists for organisms was due primarily to Linnaeus. Organisms are grouped at each level on the basis of similarities. As the hierarchy is ascended (shown below), the similarities become more general. A well-known mnemonic is given with the hierarchy:

| | |
|---|---|
| King | Kingdom |
| Phillip | Phyllum |
| Came | Class |
| Over | Order |
| For | Family |
| Green | Genus |
| Stamps | Species |

All organisms are given a two-component Latin name. The first is the genus (capitalized), and the second is the species (not capitalized), e.g. Homo sapiens.

2.21.1.4      Major Adaptive Evolutionary Changes in Vertebrates

Chordates are distinguished by (1) a dorsal, hollow nerve cord, (2) gill slits in the throat region, and (3) a notochord. Chordates are divided into invertebrate chordates (tunicates, acorn worms, cephalochordates or amphioxus) and vertebrates. Vertebrates have a vertebral column, closed circulatory system (enabling large growth), a better developed nervous system and improved sensory apparatus. Fishes include the Agnatha (jawless, e.g. lampreys), Chondrichthyes (e.g., sharks, all cartilage except inner ears) and Osteichthyes (bony fishes). The pectoral fins, pelvic fins and lateral line system are important for balance. Lobe fin fishes (or crossopterygians, e.g. latimeria) invaded land, had lungs, had stubby fins (bones into fins--was a crucial step for land invasion) and gave rise to the amphibians. <u>Amphibians</u> (frogs, toads, salamanders) are still tied to water because their eggs are easily dessicated. <u>Reptiles</u> (snakes, turtles, lizards, crocodiles and alligators) arose from amphibians. Total land life was possible because of the amniotic egg which wouldn't dessicate and which had a sufficient food supply. Reptiles are also advanced beyond amphibians by (1) internal fertilization by copulation, (2) ventricle of heart is partly divided to separate oxygenated and unoxygenated blood, (3) ribs aid in respiration, and (4) the brain has small cerebral hemispheres. The pterosaurs (extinct) gave rise to the birds. <u>Aves</u> (birds) can fly because of special feathers (modified reptile scales, large quills for flying surface, fanlike tail feathers for stabilization, contour and down feathers for insulation), light skeleton and a special breastbone for flight muscles, warm-blooded, efficient respiration with the four-chambered heart, advanced sight and muscular coordination by the brain. <u>Mammals</u> arose from a different type of reptile than did the birds. Key distinguishing features of mammals are: (1) internal development of young and nutrition by mammary glands, (2) jaw is strengthened and teeth are differentiated, (3) a diaphragm is present to separate thorax and abdomen and is used in breathing, (4) legs are swung underneath the body, and (5) the brain is greatly enlarged.

2.21.1.5        <u>Population Growth</u>

Although many factors affect the ultimate growth of a population (species), four factors can be used to describe the growth rate (R). These are the birth rate (B), the death rate (D), the carrying capacity (C), and the number of individuals in the population (N). B is the rate of live births per unit population (e.g., 5/1000 means 5 live births per 1000 individuals). D is similarly defined. Both are dependent on the age of the population and the reproductive capacity of the population. Very old or young populations will have high D. C represents the number of individuals the environment is able to support. C is independent of the R of the population, but over time the total N can affect its value (e.g., by using up the food supply). The maximum growth rate may vary as the C of particular environments varies. The equation linking these four factors is:

$$R = (B - D) \times \left( \frac{C - N}{C} \right) \times N.$$

Note that B - D is the intrinsic growth rate (IGR) of the population. The key points to remember are:

(1) R is directly proportional to IGR;
(2) R is directly proportional to N;
(3) when N is small, the term C-N/C is about one and growth is exponential;
(4) when N approaches and equals C, the term C-N/C is zero and the population is in zero growth (mild fluctuations may occur);
(5) the C-N/C factor results in the logistic (S shaped) growth curve for populations.

146

Growth curves are:

EXPONENTIAL (no constraints on growth)

$$\frac{C - N}{C} = 1$$

Population (N) vs Time — exponential growth curve

LOGISTIC

(N) vs Time — logistic curve, with labels: C, zero growth, deceleration, maximal growth, acceleration (exponential phase)

Note the maximal growth rate occurs in approximately the center of the curve (logistic). The maximal growth rate of the exponential growth curve is not reached as it is always increasing (and is never realized except for very short periods and then the logistic curve will intervene). The point of maximal growth is also the point of optimal yield of a population. This means to get the greatest number of individuals (including more mature) out of a population, the population size (N) should be kept near this point. It is always near the center of the logistic growth curve.

Age distributions of populations are important in understanding and predicting changes in population growth. Age distribution curves may be done in many different graphic representations. One example is (with different distributions):

Age brackets: 80 +, 60 - 79, 40 - 59, 20 - 39, 0 - 19

← NUMBER OF INDIVIDUALS →

relatively balanced population

excessively young population

excessively old population

Survivorship of the population may also be graphically represented as:

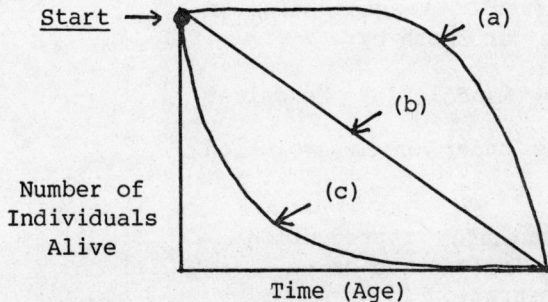

Start → ; curves labeled (a), (b), (c); Number of Individuals Alive vs Time (Age)

(a) individuals live to older ages, many younger & older
(b) death rates same at all ages, equal representation of all ages
(c) younger die at high rates, few older in population

147

The factors limiting population growth may be divided into density dependent (DD) and density independent (DI) effects. DD effects (as population grows, these are more important) include space, food, diseases, predation, and other competitive factors. DI effects include weather, natural disasters, and aging. The limitations on population growth can be overcome by emigration (relocation to alleviate DD effects), migration (relocating annually to maximize environments), evolution of different characteristics, or undergoing population cycles (increases and decreases in population size on a regular basis by mechanisms unknown, e.g., the lemmings). If unsuccessful, the population may become extinct.

## 2.21.2    QUESTIONS TO REVIEW EVOLUTION AND COMPARATIVE ANATOMY

(1)    Select the correct statement:

   (a)    Phenotypic differences alone serve as a basis for evolution.
   (b)    Phenotypic differences serve as a basis for evolution when they reflect somatic cell genetic differences.
   (c)    Phenotypic differences serve as a basis for evolution when they reflect germ cell genetic differences.
   (d)    None of the above.

(2)    The ultimate source of all new genes in a population is due to:

   (a)  mitosis   (b)  mating   (c)  meiosis   (d)  mutation

(3)    Mutations tend to be:

   (a)  recessive      (b)  dominant      (c)  codominant

(4)    Mutations do not affect evolutionary change primarily because they are:

   (a)  expressed   (b)  recessive   (c)  too rare   (d)  random

(5)    "Under certain conditions the gene frequencies and genotypic frequencies remain constant from generation to generation in sexually reproducing populations" was put forth by:

   (a)  Dalton   (b)  Hardy-Weinberg   (c)  Mendel   (d)  Mendeleev

(6)    All of the following are conditions under which evolution would not occur except:

   (a)  large populations        (b)  nonrandom reproduction
   (c)  no mutations             (d)  no immigration or
                             emigration

(7)    Genetic drift may lead to evolution in populations that are:

   (a)  any size      (b)  large      (c)  small

(8)   Which is <u>not</u> considered as part of the evolutionary concept of the reproductive process?

    (a)   mate selection and mating behavior
    (b)   embryo development
    (c)   growth of young to reproductive maturity
    (d)   all of the above are part of the reproductive process


(9)   Darwin's idea of natural selection is the same as:

    (a)   polyploidy        (b)   mutation pressure
    (c)   genetic drift      (d)   nonrandom reproduction


(10)  Natural selection results in:

    (a)   increased favorable gene combinations
    (b)   decreased unfavorable gene combinations
    (c)   both
    (d)   neither


(11)  Selection pressure depends on:

    (a)   nonrandom reproduction
    (b)   environmental factors
    (c)   both
    (d)   neither


(12)  The first step in the formation of a new species is:

    (a)   reproductive isolation
    (b)   geographic isolation
    (c)   both occur together


(13)  Populations that are separated by geographic barriers will tend to differ because

    (a)   gene frequencies usually differ between them;
    (b)   mutations vary between populations;
    (c)   there are different evironmental pressures;
    (d)   all of the above.


(14)  Structures that have different functions but arose from a common structure are called:

    (a)   convergent      (b)   divergent
    (c)   analogous      (d)   homologous


(15)  Assuming all other factors are constant, which situation will not result in an increase in the population growth rate?

    (a)   increase in the total individuals in the population near the carrying capacity
    (b)   decrease in the death rate
    (c)   increase in the birth rate
    (d)   increase in the intrinsic growth rate

(16) Important features in the development of mammals are:

   (1)  internal development of young
   (2)  jaw is strengthened and teeth differentiated
   (3)  diaphragm
   (4)  legs underneath body
   (5)  brain greatly enlarged

   (a)  1, 3, 5                  (b)  1, 3, 4, 5
   (c)  1, 2, 3, 5               (d)  all of the above

(17) A factor which would be detrimental to the flight of birds is

   (a)  light skeleton;
   (b)  advanced sight and muscle coordination;
   (c)  three-chambered heart;
   (d)  large quill feathers or fan-like tail feathers.

(18) Reptiles differ from amphibians by all of the following
     except:

   (a)  amniotic egg
   (b)  internal fertilization by copulation
   (c)  complete four-chambered heart
   (d)  ribs aid in respiration

(19) The primary reason amphibians are still tied to the water is

   (a)  lungs are inadequate;
   (b)  they are cold blooded;
   (c)  eggs are easily dessicated;
   (d)  they need to breathe through moist skin.

(20) A fish manager wants to increase the productivity of a lake.
     He desires greater catches of fish and larger sized fish. He
     wants to maintain this over a long period of time. This
     increase will be accomplished best by:

   (a)  increasing the bait (food) available to the fish
   (b)  keeping the fish population near the maximal growth rate
        point
   (c)  restricting the number of fish caught for several years
   (d)  stocking the lake with reproductive size fish this year

(21) Which type of heart can separate oxygenated and deoxygenated
     blood completely?

   (a)  two chambers            (b)  three chambers
   (c)  four chambers           (d)  all can

(22) Diaphragms are muscles used in the act of breathing.  Which of
     the following utilizes a diaphragm to breathe?

   (a)  amphibians             (b)  reptiles
   (c)  birds                  (d)  none of the above

150

(23) What is the correct hierarchy (from highest to lowest) of the given levels of taxonomy?

    (a) class, order, family, genus
    (b) order, family, genus, class
    (c) family, genus, class, order
    (d) family, class, order, genus

(24) Organisms are given a two-component scientific name. The first part is the:

    (a) class    (b) order    (c) species    (d) genus

## 2.21.3 ANSWERS TO QUESTIONS IN SECTION 2.21.2

( 1) c   (2) d   (3) a   (4) d   (5) b   (6) b   (7) c
( 8) d   (9) d   (10) c   (11) c   (12) b   (13) d   (14) d
(15) a   (16) d   (17) c   (18) c   (19) c   (20) b   (21) b
(22) d   (23) a   (24) d

## 2.21.4 DISCUSSION OF ANSWERS TO QUESTIONS IN SECTION 2.21.2

QUESTIONS #1 - #19 Adequately discussed in section.

QUESTION #20 (Answer: b) The point of optimal yield is at the maximum growth rate (MGR). If the MGR can be determined and the population kept at this level, the lake will produce the greatest yield.

Increasing the food (that is, the carrying capacity) will not increase the yields per se. If the amount of fish caught is restricted, the lake will approach the carrying capacity, and zero growth rate and the yield will decrease. Adding more fish may overload the carrying capacity, and, of itself, may not increase the yield. Arguments for each choice may be made; the best answer is (b).

QUESTIONS #21 - #24 Adequately discussed in section.

## 2.21.5 VOCABULARY CHECKLIST FOR EVOLUTION AND COMPARATIVE ANATOMY

____ genotypic ratios
____ reproductive isolation
____ divergent evolution
____ adaptive radiation
____ genetic drift
____ homologous
____ speciation

____ population growth rate
____ birth rate
____ exponential growth
____ geographic isolation
____ convergent evolution
____ parallel evolution
____ gene pool

____ uric acid
____ analogous
____ vertebrates
____ intrinsic growth rate
____ death rate
____ logistic growth

_____ role of mutations in evolution
_____ Hardy-Weinberg Law
_____ meaning of reproduction in evolutionary terms
_____ natural selection
_____ role of environment in evolution
_____ mechanism of speciation
_____ optimal yield
_____ taxonomy
_____ carrying capacity of population
_____ major adaptive evolutionary changes in vertebrates
_____ survivorship curves
_____ density dependent effects
_____ density independent effects
_____ maximal growth rate
_____ age distributions


## 2.22     References for Review of Biology


Keeton, W.  _Biological Science_.  2nd or latest ed.  (New York:
     W. W. Norton & Co., Inc.)

     An excellent introductory text on general biology.  If any
     questions arise about material presented in this workbook, this
     textbook should be consulted first.

White, A., et al.  _Principles of Biochemistry_.  5th or latest ed.
     (New York:  McGraw-Hill Book Co.)

Wilson, W. O., et al.  _Life on Earth_.  Latest  ed.  (Sinauer
     Associates, Inc.)

# CHAPTER 3:

# REVIEW

# OF

# GENERAL CHEMISTRY

**3.1.1**    <u>REVIEW OF ATOMIC STRUCTURE</u>

<u>Bohr</u> used the theories and experimental data of Planck, Einstein and Rutherford to develop his theory of the atom.  He thought the angular momentum of the electron was in multiples of $h/2\pi$ (or $mvr=nh/2\pi$), and that electrons circulated in discrete circular orbits stabilized by having the centrifugal force on the electron equal the Coulomb force of attraction between the nucleus and the electron. From these inferences he derived the energy states of the electrons given by:

$$E = -\frac{2\pi^2 m Z^2 e^4}{n^2 h^2} \qquad n = 1,2,3,\ldots\ldots$$

$m$ = mass of electron
$e$ = charge on electron
$Z$ = atomic number (nuclear charge)
$h$ = Planck's Constant

Energy transitions occur between states with energy change equal to $h\nu$  which could be calculated from above ($h = |E_f - E_i|$).  Note that $E \propto 1/n^2$ and as n gets larger, the energy levels get closer together. Bohr was able to explain some of the hydrogen spectrum lines with his theory. Another key to his theory was that electrons in any one of the energy states  do not radiate energy. The major flaws in Bohr's theory were the discrete orbits and the determination of exact momentum of the electron concurrently.   <u>Heisenberg's uncertainty</u> <u>principle</u> stated that it is impossible to determine simultaneously the position and momentum of an electron as in Bohr's theory.  This led to the probabilistic theory of electronic structure as derived by Schroedinger.  The quantum theory and its natural quantum numbers resulted.  The quantum numbers are:

(1)    n = principal quantum number
       takes values n=1,2,3,4,5....
       higher n means higher total energy of electron
       defines <u>shells</u> of the atom

       1 = K, 2 = L, 3 = M, 4 = N, etc.

(2)    $\ell$ = angular momentum quantum number
       higher $\ell$ means higher angular momentum of electron
       angular momentum is limited by the total energy (n)
       $\ell$ = 0,1,2....n-1
       <u>defines orbitals</u> of atom (along with n)
       0 = s, 1 = p, 2 = d, 3 = f, etc.

(3)    $m_\ell$ = magnetic quantum number
       orientation of the electron's magnetic field in an external field--limited by the angular momentum ($\ell$)
       $m_\ell$ = $\ell$,  $\ell$-1,...0,....,-$\ell$ +1, -$\ell$
       (i.e., takes all values between + $\ell$ and -$\ell$) determines spatial orientation of orbitals and, consequently, the <u>number</u> of orbitals of type $\ell$

(4)     $m_s$ = spin quantum number

        does not arise from solution of the Schroedinger equation

        the spin of an electron in its axis also generates a
        magnetic field which can orient two ways with an
        external field

        values have been chosen as  $+\frac{1}{2}$, $-\frac{1}{2}$ for the direction of
        spin.

Each electron in an atom has a set (n, $\ell$, $m_\ell$, $m_s$) of quantum numbers
that uniquely defines it.  <u>Pauli's Exclusion Principle</u> states that
no two electrons in the same atom may have the same set of quantum
numbers.  Only a certain number of electrons is allowed for each
quantum number:

  n:  a maximum of 2 $n^2$ electrons
      for n = 1, get 2 electrons
      for n = 2, get 8 electrons
      for n = 3, get 18 electrons

  $\ell$:  a maximum of 4$\ell$ +2 electrons
      for $\ell$ = 0 (s orbital), get 2 electrons
      for $\ell$ = 1 (p orbital), get 6 electrons
      for $\ell$ = 3 (f orbital), get 14 electrons

  $m_\ell$ : a maximum of two electrons for each $m_\ell$

An example of how one gets these numbers is shown for n=3 (maximum
numbers of electrons are in parentheses) in Fig. 3.1.

| n | $\ell$ | $m_\ell$ | $m_s$ |
|---|---|---|---|
| 3 (18) | 0(2) | 0(2) | +1/2,−1/2 |
|  | 1(6) | +1(2) | +1/2,−1/2 |
|  |  | 0(2) | +1/2,−1/2 |
|  |  | −1(2) | +1/2,−1/2 |
|  | 2(10) | +2(2) | +1/2,−1/2 |
|  |  | +1(2) | +1/2,−1/2 |
|  |  | 0(2) | +1/2,−1/2 |
|  |  | −1(2) | +1/2,−1/2 |
|  |  | −2(2) | +1/2,−1/2 |

**Fig. 3.1 – Example of the Quantum Number Relationships**

Each orbital is symbolized by using the n and $\ell$ quantum numbers as
follows:

                    1s, 3p, 5f
               n ↗            ↖ $\ell$.

The <u>orbitals are filled</u> in sequence, from the lowest energy to the
highest energy.  The pattern of orbitals filled is called the
<u>electron configuration</u>.  The sequence is not that expected because
some orbitals, especially those with s($\ell$ =0), penetrate (get closer
to the nucleus than others) and are consequently lowered in energy
more and are filled first. A useful way to remember the sequence is
to add the n and $\ell$ numerical values.  The lowest sum is filled
first.  In the case of a tie, the lowest n value is filled first
(remember s = 0, p = 1, d = 2, f = 3).  For example: 1s 2s 2p 3s 3p
3d 4s vs. 1s 2s 2p 3s 4s 3d.  In the first configuration 3d is written
before 4s.  Using the rule for 3d, n(=3) + d(=2) = 5, whereas for 4s,
n(=4) + s(=0) = 4; therefore second configuration should be used.

155

The orbitals are filled by knowing the number of electrons in the atom (if neutral, this is the atomic number), and then filling each orbital sequentially up to its maximum number of electrons. For example:

$$Al = 13: \quad 1s^2\ 2s^2\ 2p^6\ 3s^2\ 3p^1.$$
$$Ca = 20: \quad 1s^2\ 2s^2\ 2p^6\ 3s^2\ 3p^6\ 4s^2.$$

If the atom is charged, the extra electrons (if negative) are added or the lost electrons (if positive) are removed. For example:

$$Al^{+3}\ (AN = 13): \quad 1s^2\ 2s^2\ 2p^6$$
$$O^{-2}\ \ (AN = 8): \quad 1s^2\ 2s^2\ 2p^6.$$

Fig. 3.2 shows another way to remember the sequence of filling:

The sequence: 1s 2s 2p 3s 3p 4s 3d 4p 5s, etc.

**Fig. 3.2 – A Way of Remembering the Sequence of Filling of Orbitals**

Hund's rule describes the way electrons are to be put into each orbital $(n, \ell)$. Electrons go into each orbital of same energy $(m_\ell)$ with parallel spins (same $m_s$) until each orbital is half filled (i.e., all electrons unpaired), then they are paired (put in the same orbital with opposite $m_s$'s) (Fig. 3.3).

**Fig. 3.3 – Hund's Rule**

156

Orbitals (Fig. 3.4) are determined by the n, $\ell$, and $m_\ell$ numbers. The n and $\ell$ are important for determining the energy and shape of the orbital. The $m_\ell$ determines the orientation (direction in space) of the orbitals. Remember that an orbital describes the probability of an electron being in a region of space; it is not the electron spread out.

Fig. 3.4 - Orbitals

The ground state of the electrons of an atom is when the electrons are in the lowest energy states available to the electrons. For example, the ground state of the aluminum was

$$1s^2 \; 2s^2 \; 2p^6 \; 3s^2 \; 3p^1.$$

An excited state of the atom occurs when one or more electrons occupy orbitals (energy levels) other than the lowest available to the atom. This occurs by "exciting" the electron (by input of some type of energy) to the higher state. For example, for the aluminum:

$$1s^2 \; 2s^2 \; 2p^6 \; 3s^2 \; 3p^1 \xrightarrow{energy} 1s^2 \; 2s^2 \; 2p^6 \; 3s^0 \; 3p^3$$

both 3s electrons are now in the higher energy level 3p.

For the electrons, the higher the n or $\ell$ quantum numbers, the higher the energies. When electrons shift between the different orbitals, energy is absorbed or emitted as a frequency of light. When energy is emitted (the electron moves from higher orbitals to lower orbitals, i.e., closer to the nucleus in general), a bright band appears at that frequency (or wavelength) in a spectrum (the continuum of all frequencies or wavelengths)--this results in emission spectra. When energy is absorbed by the electron (as must occur in the example above), a dark band appears at that frequency because energy is removed from the spectrum. This results in absorption spectra. Look at the spectrum as a source of light containing all the frequencies (wavelengths) representing different energies. As this passes through a substance, energy may be added (by emission from atoms) and certain frequencies become more intense (brighter) or energy may be removed (by absorption by atoms) and certain frequencies become less intense (less bright).

3.1.2      QUESTIONS TO REVIEW ATOMIC STRUCTURE

(1)   All of the following were theorized by Bohr in his description of the atom except:

      (a) angular momentum of electrons in multiples of $h/2\pi$
      (b) electrons circulate in discrete circular orbits
      (c) energy of each electron is inversely proportional to $n^2$
      (d) electrons radiate energy continuously in a given orbit

(2)   The statement, "it is impossible to determine simultaneously the position and momentum of an electron," is attributable to:

      (a) Heisenberg                    (b)   Einstein
      (c) Planck                        (d)   Schroedinger

(3)   The following shape represents what type of orbital?

      (a) p       (b) s       (c) d       (d) f

(4)   The letters s,p,d and f are used to represent which quantum numbers?

      (a) angular momentum ($\ell$)      (b)   principal (n)
      (c) magnetic ($m_\ell$)            (d)   spin ($m_s$)

158

(5)    The magnetic quantum number (QN) has its values limited
       <u>directly</u> by the value of:

       (a) principal QN                    (b)  angular momentum QN
       (c) spin QN                         (d)  none of the above


(6)    Hund's Rule:

       (a) Electrons go into orbitals with parallel spins until all
           the orbitals of the same energy are half filled, then they
           go into suborbitals with anti-parallel (opposite) spins.
       (b) Two electrons in the same atom cannot have the same four
           quantum numbers.
       (c) There is a maximum of two electrons in any orbital.
       (d) None of the above.


(7)    Pauli's Exclusion Principle states that:

       (a) The position and momentum of an electron cannot be
           simultaneously determined.
       (b) Electrons with the same spin cannot go into the same
           orbital.
       (c) No two electrons in an atom may have the same set of the
           four quantum numbers.
       (d) None of the above.


(8)    When an atom emits energy as light, bands in the spectrum will
       appear:

       (a) brighter     (b)  darker     (c)  remain the same


(9)    The maximum number of electrons in an orbital with
       $m_\ell$ (magnetic quantum number) = -3 is:

       (a) 6     (b)  4     (c)  3     (d)  2


(10)   The maximum number of electrons in a shell with n (principal
       quantum number) = 3 is:

       (a) 6     (b)  8     (c)  18     (d)  32


159

(11) The maximum number of electrons in an orbital with $\ell$ (angular momentum quantum number) = 3 is

(a) 6    (b) 10    (c) 14    (d) 18

(12) An element with atomic number = 22 has how many electrons in the 2p orbital?

(a) 6    (b) 4    (c) 3    (d) 1

(13) The electron configuration of magnesium (Mg) with atomic number 12 is:

(a) $1s^2$ $2s^2$ $2p^6$ $3s^2$
(b) $1s^2$ $2s^2$ $3s^2$ $3p^6$
(c) $1s^2$ $2s^2$ $2p^2$ $3s^2$ $3p^2$ $3d^2$
(d) None of the above

(14) Sodium has an atomic number = 11. The electron configuration of the sodium ion ($Na^{+1}$) is:

(a) $1s^2$ $2s^2$ $2p^6$ $3s^2$
(b) $1s^2$ $2s^2$ $2p^5$ $3s^2$
(c) $1s^2$ $2s^2$ $2p^6$ $3s^1$
(d) $1s^2$ $2s^2$ $2p^6$

Use the following information for Questions #15-#17

The atomic number of manganese (Mn) is 25.

(15) The electron configuration of the ground state is:

(a) $1s^2$ $2s^2$ $2p^6$ $3s^2$ $3p^6$ $3d^7$
(b) $1s^2$ $2s^2$ $2p^6$ $3s^2$ $3p^6$ $4s^2$ $4p^5$
(c) $1s^2$ $2s^2$ $2p^6$ $3s^2$ $2d^{10}$ $3p^3$
(d) None of the above

(16) An excited state of the atom may be:

(a) $1s^2$ $2s^2$ $2p^6$ $3s^2$ $3p^6$ $4s^1$ $3d^6$
(b) $1s^2$ $2s^2$ $2p^6$ $3s^2$ $3p^6$ $4s^2$ $3d^5$
(c) $1s^2$ $2s^2$ $2p^6$ $2d^{10}$ $3s^2$ $3p^3$
(d) None of the above

(17) In going from $1s^2$ $2s^2$ $2p^6$ $3s^2$ $3p^6$ $4s^2$ $3d^5$ to $1s^2$ $2s^2$ $2p^6$ $3s^2$ $3p^6$ $4s^1$ $3d^6$, the atom would _____ energy.

    (a) absorb    (b) emit    (c) not change energy states

## 3.1.3    ANSWERS TO QUESTIONS IN SECTION 3.1.2

(1) d  (2) a  (3) a  (4) a  (5) b  (6) a  (7) c
(8) a  (9) d  (10) c  (11) c  (12) a  (13) a  (14) d
(15) d  (16) a  (17) a

## 3.1.4    DISCUSSION OF ANSWERS TO QUESTIONS IN SECTION 3.1.2

QUESTIONS #1-#8:  Adequately discussed in Section.

QUESTION #9  (Answer:  d)  All orbitals contain a maximum of two electrons.

QUESTION #10  (Answer:  c)  Using the formula given in Section, $2n^2 = 2(3)^2 = 2(9) = 18$.  See example in Section for alternative method to determine it.

QUESTION #11  (Answer:  c)  Using the formula given in the Section, $4\ell + 2 = 4(3) + 2 = 12 + 2 = 14$.

QUESTION #12  (Answer:  a)  There are 22 electrons (from the AN = 22 and the atom is neutral).  The electron configuration is:

$1s^2$ $2s^2$ $2p^6$ $3s^2$ $3p^6$ $4s^2$ $3d^2$

It might have been clear that the 2p orbital would have been filled. So, the answer would be a filled p orbital which has six electrons.

QUESTION #13  (Answer:  a)  There are 12 electrons in the neutral atom because AN = 12.  The sequence of filling is:

1s  2s  2p  3s  3p  4s  3d

The s has a maximum of 2 electrons, and the p has a maximum of 6 electrons.  The electron configuration is:

$1s^2$ $2s^2$ $2p^6$ $3s^2$.

QUESTION #14  (Answer:  d)  There are 10 electrons in the sodium ion.  In the neutral atom there are 11 (from atomic number = 11). Since the ion is a positive one, there must be one less electron available.  The electron configuration is then:

$1s^2$ $2s^2$ $2p^6$.

QUESTION #15  (Answer:  d)  The ground state is when the electrons are in the lowest energy levels available.  The sequence of filling for 25 electrons is:

$$1s^2 \quad 2s^2 \quad 2p^6 \quad 3s^2 \quad 3p^6 \quad 4s^2 \quad 3d^5$$

So, none of the answers given is correct.

QUESTION #16  (Answer:  a)  An excited state occurs when electrons in the ground state orbitals are "excited" to higher energy orbitals.  In (a), a 4s electron is excited to a 3d electron.

QUESTION #17  (Answer:  a)  Here the 4s electron  is  being excited to become a 3d electron. Since 3d electrons are of higher energy than 4s (due to the penetrance of this orbital and consequent lowering of its energy), it would require energy to move 4s to 3d levels. Therefore, the atom must absorb this energy.

3.1.5        VOCABULARY CHECKLIST FOR ATOMIC STRUCTURE

| | |
|---|---|
| ____ Heisenberg's Uncertainty Principle | ____ absorption spectra |
| ____ Bohr | ____ excited states |
| ____ Pauli's Exclusion Principle | ____ emission spectra |
| ____ orbital | ____ n |
| ____ shell | ____ $\ell$ |
| ____ Hund's rule | ____ $m_\ell$ |
| ____ ground states | ____ $m_s$ |

3.1.6        CONCEPTS,  PRINCIPLES,  ETC.  CHECKLIST  FOR  ATOMIC STRUCTURE

____ Bohr theory of atomic structure
____ quantum numbers and filling of electron orbitals (electronic structure)
____ relation of spectra to atomic structure

**3.2        Periodic Table**

**3.2.1        REVIEW OF THE PERIODIC TABLE**

The periodic table is an orderly arrangement of elements by their
atomic numbers based on the quantum theory of the atom.  Mendeleev
was the first to arrange elements by their atomic numbers.  Features
of the organization of the chart are (see also Fig. 4.5):

(1)    Rows or periods represent the principal quantum number (n) and
       have values from n = 1 to n = 7.  Each period is the sequential
       filling of the orbitals within a shell.

(2)    Columns or groups represent elements with the same electron
       configuration in the outermost shell.  There is the A set of
       elements called representative, and these have the s and/or p
       orbitals as the outermost.  The nonrepresentative, or B set,
       elements have the d or f orbitals as the outermost.  The Roman
       Numerals (I, II, etc.) give the number of electrons in the
       outermost orbitals.  From this, the electron configuration and
       valence can be determined.  For the VI A group, for example,
       there are six electrons in s and p orbitals.  This gives an
       $s^2p^4$.  Remember that second period atoms prefer the octet
       state  and that they will gain or lose electrons to reach it,
       whichever is easier.  The common valence in VI A is -2 because
       it is easier to gain 2 electrons to go to $s^2 p^6$ (octet) than to
       lose 6 electrons and go to $s^0 p^0$ (which would be the next lower
       octet) and have a + 6 valence.  Elements in the same group tend
       to have similar chemical properties.

(3)    The different blocks represent the angular momentum quantum
       number ($\ell$).  The number of spaces from left to right in each
       block is the maximum number of electrons for each quantum
       number: s has a maximum of 2, p has a maximum of 6, d has a
       maximum of 10, and f has a maximum of 14.

(4)    The magnetic quantum number ($m_\ell$) and spin quantum number ($m_s$)
       are not represented on the chart.

(5)    Representative    elements,    transition    elements,    inner
       transition elements (actinides, lanthanides), inert gases and
       other special groups are labeled on the chart (Fig. 3.5).

**Fig. 3.5 – The Periodic Chart**

The <u>periodic properties</u> are properties of the elements which vary in a more or less regular pattern as a function of the atomic numbers, and, hence, electron configuration. Most can be understood by understanding that:

(1) As one reads from left to right in a given period, the nuclear pull on the outermost electrons increases. This causes the electrons to be bound tighter and to be closer to the nucleus.

(2) As one reads down a given column, the outermost electrons are bound less tightly because more electrons are between the nucleus and the outermost electrons, and because a shell has been completed and this effectively shields the outer electrons.

Based upon the above discussion, the gross atomic trends of the periodic properties from the chart can be understood. These are:

(1) <u>Ionization energy (IE)</u> – The energy (or voltage) required to ionize a gaseous atom, i.e., take the outermost electron away from the atom. The higher the IE, the more difficult it is to remove an electron, and this means the nucleus is holding on tighter. IE increases, generally, from left to right in a period, and it decreases from top to bottom in a group.

(2) <u>Electron Affinity (EA)</u> – The energy released when an electron is moved from infinity into the lowest energy vacant orbital in the gaseous atom. The stronger the nuclear attraction for electrons, the higher the EA (absolute value). The EA is subject to configuration variations (Be $2s^2 <$ Li $2s^1$ but $C > B$) and repulsion of electrons in the same energy level ($F < Cl$ but $Br < Cl$). No overall trend is observed.

(3) <u>Electronegativity (E)</u> – The relative attraction of the nucleus for the electrons in a chemical bond. Not measured directly, but it can be indirectly obtained from EA, IE and/or bond energies. The E increases from left to right in a period and decreases from top to bottom in a group--this is similar to IE.

164

(4)   **Atomic Radius (AR)** - The distance from the middle of the nucleus to the "outermost limit" of the electrons.  The AR is determined by using x-rays on bonded atoms.  The AR decreases from left to right in a given period and increases from top to bottom in a given group.

Additional trends of properties can be inferred from the above basic properties.  These are:

(1)   **Metallic character (MC)** - The key feature of a metal is high mobility of electrons.  This requires a low IE and/or a low EA. This means MC decreases from left to right in a period but increases from top to bottom in a group.  In the chart, the metals are to the left and bottom, and the non-metals are in the top and right.  Between is a region of transition called the semi-metals.

(2)   **Oxidation State (OS)** - The OS depends on IE and EA.  Low IE elements tend to have positive OS, and high EA elements tend to have negative OS.  Metals tend to have positive OS, and non-metals tend to be negative.  Determination of OS (valence) from the chart is given above.  In general, note that the OS of the transition (d orbital) elements tend to be variable but positive.  And the OS of the inner transition elements (f-orbitals) tend to be +3.

(3)   **Chemical Activity (CA)** - This depends on the ease of removing an electron (low IE) or the ease of adding an electron (high EA).  Either situation leads to high CA.  Hence, CA trends are not usually discussed across a period (because the balance of IE and EA changes), but trends are meaningful for groups.  On the left side of the chart, CA increases as you go down the chart in a given group (because IE decreases).  On the right side of the chart, CA increases as you go up the chart in a given group (because EA generally increases).

(4)   **Acidity Trends** - See Section 3.11.1.

(5)   **Hydrogen Bonding (HB)** - HB exists for F, O, N and Cl but would theoretically increase as one ascended a given group.

3.2.2      **QUESTIONS TO REVIEW THE PERIODIC TABLE**

(1)   The periodic table is based upon:

    (a) atomic weights        (b)  mass number
    (c) neutron number       (d)  atomic number

(2)   The periods of the periodic table are _____ and represent the _____ quantum number.

    (a) horizontal; principal   (b)  horizontal; angular momentum
    (c) vertical; principal     (d)  vertical; angular momentum

(3)    Groups of the periodic table:

(a) represent the magnetic quantum number;
(b) represent elements with the same outer electron configuration;
(c) are horizontal;
(d) all of the above are correct.

(4)    Which of the following quantum numbers is not represented on the periodic chart?

(a) principal                    (b)    angular momentum
(c) magnetic                     (d)    all are

(5)    The transition elements have the __-orbital as the outermost.

(a) s        (b) p        (c) d        (d) f

(6)    Inert gases

(a) have incomplete shells;
(b) are found in the same period;
(c) are found at the beginning of a period;
(d) are found in the same group.

(7)    All of the following are correct except:

(a) The nuclear attraction for the outermost electrons decreases from right to left in a given period.
(b) In moving down a given column, the outermost electrons are bound less tightly.
(c) Half-filled or completely filled orbitals have more stability than other incompletely filled orbitals.
(d) All of the above are correct.

(8)    The energy required to ionize a gaseous atom is called the:

(a) ionization energy            (b)    electron affinity
(c) electronegativity            (d)    none of the above

(9)    The relative attraction of the nucleus for the electrons in a chemical bond is called the:

(a) ionization energy            (b)    electron affinity
(c) electronegativity            (d)    none of the above

(10)   The energy released when an electron is moved from infinity into the vacant orbital with the lowest energy:

(a) electron affinity            (b)    electronegativity
(c) ionization energy            (d)    none of the above

(11)   The ionization energy

(a) generally increases from left to right in a period;
(b) does not change in a period;
(c) increases from top to bottom in a group;
(d) does not change in a group.

(12)   The electron affinity

(a) decreases from left to right in a period;
(b) measures the attraction of the atom for electrons;
(c) increases from top to bottom in a group;
(d) variations follow no overall trend.

(13)   The electronegativity

(a) is measured directly from physical characteristics;
(b) does not vary in a group;
(c) decreases from left to right in a period;
(d) decreases from top to bottom in a group.

(14)   The atomic radius

(a) is calculated from bond energies;
(b) decreases from left to right in a period;
(c) decreases from top to bottom in a group;
(d) all of the above.

(15)   Metallic character

(a) depends upon the mass number;
(b) decreases from bottom to top in a group;
(c) requires a high ionization energy and a high electron affinity;
(d) decreases from top to bottom in a group.

(16)   Oxidation states (OS):

(a) high ionization energy elements have positive OS
(b) metals tend to have negative OS
(c) low electron affinity elements tend to have positive OS
(d) non-metals tend to have negative OS

(17)   Chemical activity

(a) increases as ionization energy increases;
(b) decreases as electron affinity decreases;
(c) in groups on the left side of the chart, chemical activity increases as you read down the chart.

(18)   Phosphorus (P) is in group VA; the electron configuration of its outermost shell is

(a) $s^2 \ p^3$                       (b)  $p^5$
(c) $d^5$                             (d)  cannot be determined

(19)   Bromine (Br) is in group VII A; its most common oxidation state (OS) is probably:

(a) +1                                (b)  -1
(c) -2                                (d)  cannot be determined

(20)   The electron configuration of selenium is:
       $1s^2 \ 2s^2 \ 2p^6 \ 3s^2 \ 3p^6 \ 4s^2 \ 3d^{10} \ 4p^4$. It is probably in what group?

(a) VI A                              (b)  IV A
(c) VI B                              (d)  need more information

(21)  The atomic number of chlorine is 17.  It is in what group?

    (a) VII A                        (b)  IV A
    (c) I A                           (d)  cannot be determined by trends

(22)  Fluorine (F) has an atomic number (AN) = 9 and chlorine (Cl) has an AN = 17.  Which has the highest electron affinity?

    (a)  both are equal             (b)  Cl
    (c)  F                      (d)  cannot be determined

(23)  Sodium (Na) has an atomic number (AN) = 11 and aluminum (Al) has an AN = 13.  Which has the highest ionization energy?

    (a)  both are equal             (b)  Na
    (c)  Al                      (d)  cannot be determined

(24)  Oxygen (O) has an atomic number (AN) = 8 and sulfur (S) has an AN = 16.  Which has the greatest electronegativity?

    (a)  S                        (b)  O
    (c)  both are equal             (d)  cannot be determined

(25)  The atomic number (AN) of magnesium (Mg) is 12, and the AN of sulfur (S) is 16.  Which has the larger atomic radius?

    (a)  Mg                      (b)  S
    (c)  both are equal             (d)  cannot be determined

(26)  Lithium (Li) has an atomic number (AN) = 3 and potassium (K) has an AN = 19.  Which has the greater metallic character?

    (a)  both are equal             (b)  Li
    (c)  K                       (d)  cannot be determined

(27)  Berylium (Be) has an atomic number (AN) = 4, and strontium (Sr) has an AN = 38.  Which has the greater chemical activity?

    (a)  both are equal             (b)  Sr
    (c)  Be                    (d)  cannot be determined

(28)  Magnesium (Mg) has an atomic number (AN) = 12 and Bromine (Br) has an AN = 35.  Which has the greater chemical activity?

    (a)  both are equal             (b)  Mg
    (c)  Br                    (d)  cannot be determined

3.2.3      ANSWERS TO QUESTIONS IN SECTION 3.2.2

(1 ) d  (2) a  (3) b  (4) c  (5) c  (6) d  (7) d
(8 ) a  (9) c  (10) a  (11) a  (12) d  (13) d  (14) b
(15) b  (16) d  (17) c  (18) a  (19) b  (20) a  (21) a
(22) d  (23) c  (24) b  (25) a  (26) c  (27) b  (28) d

QUESTIONS #1-#17:  Adequately discussed in Section.

QUESTION #18  (Answer: a)  The $\underline{A}$ means the p is a representative element and that its outermost shell contains s and p orbitals.  The V means there are 5 electrons, and these give the following electron configuration, $s^2$ $p^3$.

QUESTION #19  (Answer:  b)  Since Br is in group VII A the electron configuration of its outermost shell is $s^2$ $p^5$.  The closest octet is $s^2$ $p^6$, and this requires an extra electron to give it an OS of -1.

QUESTION #20  (Answer:  a)  Since the outermost incomplete orbitals are $\underline{s}$ and $\underline{p}$ (the d orbital is complete), the selenium is an $\underline{A}$ element.  The $\underline{s}$ and $\underline{p}$ contain 2 + 4 = 6 electrons.  This means selenium is group VI A.

QUESTION #21  (Answer:  a)  The electron configuration of chlorine is $1s^2$ $2s^2$ $2p^6$ $3s^2$ $3p^5$.  The outermost incomplete orbitals are $\underline{s}$ and $\underline{p}$--this makes it $\underline{A}$ (representative).  There are 2 + 5 = 7 electrons in the $\underline{s}$ and $\underline{p}$ orbitals--this makes it a VII.  So it is group VII A.

QUESTION #22  (Answer: d)  EA has no overall trend useful for predictions.

QUESTION #23  (Answer:  c)  The electron configuration of Na is $1s^2$ $2s^2$ $2p^2$ $3s^1$ and Al is $1s^2$ $2s^2$ $2p^6$ $3s^2$ $3p^1$.  This places them in the same period--highest $\underline{n}$ number is 3 in each.  Ionization energy (IE) increases from left to right on the table.  Then Al has a higher IE than Na.

QUESTION #24  (Answer:  b)  O has an electron configuration of $1s^2$ $2s^2$ $2p^4$, and sulfur has an electron configuration of $1s^2$ $2s^2$ $2p^6$ $3s^2$ $3p^4$.  This places both in group VI A.  In a group, the electronegativity decreases from top to bottom.  Then O has the greater electronegativity.

QUESTION #25  (Answer: a)  The electron configurations are: Mg = $1s^2$ $2s^2$ $2p^6$ $3s^2$; S = $1s^2$ $2s^2$ $2p^6$ $3s^2$ $3p^4$.  They are, therefore, in the same period.  The atomic radius decreases from left to right in a period.  Then Mg is larger than S.

QUESTION #26  (Answer:  c)  The electron configurations are:  Li = $1s^2$ $2s^1$; K = $1s^2$ $2s^2$ $2p^6$ $3s^2$ $3p^6$ $4s^1$.  Therefore, both are in group IA.  In a group the metallic character increases from top to bottom.  Then K has more metallic character than Li.

QUESTION #27  (Answer: b)  The electron configurations are: Be = $1s^2$ $2s^2$; Sr = $1s^2$ $2s^2$ $2p^6$ $3s^2$ $3p^6$ $4s^2$ $3d^{10}$ $4p^6$ $5s^2$.  Therefore, they are both in group II A.  In a group on the left side, the chemical activity increases from top to bottom.  Then Sr is more reactive than Be.

QUESTION #28  (Answer: d)  The electron configurations are: Mg = $1s^2$ $2s^2$ $2p^6$ $3s^2$; Br = $1s^2$ $2s^2$ $2p^6$ $3s^2$ $3p^6$ $4s^2$ $3d^{10}$ $4p^5$.  This means they are neither in the same group nor period and cannot be compared by general periodic trends.

## 3.2.5     VOCABULARY CHECKLIST FOR THE PERIODIC TABLE

____ periods
____ groups
____ representative elements
____ octet state
____ periodic properties
____ oxidation state

____ ionization energy
____ electron affinity
____ electronegativity
____ atomic radius
____ metallic character
____ chemical activity

## 3.2.6     CONCEPTS, PRINCIPLES, ETC. CHECKLIST FOR THE PERIODIC TABLE

____ basis for the periodic table
____ organization of the table, especially the relation to the quantum numbers
____ general basis for the variation of the periodic properties
____ variation of the periodic properties within groups and periods

## 3.3     Gas Phase

## 3.3.1     REVIEW OF THE GAS PHASE

The metric _pressure_ units are mmHg = torr. The English system uses atmospheres (atm). The conversion is 760 torrs = 1 atm. See Section 5.5.1 for temperature scales.

Gases have relatively high translational kinetic energies per molecule as compared with liquids. Gases take the shape of the container they are in, like liquids; but, unlike liquids, they completely fill any container. The _key characteristics_ of gases are the pressure (P), the volume (V), the temperature (T), and the quantity (moles = n). Gases are broadly considered as ideal or non-ideal. An _ideal gas_ has no intermolecular forces, and the gas molecules occupy no volume (they are points in space). This means the gases should have low density. In general, at high temperatures and low pressures, most gases can be considered to be ideal. A _non-ideal gas_ has intermolecular forces, and the molecules do have a finite volume. Laws covering the behavior of ideal gases will be covered first.

_Boyle's Law_ states that pressure and volume are inversely related ($P \propto 1/V$), i.e., as the pressure increases, the volume decreases and vice versa. _Charles' (Gay-Lussacs) Law_ states that the temperature and volume are directly related, i.e., as the temperature increases, the volume increases and vice versa. These laws are combined to give the _Ideal Gas Law_ which is:

$$PV = nRT$$

P = pressure, V = volume, n = moles, T = absolute temperature
R = Ideal gas constant = 0.0821 $\ell$-atm/°K-mole

Another useful way of writing the Ideal Gas Law is,

$$\frac{PV}{T} = \text{constant or,}$$

$$\frac{P_1V_1}{T_1} = \frac{P_2V_2}{T_2}$$

Also, note that 22.414 liters of an ideal gas at S.T.P. (Standard Temperature and Pressure--273°K and 1 atmosphere pressure) represent 1 mole of that gas. Avogadro's Principle is also important for solving problems and states that equal volumes of ideal gases at the same temperature and pressure contain the same number of moles (or molecules). Dalton's Law states that the total pressure ($P_t$) of a mixture of gases is equal to the sum partial pressures ($P_i$) of the gases:

$$P_t = P_1 + P_2 + P_3 + \ldots$$

The partial pressure ($P_i$) of a gas in a mixture of gases is determined as follows:

$$P_i = X_i P_t$$
$P_t$ = total pressure
$X_i$ = mole fraction of gas in the mixture

$$X_i = \frac{n_i}{n_1 + n_2 + n_3 + \ldots} = \frac{n_i}{\Sigma n_i}$$

$n_i$ = moles of a gas
$\Sigma n_i$ = sum of the moles of all gases.

The Kinetic Theory of Gases attempts to decribe the energy characteristics of gases as a whole by analyzing the motion and mass characteristics (e.g. forces, momentum) of individual molecules. It has its limitations but important results of it are:

(1)    Boyle's Law, Charles' Law, and the Ideal Gas Law are derivable from it;

(2)    P and V can be related to the Kinetic energy of molecules,
        $PV = 2/3\ NE_k$ (on a molecular scale)
        N = # of molecules, $E_k$ = translation energy/molecule
        or, $E_k = (3/2)\ RT$ (on a mole scale)
        also at a given temperature, all molecules have the same average $E_k$;     $PV = \frac{2}{3} N \left( \frac{3}{2} RT \right)$

(3)    Graham's Law of Diffusion can be determined from $E_k$ as follows:

        $E_{k_1} = E_{k_2}$ i.e., the average $E_k$s are equal
        1, 2 = molecules
        also, $\frac{1}{2}m_1v_1^2 = \frac{1}{2}m_2v_2^2$     (see Section 5.4.1)
        after solving, get

$$v_1/v_2 = \sqrt{m_2} / \sqrt{m_1} = \sqrt{m_2/m_1}$$

v = velocities of diffusion (e.g., mls/min)
m = molecular weights or densities.

(4)    Values for Heat Capacities of Monatomic Gases (see Section 5.5.1).

$$Cv = \frac{3}{2} R$$
$$Cp = Cv + R$$
$$Cp/Cv = 1.67$$
$$R = 1.99 \text{ cals/mole-}^\circ k$$

One of the simpler equations for nonideal gases is the <u>van der Waals equation</u> which takes into account the false assumptions of ideal gases:

$$\left( P + \frac{n^2 a}{v^2} \right) (V - nb) = nRT$$

a, b are constants
$n^2 a/v^2$ corrects for intermolecular forces
nb corrects for the volume occupied by gas molecules.

Note that if the density is very low, then $V \gg nb$ and $n^2 a/v^2 \to 0$, and the Ideal Gas Law results. The effect of the intermolecular forces is to decrease the pressure of the gas. The effect of the volume of molecules is to increase the volume occupied by the gas. The terms above bring the pressure and volume back to ideal levels.


### 3.3.2    QUESTIONS TO REVIEW THE GAS PHASE

(1)    The variables used to describe gases include all except:

(a) pressure                      (b)  volume
(c) moles                         (d)  all of the above

(2)    All of the following are characteristics of ideal gases except:

(a) absence of intermolecular forces
(b) nonideal gases may exhibit ideal behavior at high pressure and low temperatures
(c) the molecules occupy no space
(d) all of the above are correct

(3)    Boyle's Law states that

(a) volume varies inversely as temperature;
(b) volume varies directly as temperature;
(c) pressure varies inversely as volume;
(d) pressure varies directly as volume.

(4)    Charles' Law states that

(a) volume varies inversely as temperature;
(b) volume varies directly as temperature;
(c) pressure varies inversely as volume;
(d) pressure varies directly as volume.

(5)    All are expressions for the Ideal Gas Law except:

(a) $PV = nRT$                     (b) $\frac{PV}{T} = \text{constant}$

(c) $\frac{P_1 V_1}{T_1} = \frac{P_2 V_2}{T_2}$        (d) $\left( P + \frac{n^2 a}{v^2} \right) (V - nb) = nRT$

(6)    One mole of an ideal gas at STP has all of the following
       characteristics except:

       (a) volume = 1 liter          (b)  temperature = $273^\circ$ K
       (c) pressure = 1 atmosphere   (d)  all of the above are correct

(7)    Each gas in a mixture exerts a pressure.  The total pressure of
       all the gases in the container is

       (a) less than the sum of the separate pressures of each gas;
       (b) more than the sum of the separate pressures of each gas;
       (c) equal to the sum of the separate pressures of each gas;
       (d) the sum is variable.

(8)    The correct expression for the partial pressure ($P_A$) of $n_A$
       moles of a gas in a mixture of gases with a <u>total</u> of $n_T$ moles
       and a total pressure = $P_T$ is

       (a) $P_A = (n_A + n_T) P_T$              (b)  $P_A = (n_T - n_A) P_T$
       (c) $P_A = n_A P_T$                      (d)  $P_A = (n_A/n_T) P_T$

(9)    All of the following are conclusions of the Kinetic Theory of
       Gases except

       (a) derivation of the van der Waals equation;
       (b) derivation of Boyle's and Charles' Law;
       (c) relation of average kinetic energy of gases to
           temperature;
       (d) Graham's Law of Diffusion.

(10)   In the van der Waals equation for  nonideal gases,

$$\left(P + \frac{n^2 a}{V^2}\right)(V - nb) = nRT,$$

       It is <u>not true</u> that

       (a) $\dfrac{n^2 a}{V^2}$ corrects for intermolecular forces;

       (b) nb corrects for the volume occupied by gas molecules;
       (c) at high densities the equation reduces to the Ideal Gas
           Law;
       (d) all of the above are correct.

(11)   The pressure on a sample of gas is tripled, the volume is

       (a) 9 times the original        (b)  3 times the original
       (c) 1/3 of the original         (d)  1/9 of the original

(12)   If the temperature on a gas is increased by a factor of 4, the
       volume is

       (a) increased by a factor of 16;
       (b) increased by a factor of 4;
       (c) increased by a factor of 2;
       (d) decreased by a factor of 4.

(13)   One mole of an ideal gas occupies 3 liters at $37^\circ$C.
       Approximately what pressure, in atmospheres, does the gas
       exert?

       (a) 1.1 atm                     (b)  4.2 atm
       (c) 8.5 atm                     (d)  12.3 atm

173

$$V = \frac{nRT}{P} = \frac{0.08 \cdot 300}{}$$

(14) What volume will 2 liters of a gas at 27°C and 2 atm occupy at S.T.P.?

    (a) 3.6 liters                   (b) 5.1 liters
    (c) 1.1 liters                   (d) cannot be determined

(15) Two moles of an ideal gas occupy what volume at S.T.P.?

    (a) 22.4 liters                (b) 44.8 liters
    (c) 67.2 liters                (d) cannot be determined

(16) It is found that 2 grams of a vaporized liquid occupy 0.82 liters at S.T.P. What is the molecular weight of the gas?

    (a) 13.5 grams                 (b) 27 grams
    (c) 54 grams                   (d) cannot be determined

(17) A container of pure oxygen has a pool of water at its bottom. The atmospheric pressure is 760 torrs and equals the total pressure of the container. If the temperature is 37°C and the vapor pressure of water is 47 torrs at this temperature, what is the pressure of the dry oxygen?

    (a) 700 mm Hg                 (b) 684 mm Hg
    (c) 807 mm Hg                 (d) 713 mm Hg

(18) A mixture of 2 moles of $O_2$, 3 moles of $N_2$, and 5 moles of $H_2$ exerts a pressure of 700 torrs. The partial pressure of $N_2$ is:

    (a) 700 torrs                  (b) 210 torrs
    (c) 490 torrs                  (d) 760 torrs

(19) A mixture of 5 moles of $O_2$, 4 moles of $N_2$, and 1 mole of CO is collected above water at a temperature of 27°C. The total pressure is 760 torrs and the vapor pressure of water at 27°C is 27 torrs. What is the partial pressure exerted by $O_2$?

    (a) 76 torrs                   (b) 100 torrs
    (c) 367 torrs                  (d) 380 torrs

(20) Oxygen (molecular weight = 32) diffuses at a rate of 10 mls/min. Under the same conditions of temperature and pressure, how fast will hydrogen (molecular weight = 2) diffuse?

    (a) 20 mls/min                 (b) 40 mls/min
    (c) 160 mls/min              (d) need more information

3.3.3     ANSWERS TO QUESTIONS IN SECTION 3.3.2

(1) d   (2) b   (3) c   (4) b   (5) d   (6) a   (7) c
(8) d   (9) a   (10) c   (11) c   (12) b   (13) c   (14) a
(15) b   (16) c   (17) d   (18) b   (19) c   (20) b

QUESTIONS #1-#10:  Adequately discussed in Section.

QUESTION #11  (Answer:  c)  This is a direct application of Boyle's Law.  Volume varies inversely as pressure.  So, if pressure is increased by a factor of 3, the volume is decreased by a factor of 3. That is, the volume is 1/3 of the original.

QUESTION #12  (Answer:  b)  A direct application of Charles' Law. Volume varies directly as temperature.  Since temperature is increased by a factor of 4, the volume is increased by a factor of 4.

QUESTION #13  (Answer:  c)  This problem deals with one gas under one set of n-P-V-T; this suggests that the equation to use is PV = nRT.  Solving for pressure, one gets,

$$P = nRT/V$$

The value of R is required.  By knowing the units used, this can be determined as follows:

$$R = \frac{PV}{nT} = \frac{(1 \text{ atm})(22.4 \text{ liters})}{(1 \text{ mole})(273°K)} = 0.082 \frac{\text{atm-liters}}{\text{mole-°K}}$$

(Because 1 mole of an ideal gas at STP--273°K, 1 atm--occupies 22.4 liters.)

Also, remember, that the temperature is the absolute temperature: $T = 37° + 273° = 310°K$
Then,

$$P = \frac{(1)(0.082)(310)}{(3)} \approx 8.2 \text{ atms}$$

note $\frac{310}{3} \approx 100$ and then $(100)(0.082) \approx 8.2$.

Note the approximations made.  The 8.2 is closest to 8.5 atms.

QUESTION #14  (Answer:  a)  Note that this problem requires the gas be compared at two different conditions of P-V-T; the best equation to use in this instance is,

$$\underset{\text{(STP)}}{\frac{P_2 V_2}{T_2}} = \underset{\text{(Original)}}{\frac{P_1 V_1}{T_1}} .$$

Solving for $V_2$,

$$V_2 = V_1 \left(\frac{T_2}{T_1}\right)\left(\frac{P_1}{P_2}\right) = (2)\left(\frac{273}{300}\right)\left(\frac{2}{1}\right) \approx 3.6$$

$T_1 = 27 + 273 = 300$

the approximation is made as follows

$$\frac{273}{300} \approx \frac{270}{300} \approx \frac{27}{30} \approx \frac{9}{10}$$

then, $(2)\left(\frac{9}{10}\right)(2) = \frac{36}{10} = 3.6$

QUESTION #15  (Answer:  b)  Since one mole of an ideal gas occupies 22.4 liters at STP, two moles would occupy twice as much or 2x22.4 = 44.8 liters.

QUESTION #16  (Answer:  c)  First the number of moles is determined. Since the substance is a gas and there is one set of PV-T conditions use:

$$PV = nRT.$$

Solving for n,  $\quad n = \dfrac{PV}{RT} = \dfrac{(1)(0.82)}{(0.082)(273)} \approx \dfrac{1}{27}$

the approximation for n is as follows

$\dfrac{0.82}{0.082} = 10$, then  $\dfrac{10}{273} \approx \dfrac{10}{270} \approx \dfrac{1}{27}$ .

The definition of moles (n) is (Section 3.6.1):

$$\text{moles} = \dfrac{\text{weight}}{\text{molecular weight}} \quad \text{or,}$$

$$\text{molecular weight} = \dfrac{\text{weight}}{\text{moles}} \approx \dfrac{2}{1/27} \approx (2)\left(\dfrac{27}{1}\right) \approx 54 \text{ gms.}$$

alternate:  Since n = wt/mw, PV = (wt/mw)RT; mw = wt(RT/PV).

QUESTION #17 (Answer: d) The only point of this problem is to stress that when gases are collected over a liquid (e.g. water), the vapor pressure of that liquid must be subtracted from the total pressure to get the pressure of the gases without the added effect of the liquid's vapor pressure.   The vapor pressure varies with temperature.  Note that the total pressure of the gases is still the sum of the partial pressures (Dalton's Law),

$$P_{tot} = P_{O_2} + P_{H_2O} \text{ vapor}$$
$$P_{O_2} = P_{tot} - P_{H_2O} \text{ vapor} = 760-47 = 713.$$

QUESTION #18 (Answer:  b)  This is a direct application of Dalton's Law of partial pressures.  The partial pressure of $N_2$ ($P_{N_2}$) is,

$$P_{N_2} = X_{N_2} P_T$$
$$P_T = 700 \text{ torrs}$$
$$X_{N_2} = \dfrac{n_{N_2}}{n_{N_2} + n_{O_2} + n_{H_2}} = \dfrac{3}{3+5+2} = \dfrac{3}{10}$$
$$P_{N_2} = \dfrac{3}{10}(700) = 210 \text{ torrs.}$$

QUESTION #19 (Answer: c) This is just a combination of the principles of questions #17 and #18.  First, the effect of the water vapor on the total pressure is taken into account:

$P_T$ (Total pressure of gases) = total pressure - water vapor pressure

$$P_T = 760 - 27 = 733 \text{ torrs.}$$

Then Dalton's Law is applied using this 733 torrs:

$$P_{O_2} = X_{2} P_T$$
$$X_{2} = \dfrac{n_{O_2}}{n_{O_2} + n_{N_2} + n_{CO_2}} = \dfrac{5}{5+4+1} = \dfrac{5}{10} = \dfrac{1}{2}$$
$$P_{O_2} = \left(\dfrac{1}{2}\right)(733) = 367 \text{ torrs.}$$

QUESTION #20  (Answer:  b)  In general, the lighter gas will diffuse faster.  Using the formulation of Graham's Law of Diffusion,

$$\frac{V_{H_2}}{V_{O_2}} = \sqrt{\frac{MW_{O_2}}{MW_{H_2}}}$$

$$\frac{V_{H_2}}{10} = \sqrt{\frac{32}{2}} = \sqrt{16} = 4$$

$$V_{H_2} = (10)(4) - 40 \text{ mls/min.}$$

3.3.5        VOCABULARY CHECKLIST FOR THE GAS PHASE


____  pressure                    ____  Dalton's Law
____  ideal gas                   ____  partial pressure
____  nonideal  gas               ____  mole fraction
____  Boyle's Law                 ____  Graham's Law of
____  Charles' Law                      Diffusion
____  Avogadro's Principle        ____  van der Waals
                                        Equation


3.3.6        CONCEPTS, PRINCIPLES, ETC. CHECKLIST FOR THE GAS PHASE


____  characteristics of ideal gases
____  concept of partial pressures
____  Ideal Gas Law
____  Kinetic Theory of Gases
____  volume-mole relationship of ideal gas at STP
____  characteristics of  nonideal gases


3.4        Condensed Phases


3.4.1        REVIEW OF THE CONDENSED PHASES


The condensed phases are the liquids and the solids as opposed to the vaporized phase (i.e. gas).  The intermolecular forces are forces that exist between the molecules of the liquid or solid.  These forces depend upon the chemical characteristics of the molecules and play a large part in determining the physical behavior (e.g., phase changes, solubility) of the liquid or solid.  The types of forces that exist between molecules are van der Waals, hydrogen bonds, and hydrophobic.  Van der Waals forces are very weak attractive forces due to the net attraction between the nucleus of one atom and the electrons in another.  These forces are effective only over short distances and increase as the molecular weights increase, i.e., as the number of atoms or electrons in a molecule increases.  This type of van der Waals force merges with the slightly stronger forces (may also be considered van der Waals) that exist between polar molecules or between molecules that are inducible (i.e., a separation of charge in a molecule can be induced by the presence of a second).  Polar molecules are those made up of elements differing in

177

electronegativity, e.g.,

$$\overset{\delta^+}{C} - \overset{\delta^-}{O}, \quad \overset{\delta^+}{C} - \overset{\delta^-}{Cl},$$ and are asymmetric in geometry.

Hydrogen bonds are weak attractive bonds, but stronger than van der Waals, between the hydrogens on chlorine, fluorine, nitrogen or oxygen and the nonbonding electrons on these same elements. These are the only elements for which hydrogen bonding exists. Bonding becomes stronger when the electronegativity of the atoms increases and when the hydrogen bond can have a 180° orientation. (Fig. 3.6.)

**Fig. 3.6 – Hydrogen Bonding**

Hydrophobic bonds are weak attractive bonds between molecules that are nonpolar (no net separation of charges in molecules). These bonds exist because nonpolar molecules (e.g. hydrocarbons, fats, aromatics) decrease the entropy (see Section 3.8.1) of water when the molecules are apart. When these nonpolar molecules come together and form hydrophobic bonds, the entropy increases and the free energy is lowered and the bonds become stable. Ionic forces exist between ions, i.e., positive and negative ions. These can be very strong forces and are exemplified in ionic solids (e.g. NaCl, table salt). Ionic forces are due to Coulomb forces (see Section 5.7.1).

The weak forces (van der Waals, hydrogen bonds and hydrophobic), although very weak individually, are very strong when many exist between molecules as in proteins or nucleic acids. A large part of the stability of these and other polymers is due to the multitude of these weak forces. When solids melt or liquids evaporate, these are the forces that must be overcome. The greater the number of these intermolecular bonds, or the more different types these bonds present, the greater the stability of the substance and the more difficult it is to melt or evaporate. Temperature increases tend to disrupt these weak intermolecular forces easily, especially when they are few in number.

Also, molecules of similar types (e.g. hydrophobic or polar or with hydrogen bonding) tend to be soluble in each other because the forces are similar. Similarly, molecules of different types, especially polar versus nonpolar, tend to be insoluble.

The basic organization of ionic crystals is based on attempts to maximize the stability of the crystal by maximizing the attractive forces betwen cations (positive) and anions (negative) and minimizing the repulsive forces between ions of the same charge. Hence, anions and cations try to be as close together as possible, while minimizing anion-anion repulsion.

3.4.2    QUESTIONS TO REVIEW CONDENSED PHASES

(1)    Which of the following is not considered as an intermolecular
       force between molecules?

       (a) covalent bonds          (b)  hydrogen bonds
       (c) hydrophobic bonds       (d)  van der Waals forces

(2)    Van der Waals forces depend upon

       (a) repulsion of the molecules from water;
       (b) Coulomb attractions between ions;
       (c) attraction between the nucleus of one atom and the
           electrons of another;
       (d) none of the above.

(3)    All of the following factors increase the strength of van der
       Waal forces between molecules except by an

       (a) increase in the molecular weight of the molecules;
       (b) increase in the number of atoms in the molecule;
       (c) increase in the number of electrons in the molecule;
       (d) increase in the ionic strength of the molecule.

(4)    The weakest (in strength) of the following intermolecular
       forces is:

       (a) hydrogen bonding
       (b) the typical van der Waals
       (c) forces between polar molecules
       (d) ionic

(5)    Hydrogen bonds are possible between all the following elements
       except:

       (a) carbon          (b)  nitrogen
       (c) oxygen          (d)  fluorine

(6)    Hydrophobic bonds

       (a) are interactions between polar molecules;
       (b) do not occur for hydrocarbons;
       (c) are due to an increase in entropy of the system;
       (d) all of the above.

(7)    The strongest of the forces between molecules is:

       (a) van der Waals          (b)  hydrogen bonding
       (c) hydrophobic            (d)  polar

(8)    For the three atoms involved in the hydrogen bond (e.g., $-\ddot{A}$:
       and $H-\ddot{B}-$ ), the angle that allows the greatest strength (using
       H as the vertex) is:

       (a) less than 90°          (b)  90°
       (c) 90° to 180°            (d)  180°

179

(9)    The stability of some polymers may be due to

       (a) many of the weak intermolecular forces (bond);
       (b) a few of the weak intermolecular bonds;
       (c) cannot be due to the weak intermolecular bonds;
       (d) none of the above.


3.4.3        ANSWERS TO QUESTIONS IN SECTION 3.4.2


(1) a   (2) c   (3) d   (4) b   (5) a   (6) c   (7) d
(8) d   (9) a


3.4.4        DISCUSSION OF ANSWERS TO QUESTIONS IN SECTION 3.4.2


All questions adequately discussed in the Section.


3.4.5        VOCABULARY CHECKLIST FOR CONDENSED PHASES


       intermolecular forces
       van der Waals forces
       polar molecules
       hydrogen bonds
       hydrophobic bonds
       ionic forces


3.4.6        CONCEPTS, PRINCIPLES, ETC. CHECKLIST FOR CONDENSED
             PHASES


       weak intermolecular forces
       general idea of ionic forces in crystals
       role of weak forces in stability of molecules
       role of weak forces in phase changes and solubility

**3.5**      **Phase Equilibria**


**3.5.1**      <u>REVIEW OF PHASE EQUILIBRIA</u>


**3.5.1.1**      <u>Review of Phase Equilibria</u>


The <u>three phases</u> are gases, liquids and solids.  Following are the conversions between the three states:

energies:     $\Delta H_f$         $\Delta H_v$
           f=fusion   v=vaporization


<u>As a substance moves from solid to liquid to gas</u>, several changes occur:  (1) the molecules become more disordered, (2) the kinetic energy of the molecules increase, (3) the intermolecular forces become weaker, and (4) the molecules become farther separated (density decreases).

The relative sizes of the heats of phase changes ( $\Delta H_v > \Delta H_f$) imply that the liquid state is more like the solid state than the gaseous state.  When going in the forward direction, heat must be put into the system and the surroundings become cooler (e.g. vaporization of sweat cools the body).  When going in the reverse direction, heat is given off from the system and the surroundings become warmer (e.g., condensation of water vapor from the air warms the body).  <u>Brownian motion</u> (e.g. the random motion of a pollen grain due to collision with the liquid molecules) is evidence for the motion and kinetic energies of liquid molecules.  Molecules have a range of kinetic energies.  The number in a given energy range ( $\Delta E$) is proportional to $e^{-\Delta E/kT}$ (from the Boltzman distribution).  Those molecules above a certain kinetic energy level can escape into the vapor phase (i.e. evaporate).  To evaporate, the molecules must have enough energy to overcome the intermolecular forces (the stronger the attractive forces, the more energy required--see Section 3.4.1 for intermolecular forces).  The molecules that evaporate become gases and exert a pressure called the <u>vapor pressure</u>.  Solids also have a vapor pressure based on a similar argument.  Generally, substances with stronger intermolecular attractive forces have lower vapor pressures.  Substances with weak intermolecular forces tend to have high vapor pressures.  Note:  as the temperature increases, the average kinetic energy per molecule increases, and the liquid (or solid) evaporates faster (Fig. 3.7).

$T_2 > T_1$

$E_k$ = energy level needed for evaporation (molecules to the right of it will evaporate)

Note: as Temperature (T) increases ($T_1 \rightarrow T_2$) more molecules have $E_k$'s high enough to evaporate.

**Fig. 3.7 – Kinetic Energy of Molecules**

The <u>boiling point</u> (BP) of a liquid is the temperature at which the vapor pressure of the liquid equals the atmospheric (opposing) pressure. For the standard BP, this pressure is taken to be one atmosphere. Note, as the atmospheric pressure decreases, the liquid can boil at lower temperatures. Boiling points have great dependence upon intermolecular forces. Remember that nonpolar molecules have weaker forces. Note that symmetric molecules tend to have smaller intermolecular attractive forces also. The <u>freezing point</u> (FP) of the liquid (or melting point, MP, of the solid) is that temperature at which the vapor pressure of the solid equals the vapor pressure of the liquid.

Another way of describing the relationships above is the <u>phase diagram</u> (Fig. 3.8).

(a) Water

(b) Carbon Dioxide

**Fig. 3.8 – Phase Diagrams: Water (a) and Carbon Dioxide (b)**

(1)    this is a plot of <u>pressure (P) versus temperature (T)</u>,
(2)    TP = <u>Triple point</u> which is the value of P and T where solid, liquid and gas all coexist in equilibrium,
(3)    <u>regions</u> marked solid, liquid and gas signify the existence of only that phase,
(4)    the <u>lines</u> represent the coexistence of two phases in equilibrium and the vapor pressures (below)
        AD = solid and liquid in equilibrium, transition is melting (freezing)
        BD = solid and gas in equilibrium, transition from solid to gas is called sublimation (reverse is condensation)
        CD = liquid and gas in equilibrium, transition is vaporization (condensation),
        CD = vapor pressure of the liquid at different temperatures
        BD = vapor pressure of the solid at different temperatures
(5)    Note that all the lines except AD for $H_2O$ have <u>positive slopes</u>. This means that as the pressure is increased on solid $H_2O$ (ice), its melting point decreases and ice can melt at a lower temperature. This is the basis for ice skating.
(6)    <u>The location of the 1 atmosphere of pressure relative to the TP</u> determines if a solid melts at atmospheric pressure or

sublimes.  If 1 atm is above the TP, get solid ⟶ liquid as for water.  If the 1 atm is below the TP get solid ⟶ gas (sublimation) as for $CO_2$.


3.5.1.2    Review of Colligative Properties and Freezing Point Depression


A solute added to a pure liquid changes some properties of that liquid.  The effect of a solute on a pure liquid depends, primarily, on the relative number of particles present and not their identity.  Properties that are affected by the number of particles present and not by the characteristics of the particles are called colligative properties (boiling point elevation, freezing point depression, vapor pressure and osmotic pressure).  See Section 2.5.1.1 for osmosis.  The effect of the number of solute particles (usually non-volatile, so there is no contribution to the overall vapor pressure) on the boiling point (BP) and freezing point (FP) can be understood by considering their effect on vapor pressure (VP) and using the phase diagram.  When a solute is dissolved in a pure liquid, the solute molecules are bound by liquid molecules.  This represents an increase in potential energy which must be overcome by kinetic energy if the molecules are to escape.  This causes fewer to have enough kinetic energy to escape into the vapor phase, resulting in a lowering of the VP (Fig. 3.9).

**Fig. 3.9 - Effect of Solutes on BP and FP**


AB = original VP line of the liquid
CB = original FP line of the solid
A'B' = lowering of the VP of the liquid by added solute
C'B' = lowering the FP of the solid by the solute
ΔBP = BP' - BP = boiling point elevation
FP = original freezing
FP' = new FP caused by solute
ΔFP = FP' - FP = freezing point depression

Equations can be derived by thermodynamics to calculate the effect of a solute on the FP or BP of a liquid.  These are (simplified):

$$\Delta T = +k_b m$$
$$\Delta T = -k_c m$$
ΔT = elevation (for BP) or depression (for FP) of BP or FP respectively
$$m = \text{molality} = \frac{\text{moles of solute particles}}{\text{kilogram of solvent}}$$

Note that the equation calls for moles of solute particles.  This means that if a solute dissociates (e.g. NaCl), the moles of particles are greater than the moles of solute.  If the solute dimerizes, the moles of particles are less.  An alternative way to write the formula to take this into account is:

$$\Delta T = -i \; k_f \; m$$
i = # of particles the solute dissociates into

$$m = \frac{\text{moles of solute}}{\text{kilogram of solvent}}$$

$k_b$ = boiling point elevation constant--depends on the pure liquid being used.
$k_b$ = 0.51 for $H_2O$
$k_f$ = freezing point depression constant depends on the pure liquid being used
$k_f$ = 1.86 for $H_2O$

The above equations can be used for a variety of purposes:

(1)   K's can be calculated,

$$k = \frac{\Delta T}{m}$$

(2)   The number of actual particles can be inferred--make a known m for a liquid with a known k and calculate the expected $\Delta T$.  If $\Delta T$ (by experiment) is greater than that calculated, then more particles than expected were present and the solute must have dissociated.  If $\Delta T$ (by experiment) is less than that calculated, then fewer particles than expected were present, and the solute must have aggregated (e.g. dimerized).  The actual molality of the particles can then be calculated because $\Delta T$ (from experiment) and k are known.

(3)   Most often, the equations are used to estimate molecular weights = MW (given that corrections are made for dissociation or aggregation)

take a liquid with a known k
dissolve x grams of solute (MW unknown)
  in y kg's of the liquid (solvent)
then determine the $\Delta T$ experimentally
the MW is found by going through these calculations

(a)   $m = \frac{\Delta T}{k}$        $\Delta T$, k are known

(b)   $m = \frac{\text{moles of solute}}{\text{kg of solvent}} = \Delta T / k$

(c)   m = (g solute/ MW solute)/Kg of solvent = $\Delta T / k$

(d)   MW solute = (g solute)(k)/(Kg solvent)($\Delta T$)

3.5.2        <u>QUESTIONS TO REVIEW PHASE EQUILIBRIA</u>

(1)   The conversion of a gas to a liquid is called:

(a) melting                    (b)  vaporization
(c) freezing                   (d)  condensation

184

(2)   As a solid changes to a liquid, all of the following occur except

   (a) molecules become more disordered;
   (b) kinetic energy of the molecules decreases;
   (c) intermolecular forces become weaker;
   (d) molecules become farther separated.

(3)   The liquid state is more like the _____ state than the _____ state.

   (a) gas; solid
   (b) solid; gas
   (c) equally similar to both

(4)   Vaporization of a liquid from the skin will cause the skin to become:

   (a) cooler
   (b) warmer
   (c) no change in temperature

(5)   Which of the following liquids will have the highest vapor pressure?

   (a) strong intermolecular forces
   (b) weak intermolecular forces
   (c) intermolecular forces have no effect on vapor pressure

(6)   As the temperature of a substance increases, the average kinetic energy per molecule

   (a) decreases
   (b) increases
   (c) is not affected
   (d) cannot be determined

(7)   As the atmospheric pressure decreases, the boiling point of a liquid

   (a) cannot be determined      (b)  is not affected
   (c) increases                 (d)  decreases

Use the following data for questions #8-#12.

Phase Diagram for a Compound

(8)   Gas is represented by:

   (a) 1     (b) 3     (c) 4     (d) 7

185

(9)     The vapor pressure of the liquid is represented by:

(a)  3     (b)  4     (c)  6     (d)  7

(10)    The triple point is:

(a)  1     (b)  4     (c)  5     (d)  7

(11)    Liquid can exist only in region _____.

(a)  1     (b)  2     (c)  3     (d)  5

(12)    At atmospheric pressure the solid phase of this substance will
only:

(a)  remain a solid             (b)   melt
(c)  freeze                     (d)   vaporize

(13)    Colligative properties depend upon

(a) the chemical properties of the solute;
(b) the physical properties of the solute;
(c) the chemical properties of the solvent;
(d) the number of solute particles present in solution.

(14)    Examples of colligative properties include all except:

(a) boiling point elevation     (b)   solubility
(c) vapor pressure              (d)   osmotic pressure

(15)    The effect of a solute on the vapor pressure of a liquid is to:

(a) have no effect              (b)   increase it
(c) decrease it                 (d)   cannot be determined

(16)    The equation relating the freezing point depression ($\Delta T$) with
the freezing point constant ($k_f$) and the molality (m) of the
solution is (excluding the minus sign and i):

(a) $\Delta T = k_f/m$          (b)   $\Delta T = m/k_f$
(c) $\Delta T = 1/k_f m$        (d)   $\Delta T = k_f m$

Use the following for Questions #17 to #19:

Five grams of a compound with a molecular weight of 80 is placed in
500g of a liquid which has a normal freezing point of 58.5°C.  The
freezing point of the solution is now 57°C.  Next, 2g of an unknown
compound is placed in 250g of the same liquid, and the freezing point
is now 58°C.

(17)    What is the freezing point depression constant ($k_f$) of the
liquid?

(a)  12    (b)  6     (c)  3     (d)  1.5

(18)    What is the expected molecular weight of the unknown compound
by freezing point analysis?

(a)  192   (b)  96    (c)  48    (d)  cannot be determined

186

(19) A mass spectograph analysis shows the true molecular weight of the compound to be 384. What inference can be made about the compound's behavior in the liquid?

(a) it dissociates      (b) it forms dimers
(c) it forms tetramers    (d) no inference can be made

## 3.5.3    ANSWERS TO QUESTIONS IN SECTION 3.5.2

(1 ) d   (2) b   (3) b   (4) a   (5) b   (6) b   (7) d
(8 ) b   (9) d  (10) c  (11) b  (12) d  (13) d  (14) b
(15) c  (16) d  (17) a  (18) a  (19) a

## 3.5.4    DISCUSSION OF ANSWERS TO QUESTIONS IN SECTION 3.5.2

QUESTIONS #1-#16: Adequately discussed in Section.

QUESTION #17   (Answer: a)   Use the formula:

$$k = \Delta T / m$$

Note: the complete formula is:

$$k = \Delta T / -im$$

where i = the number of particles the substance dissociates into and the negative in the denominator offsets the negative temperature drop. If the absolute value of $\Delta T$ is taken the minus sign may be ignored, and if the molecule does not dissociate the i = 1 and may be ignored).

Then,

m = moles/Kg of solvent = (1/16)/(1/2) = (1/16)(2/1)
$$= 2/16 = 1/8$$
(moles = weight/molecular weight = 5/80 = 1/16, and
   Kgs = grams of substance/1000 grams = 500/1000 = 1/2 ).

And,

$$\Delta T = 58.5^oC - 57^oC = 1.5^oC = 1\tfrac{1}{2} = 3/2$$
(Note, if the formula,
   $k = \Delta T/-im$
is used, the $\Delta T$ must be determined as follows,
   $\Delta T = T_f - T_i = 57 - 58.5 = -1.5^oC$
     f = final, i = initial).

Finally,

$$k = (3/2)/(1/8) = (3/2)(8/1) = 24/2 = 12$$

QUESTION #18 (Answer: a) Use the results from #17 and the procedure outlined in the Section:

(a)  $m = \triangle T/k = \frac{1}{2}/12 = \frac{1}{2} \cdot 1/12 = 1/24$
     $\triangle T = 58.5 - 58 = 0.5 = \frac{1}{2}$

(b)  moles of solute = $(m)(y) = (1/24)(\frac{1}{4}) = 1/96$
     y = Kg's of solute = 250/1000 = $\frac{1}{4}$

(c)  $MW = x/$moles of solute $= 2/(1/96) = (2)(96/1) = 192$
     x = weight of solute = 2g

QUESTION #19 (Answer: a) The expected freezing point depression using the molecular weight given is

$$\Delta T = km = (12)(1/48) = 12/48 = 1/4 = 0.25^{\circ}C$$
$$m = moles/kg's \ solvents = (2/384)/(1/4) = (2/384)(4/1)$$
$$= (2)(4)/384 = 1/48$$

So, the expected $\Delta T$ is 0.25$^{\circ}$C. Since the actual is 0.5$^{\circ}$C, this means there must have been more particles present than expected, and that the compound must have dissociated, or,

$$i = \Delta T/-km = -(1/2)/-(12)(1/48) = (1/2)(48/12) = 48/24 = 2.$$

This means 2 particles per original molecule.

3.5.5        VOCABULARY CHECKLIST FOR PHASE EQUILIBRIA

____ vaporization              ____ sublimation
____ condensation              ____ colligative properties
____ heat of fusion            ____ molality
____ heat of vaporization      ____ boiling point elevation
____ Brownian motion           ____ freezing point depression
____ vapor pressure            ____ freezing point
____ boiling point             ____ phase diagram

3.5.6        CONCEPTS, PRINCIPLES, ETC. CHECKLIST FOR PHASE EQUILIBRIA

____ changes that occur during phase changes
____ interpretation of phase diagrams
____ triple point
____ colligative properties
____ freezing point depression determinations

188

**3.6**        **Chemical Compounds**

**3.6.1**        <u>REVIEW OF CHEMICAL COMPOUNDS</u>

Compounds are made of discrete individual atoms (which, however, can be divided into neutrons, protons and electrons).  These atoms then combine in specific ratios with each other, depending upon their chemical characteristics, to form compounds.  The elements (a set of atoms with the same atomic number) have a constant weight, and these weights are maintained when combined into chemical compounds (a combination of two or more elements).

A <u>mole</u> of any substance contains $6.023 \times 10^{23}$ particles <u>(Avogadro's Number)</u>.  A mole of an element contains this many atoms.  A mole of a compound contains this many molecules.  For an element, the number of moles present is,

$$\text{moles} = \frac{\text{weight of sample in grams}}{\text{atomic weight of element in grams (GAW)}}$$

$$\text{GAW} = \text{gram-atomic weight.}$$

(See Section 5.13.1 for atomic weight determination.)

For a compound, the <u>gram-molecular weight</u> (GMW) is found by adding the GAWs of all the elements that make it up (need the molecular formula).  Then, the moles of a compound is found as follows:

$$\text{moles} = \frac{\text{weight of sample in grams}}{\text{GMW}}$$

Moles can be calculated in many other ways (see below) and all of these are interconvertible via moles.  <u>Mole is important</u> because it gives the number of molecules (or atoms) in a given weight of a substance, whereas the weight itself does not.  Mole is the key to solving most quantitive mass problems in chemistry.  In general, think about how to get the number of moles, and, usually the rest of the problem will be easier to complete.

Often, the number of molecules or atoms in a given weight of a sample is not sufficient.  This is because different substances have different combining powers with each other.  That is, one molecule may be two or more times more potent than another for a specific purpose.  A familiar example should be $H_2SO_4$ (a diprotic acid) and HCl (a monoprotic acid) in terms of donation of hydrogen ions ($H^+$).  A mole would contain the same number of molecules of $H_2SO_4$ and HCl, but this does not give us their relative potency in giving $H^+$.  What is needed is a measure, like mole, which would give us the relative or equivalent effectiveness of given weights of substances for specific characteristics.  For this reason, the measure called <u>equivalents</u> was established.  When weights are converted to equivalents, one can be sure, for example, that one equivalent of an acid will react completely and equally with one equivalent of a base.  It cannot be stated, without additional information,  that one mole of an acid will react exactly with one mole of a base for the reasons above.  Note that in one equivalent of a substance there are $6.023 \times 10^{23}$ particles of interest (e.g. $H^+$ or $OH^-$ for acids and bases).  The formula for calculating equivalents is:

$$\text{equivalents} = \frac{\text{weight of sample in grams}}{\text{gram equivalent weight (GEW)}}$$

The GEW is calculated as follows:

$$\text{GEW} = \frac{\text{gram molecular weight}}{n}$$

The value of n depends on the situation. For acids, it is the number of hydrogens used in the reaction per molecule. For bases, it is the number of exchangeable $OH^-$s used in the reaction per molecule. For oxidation-reduction reactions, it depends on the number of electrons transferred by a given compound in a given reaction. For examples and further explanation of n, refer to 3.10.1, 3.11.1 and 3.12.1.

The percentage composition of compounds is the percent of the total weight of a given element in that compound:

$$\% \text{ composition of element A} = \frac{\text{total weight in grams of A}}{\text{GMW of the compound}} \times 100.$$

An example is: % of oxygen(O) in $KClO_3$ (K=39, Cl=36, O=16)

$$\% \text{ of O} = \frac{(3)(16)}{39 + 36 + 3(16)} \times 100 = 39\%.$$

Of course, the percentages of all components should sum to 100%. An empirical formula is the formula with the smallest ratio of atoms to each other. The molecular formula is the actual formula of the molecule of the substance. For example, for benzene:

structural formula

molecular formula = $C_6H_6$
empirical formula = $C_1H_1$.

Of course, it is possible for the empirical formula to be the same as the molecular formula. It is possible to determine empirical formulas if the percentage composition of the compound is known. This is done as follows:

(1)  Assume the percent of each element is the grams of each element (i.e., assume you are given 100 grams = 100% of the compound);

(2)  Divide the percentage composition of each element by its atomic weight to give the moles of each in the compound;

(3)  Divide each of these numbers by the smallest of the numbers gotten from step #2;

(4)  Determine what small number (to multiply the result of #3), usually 2-5, if any, is needed to convert the numbers from #3 into (approximately) whole numbers. These whole numbers are the ratio of the elements to each other.

What has been done is to convert weights (from percent) into moles by step #2. These moles are, themselves, the ratios of elements to each other. Steps #3 and #4 are just manipulations to get whole numbers because elements are made of atoms and not fractions of atoms. To determine the molecular formula from the empirical formula, the gram-molecular weight (GMW) must be known from some other source (can find GMW if weight of compound and number of moles is known--see below). Then determine the gram-empirical formula weight (i.e., add up the elements in the empirical formula) and then divide the GMW by the gram-empirical formula weight. The resulting number is how many times each element in the empirical formula is to be multiplied to get the molecular formula. An example is:

A compound of 2.04% H, 32.65% S, and 65.31% O has a GMW = 98 (from other experiments).
What is the empirical formula and molecular formula?

(H = 1, S = 32, O = 16)

By the steps above:

(1)   H = 2.04g      S = 32.5g      O = 65.31g

(2)   H:   2.04/1 = 2.04

      S:   32.65/32 = 1.02

      O:   65.31/16 = 4.08

(3)   H:   2.04/1.02 = 2

      S:   1.02/1.02 = 1

      O:   4.08/1.02 = 4


(4)   Not needed because already have whole numbers. Therefore, empirical formula is $H_2SO_4$.

      Then, gram-empirical formula weight is:

$$2(1) + (32) + 4(16) = 98.$$

      Then, divide gram-molecular weight by the gram-empirical formula weight:
$$98/98 = 1$$

      Then multiply each element in the empirical formula by the 1 to get the molecular formula which is the same as the empirical formula in this case.

Various means of determining the mole of substances are discussed in other Sections. The methods are:

(1) mole = weight in grams/GMW;

(2) MV = mole; M = molarity, V = liters (Section 3.10.1);
(3) NV = equivalents; N = normality, V = liters (Section 3.10.1);
(4) mV = mole; m = molality, V = kg's of solvent (Section 3.10.1);
(5) freezing point depression (or boiling point elevation) calculations (Section 3.5.1.2)
      T = km
first determine m, then use m to determine mole as in #4 above;
(6) one mole of any gas at STP occupies 22.4 liters (Section 3.3.1);

(7) at the same temperature and pressure, equal volumes of
    ideal gases contain equal numbers of moles (Avogadro's
    Principle) (Section 3.3.1);

(8) $PV = nRT$     (Section 3.3.1)
    Ideal Gas Equation;

(9) $P_1 = X_1 P_T$     (Section 3.3.1)
    $P_1$ = partial pressure of gas #1
    $P_T$ = total pressure
    $X_1$ = mole fraction of gas #1;

(10) one mole of electrons is one Faraday, a Faraday is 96,500
     Coulombs; an ampere (measure of current) is 1 Coulomb/sec
     (Section 3.12.1);

(11) Law of Dulong and Petit:
     $6.3 = (SH)(GAW)$
     SH = specific heat in cals/gram
     GAW = gram-atomic weight of element.

Note that from the moles, the gram-molecular weight can be
calculated, and that moles provide a means of conversion between the
diverse situations above.

### 3.6.2     QUESTIONS TO REVIEW CHEMICAL COMPOUNDS

(1)   A chemical compound

      (a)   is made of discrete individual atoms;
      (b)   is made of atoms (of different elements) combined with
            each other in specific ratios;
      (c)   has the weight equal to sum of the weights of the elements
            that make it up;
      (d)   all of the above.

(2)   Avogadro's number:

      (a) the number of liters that make up one mole of gas
      (b) there are $6.023 \times 10^{23}$ particles per mole
      (c) the number of molecules in a chemical compound
      (d) none of the above

(3)   Given that mole = m and the weight = w of a compound with a
      gram-molecular weight = GMW, which is the correct relationship
      between these?

      (a) $m = (w)(GMW)$              (b) $m = w/GMW$
      (c) $m = GMW/w$                 (d) $m = 1/(w)(GMW)$

(4)   Equivalents

      (a) are the same as the mole of a substance;

      (b) contain $\dfrac{6.023 \times 10^{23}}{n}$ particles, n = number of atoms under
          concern;

      (c) depend on the specific number of groups of interest, e.g.,
          $H^+$ or electrons transferred, by a molecule;

      (d) none of the above.

(5)     If equivalents = E, weight of sample = W and the gram
        equivalent weight = GEW, the correct relation between these is

        (a) E = 1/(W)(GEW)                    (b) E = GEW/W
        (c) E = W/GEW                         (d) E = (W)(GEW)

(6)     If gram-molecular weight = GMW, gram equivalent weight = GEW
        and the number of groups of interest per molecule = n, the
        correct relationship between these is:

        (a) GEW = (n)(GMW)                    (b) GEW = 1/(n)(GMW)
        (c) GEW = n/GMW                       (d) GEW = GMW/n

(7)     If the percent composition of element B in a compound = P, the
        number of atoms of element B in the compound = $n_1$, the gram
        atomic weight of element B = GAW, and the gram molecular weight
        of the compund = GMW,   then the correct relationship between
        these is:

        (a) P = (n)(GAW)/GMW  x 100          (b) P = (n)(GAW)/GMW
        (c) P = (n)(GAW)(GMW)                (d) P = GMW/(n)(GAW) x 100

(8)     All of the following formulas give moles except:

        (a) (normality) (volume) = moles

        (b) (molality) (kilograms of solvent) = moles

        (c) liters of gas at STP/22.4 = moles

        (d) (Pressure)(Volume)/(Ideal gas constant)(Temperature) = moles

(9)     Moles may be calculated from all of the following types of data
        except:

        (a) freezing point depressions
        (b) partial pressures
        (c) electrochemistry (Faradays of charge consumed)
        (d) all of the above can give moles

The following information is provided for the remainder of the
questions.  Atomic weights: H = 1, C = 12, N = 14, O = 16, F = 19,
Na = 23, Al = 27, P = 31, S = 32, Cl = 35, K = 39, Ca = 40, Cr = 52,
Fe = 56, Cu = 63, Br = 80, Ag = 108, and Pb = 207.

(10)    What is the gram-molecular weight of $NH_4Cl$?

        (a) 53      (b) 50      (c) 49      (d) none of the above

(11)    What is the gram-molecular weight of $C_6H_{12}O_6$?

        (a) 180     (b) 130     (c) 29      (d) none of the above

(12)    How many moles are 34g of $AgNO_3$?

        (a) 0.20    (b) 0.30    (c) 0.40    (d) none of the above

(13)    How many grams are there in 0.5 mole of NaOH?

        (a) 5g      (b) 20g     (c) 30g     (d) none of the above

193

(14) It is known that 5g of a compound is 0.1 mole of that substance. What is its gram-molecular weight (GMW)?

(a) 25     (b) 100     (c) 150     (d) none of the above

(15) The gram-equivalent weight (GEW) of $HNO_3$ when it acts as an acid (donation of $H^+$) is:

(a) 21     (b) 63     (c) 126     (d) none of the above

(16) The gram-equivalent weight of $H_3PO_4$ when it acts as an acid (donation of $H^+$) is approximately:

(a) 33     (b) 49     (c) 98     (d) all of the above

(17) In a reaction where $HNO_3$ is used, the nitrogen of the $HNO_3$ gains 5 electrons. The equivalent weight of $HNO_3$ in terms of its ability to exchange electrons is approximately:

(a) 3     (b) 13     (c) 63     (d) none of the above

(18) In a reaction where $KNO_3$ is used, the nitrogen gains 2 electrons. The equivalent weight of $KNO_3$ in terms of its ability to gain electrons is approximately:

(a) 21     (b) 32     (c) 63     (d) none of the above

(19) In a reaction, the Cr of $K_2Cr_2O_7$ gains 6 electrons. The equivalent weight of $K_2Cr_2O_7$ in this reaction in terms of its ability to exchange electrons is approximately:

(a) 147     (b) 49     (c) 25     (d) none of the above

(20) How many equivalents of base ($OH^-$) are there in 5g of $Al(OH)_3$ if all OHs react?

(a) 0.10     (b) 0.20     (c) 0.75     (d) none of the above

(21) Two equivalents of $H^+$ would require what weight of $H_2SO_4$?

(a) 196     (b) 98     (c) 49     (d) none of the above

(22) Approximately what percentage of $CuSO_4$ is sulfur?

(a) 20     (b) 30     (c) 40     (d) none of the above

(23) The approximate percentage of H in $(NH_4)_2SO_4$ is:

(a) 6     (b) 7     (c) 4     (d) none of the above

(24) What is the empirical formula of the following compound?

(a) $C_3H_6$     (b) $C_2H_2$     (c) $C_1H_2$     (d) none of these

194

(25) A compound contains 39.8% Cu, 20.1% S and 40.1% O.  Its empirical formula is:

(a) $CuSO_2$   (b)  $Cu_2SO_3$  (c)  $CuSO_4$   (d)  none of these

(26) A compound contains 39.9% C, 6.7% H and 53.4% O.  The empirical formula is:

(a) $CH_2O$   (b)  $C_2H_2O$  (c)  CHO    (d)  none of the above

(27) A compound contains 2.6 gms of N, 0.8 gms of H, and 6.6 gms of Cl.  The empirical formula is

(a)  $N_2H_2Cl$                     (b)  $N(HCl)_2$
(c)  $NH_4Cl$                       (d)  none of the above

(28) A compound of carbon and hydrogen contains 92.3% C.  The molecular weight (from other experiments) is known to be 52.  What is the molecular formula?

(a)  $C_2H_2$                       (b)  $C_4H_4$
(c)  $C_3H_6$                       (d)  none of these

(29) The specific heat of an element is 0.03, its gram atomic weight is:

(a)  18.9                         (b)  210
(c)  189                          (d)  need more
                                       information

3.6.3        ANSWERS TO QUESTIONS IN SECTION 3.6.2

( 1)  d   (2)  b   (3)  b   (4)  c   (5)  c   (6)  d   (7)  a
( 8)  a   (9)  d   (10)  a  (11)  a  (12)  a  (13)  b  (14)  d
(15)  b   (16)  d  (17)  b  (18)  d  (19)  c  (20)  b  (21)  b
(22)  a   (23)  a  (24)  c  (25)  c  (26)  a  (27)  c  (28)  b
(29)  b

3.6.4        DISCUSSION OF ANSWERS TO QUESTIONS IN SECTION 3.6.2

QUESTIONS #1-#9:  Adequately discussed in this Section.

QUESTION #10   (Answer:  a)   GMW = N + 4 (H) + Cl = 14 + 4(1) + 35 = 53

QUESTION #11   (Answer:  a)   GMW = 6C + 12H + 60 = 6(12) + 12(1) + 6(16)
                              = 72 + 12 + 96 = 180

QUESTION #12   (Answer:  a)   Moles = $\frac{weight}{GMW}$ = 34/169 = 0.20

                              GMW = Ag + N + 3(O) = 107 + 14 + 3(16)
                                  = 121 + 48 = 169

QUESTION #13   (Answer:  b)   weight =(moles)(GMW) = (0.5)(40) = 20 g
                              GMW = Na + O + H = 23 + 16 + 1 = 40

QUESTION #14   (Answer:  d)   GMW = weight/moles = 5/0.1 = 50.

QUESTION #15 (Answer: b) GEW = GMW/n = 63/1 = 63
GMW = H + N + 3(O) = 1 + 14 + 3(16)
= 15 + 48 = 63
n = # of exchangeable H's per molecule = 1

QUESTION #16 (Answer: d) $H_3PO_4$ can give 1, 2, or 3 protons in a reaction; therefore the reaction must be specified. $3 \times 1 + 31 + 4 \times 16 = 98$ = GMW. Then, 98/1 = 98, 98/2 = 49, $98/3 \approx 33$.

QUESTION #17 (Answer: b) $GEW = \frac{GMW}{n} = 63/5 \approx 13$
GMW = H + N + 3(O) = 1 + 14 + 3(16)
= 15 + 48 = 63
n = # of exchangeable electrons per molecule = 5

QUESTION #18 (Answer: d) $GEW = \frac{GMW}{n} = 101/2 \approx 50.$
GMW = K + N + 3(O) = 39 + 14 + 3(16)
= 53 + 48 = 101
n = # of exchangeable electrons per molecule = 2

QUESTION #19 (Answer: c) $GEW = \frac{GMW}{n} = 294/12 \approx 25$
GMW = 2(K) + 2(Cr) + 7(O) = 2(39) + 2(52) + 7(16)
= 78 + 104 + 112 = 294
n = # of exchangeable electrons per molecule
= (2)(6) = 12 because there are two Cr's per molecule

QUESTION #20 (Answer: b) $Equivalents = \frac{weight}{GEW} \approx 5/26 \approx 0.20$
$GEW = \frac{GMW}{n} = 78/3 \approx 26$
GMW = Al + 3(O) + 3(H) = 27 + 3(16) + 3(1)
= 27 + 48 + 3 = 78
n = # of exchangeable OH's per molecule = 3

QUESTION #21 (Answer: b) Weight = (GEW)(Equivalents) = (49)(2) = 98
GEW = GMW/n = 98/2 = 49
GMW = 2(H) + S + 4(O) = 2(1) + 32 + 4(16)
= 2 + 32 + 64 = 98
n = # of exchangeable H's per molecule = 2

QUESTION #22 (Answer: a) % S =(weight of S/GMW)(100) =(32/159)(100) $\approx$ 20
weight of S = (1)(S) = (1) (32) = 32
GMW = Cu +S + 4(O) = 63 + 32 + 4(16) = 95 + 64 = 159

QUESTION #23 (Answer: a) % H = (weight of H/GMW)(100) = (8/132)(100) $\approx$ 6
weight of H = 8(H) = 8(1) = 8
GMW = 2(N) + 8(H) + S + 4(O) = 2(14) + 8(1) + 32 + 4(16)
= 28 + 8 + 32 + 64 = 132

QUESTION #24 (Answer: c) The molecular formula is $C_3H_6$ (by counting all the atoms). The smallest ratio of this is $C_1H_2$.

QUESTION #25 (Answer: c) By the steps enumerated in the section,
(1) Cu 39.8 g    S = 20.1g    O = 40.1g
(2) moles Cu = 39.8/63 = 0.63
moles  S = 20.1/32 = 0.63
moles  O = 40.1/16 = 2.51
this gives $Cu_{0.63}$ $S_{0.63}$ $O_{2.51}$
(3) dividing each number by 0.63:
$Cu_{\frac{0.63}{0.63}}$    $S_{\frac{0.63}{0.63}}$    $O_{\frac{2.51}{0.63}} = Cu_1S_1O_{3.98}$
(4) not needed since $3.98 \approx 4$, and this yields $CuSO_4$

196

QUESTION # 26   (Answer:  a)   Follow the same steps as in #25,

(1) $C = 39.9g$     $H = 6.7g$     $O = 53.4g$

(2) moles C = 39.9/12 = 3.33
    moles H = 6.7/1 = 6.7
    moles O = 53.4/16 = 3.34
    this gives $C_{3.33}$     $H_{6.7}$     $O_{3.34}$

(3) dividing each number by 3.33:

$$\frac{C_{3.33}}{3.33} \qquad \frac{H_{6.7}}{3.33} \qquad \frac{O_{3.34}}{3.33} = C_1H_2O_1 \equiv CH_2O$$

(4) not needed


QUESTION #27   (Answer:  c)

(1)  just use the grams as given

   $N = 2.6g$     $H = 0.8g$     $Cl = 6.6g$

(2)  moles N = 2.6/14 = 0.19   ($\approx 0.20!$)
     moles H = 0.8/1 = 0.80
     moles Cl= 6.6/35 = 0.19 ($\approx 0.20!$)
     $N_{0.2}$        $H_{0.8}$        $Cl_{0.2}$

(3)  Divide all by 0.2
     $$\frac{N_{0.2}}{0.2} \qquad \frac{H_{0.8}}{0.2} \qquad \frac{Cl_{0.2}}{0.2} = N_1H_4Cl_1 = NH_4Cl$$

(4)  not needed


QUESTION #28   (Answer:  b)   The correct answer can be obtained just
by determining the molecular weights of the options.  The procedure
outlined in the Section is first to determine the empirical formula
and then the molecular formula from it:

(1)  $C = 92.3g$     $H = 100 - 92.3 = 7.7g$
(2)  moles C = 92.3/12 = 7.7
     moles H = 7.7/1 = 7.7
          $C_{7.7}$   $H_{7.7}$

(3)  Divide both by 7.7
     $$\frac{C_{7.7}}{7.7} \qquad \frac{H_{7.7}}{7.7} = C_1H_1 = CH$$

(4)  not needed

The gram-empirical formula weight is C + H = 12 + 1 = 13.  This goes
into the gram-molecular weight 52/13 = 4 times.  This means the
ratios of elements in the empirical formula must be multiplied by 4
and this gives

$$C_4H_4.$$

QUESTION #29   (Answer:  b)  This is a direct application of the Law
of Dulong and Petit (see Section)

   $6.3 = (SH)(GAW)$
   $$GAW = 6.3/SH = \frac{6.3}{0.03} = 210$$

_____  mole                          _____  gram atomic weight
_____  Avogadro's Number             _____  gram-equivalent weight
_____  equivalent                    _____  percent composition
_____  gram-molecular weight


3.6.6       CONCEPTS,   PRINCIPLES,   ETC.   CHECKLIST   FOR   CHEMICAL
            COMPOUNDS


_____  mole concept and calculations using moles
_____  concept of equivalents and calculations using equivalents
_____  empirical versus molecular formulas
_____  alternative methods of determining mole


3.7         **Mass Changes in Chemical Reactions - Stoichiometry**


3.7.1       REVIEW OF STOICHIOMETRY


Stoichiometry refers to the use of atomic theory to make
quantitative assessments of atoms, compounds and chemical reactions.

Chemical equations should be balanced prior to doing stoichiometric
calculations.  Balancing is by trial and error (for non-redox), and
the check is to see if there are equal numbers of each element on
each side of the equation.  A hint to aid in balancing equations is:

> balance the element(s) which appear in only one compound on
> each side of the equation, save elements which appear in more
> than one compound until last.

Practice is the key to balancing equations.  An example of a balanced
equation is:

$$N_2(g) + 3H_2(g) \longrightarrow 2NH_3(g).$$

The numbers in front of the molecules give the smallest ratios of
these molecules that will react with each other.  That is, they are
the number of moles of each that must be present to get a complete
reaction.  If there is too much (or too little) of a reactant
present, then that reactant is in excess (or is deficient), and the
reaction when finished will have some reactants left over.  The
amount and which reactant left over is calculated from the balanced
equation using the ratio of moles.  Note again that moles are the
intermediary between weights, volumes, etc. and that the numbers in
the equations reflect ratios of moles and nothing else.  Other points
will be stressed in the questions.  See Section 3.12.1 for oxidation-
reduction and disproportionation reactions.

(1)    Given the following equation, the coefficient in front of $KClO_3$ is (balance the equation):

$$KClO_3 \longrightarrow KCl + KClO_4$$

(a) 1      (b) 2      (c) 3      (d) 4

(2)    The coefficient in front of Zn in the following equation, when balanced, is:

$$Zn + HCl \longrightarrow ZnCl_2 + H_2$$

(a) 1      (b) 2      (c) 3      (d) 4

(3)    Which of the following species has the largest coefficient in the balanced equation?

$$C_{12}H_{22}O_{11} + O_2 \longrightarrow CO_2 + H_2O$$

(a) $O_2$      (b) $CO_2$      (c) $H_2O$      (d) $O_2$ and $CO_2$

(4)    What is the coefficient in front of $Ca(OH)_2$ in the following equation when balanced?

$$(NH_4)_2SO_4 + Ca(OH)_2 \longrightarrow NH_3 + H_2O + CaSO_4$$

(a) 1      (b) 2      (c) 3      (d) 4

(5)    What is the sum of coefficients in the following equation when balanced?

$$CuO + H_3PO_4 \longrightarrow Cu_3(PO_4)_2 + H_2O$$

(a) 6      (b) 7      (c) 8      (d) 9

(6)    What is the sum of coefficients in the following equation when balanced?

$$Na_2O_2 + H_2O \longrightarrow NaOH + O_2$$

(a) 5      (b) 7      (c) 9      (d) 11


Use the following unbalanced equation for questions #7 through #10.

$$N_2H_4(\ell) + N_2O_4(\ell) \longrightarrow N_2(g) + H_2O(\ell)$$

$$(H = 1, N = 14, O = 16)$$

(7)    The sum of coefficients in the balanced equation is:

(a) 4      (b) 6      (c) 8      (d) 10

(8)    How many moles of $N_2$ will be produced if 3 moles of $N_2H_4$ is used up in the reaction?

(a) 2      (b) 3      (c) 4½      (d) 9

(9) There are 8 gms of $N_2H_4$ and 92 gms of $N_2O_4$ available. What weight of water in grams can be made from this?

    (a) $4\frac{1}{2}$     (b) 9     (c) 18     (d) 36

(10) If 36g of $H_2O$ is produced in the above reaction, what volume of nitrogen is also produced assuming the reaction is at STP?

    (a) 1.5 liters                        (b) 10 liters
    (c) 33.6 liters                     (d) 44.8 liters

Use the following information for questions #11 through #14.

$$FeS(s) + O_2(g) + H_2O(\ell) \longrightarrow Fe_2O_3(s) + H_2SO_4(\ell)$$

$$(H=1, O=16, S=32, Fe=56)$$

(11) The sum of the coefficients in the balanced equation is:

    (a) 8     (b) 13     (c) 18     (d) 23

(12) If 22.4 liters of $O_2$ are allowed to react with 44g of FeS, approximately what weight of $H_2SO_4$ is produced (assume reaction run at STP)?

    (a) 98g     (b) 49g     (c) 44g     (d) 2g

(13) If 5 moles of FeS are used in the reaction, what is the maximum number of moles of $Fe_2O_3$ that can be produced?

    (a) 1.0     (b) 2.5     (c) 5.0     (d) 7.5

(14) If 98g of $H_2SO_4$ are desired, what volume of $O_2$ must be used in the reaction (assume STP)?

    (a) 50.4 liters                     (b) 22.4 liters
    (c) 11.2 liters                    (d) 1 liter

3.7.3       ANSWERS TO QUESTIONS IN SECTION 3.7.2

( 1) d   (2) a   (3) d   (4) a   (5) d   (6) c   (7) d
( 8) c   (9) b   (10) c   (11) d   (12) c   (13) b   (14) a

3.7.4       DISCUSSION OF ANSWERS TO QUESTIONS IN SECTION 3.7.2

QUESTION #1 (Answer: d) The O's appear in only one compound on each side of the equation, so balance it first. In this type of situation, simply multiply each compound by the number of atoms of the element (i.e., O in this case) in the other compound:

        unbalanced: $KClO_3 \longrightarrow KCl + KClO_4$
        balanced O: $4KClO_3 \longrightarrow KCl + 3KClO_4$

There is no apparent clear choice between K or Cl so just pick one to balance. Luckily both K and Cl are already balanced. Check by counting total number of each element on each side of the equation:

check: $4KClO_3 \longrightarrow KCl + 3KClO_4$

| | | |
|---|---|---|
| K: | 4 | 4 |
| Cl: | 4 | 4 |
| O: | 12 | 12 |

QUESTION #2 (Answer: a) Can select Zn, H or Cl because all appear in only one compound on each side. In this case, select the one that appears most complicated which is H or Cl in this case:

unbalanced: $Zn + HCl \longrightarrow ZnCl_2 + H_2$
balanced H: $Zn + 2HCl \longrightarrow ZnCl_2 + H_2$
Zn and Cl: both are balanced also

check: $Zn + 2HCl \longrightarrow ZnCl_2 + H_2$

| | | |
|---|---|---|
| Zn: | 1 | 1 |
| Cl: | 2 | 2 |
| H: | 2 | 2 |

QUESTION #3 (Answer: d)

unbalanced: $C_{12}H_{22}O_{11} + O_2 \longrightarrow CO_2 + H_2O$
balance C: $C_{12}H_{22}O_{11} + O_2 \longrightarrow 12CO_2 + H_2O$
balance H: $C_{12}H_{22}O_{11} + O_2 \longrightarrow 12CO_2 + 11H_2O$
balance O: $C_{12}H_{22}O_{11} + 12O_2 \longrightarrow 12CO_2 + 11H_2O$

check: $C_{12}H_{22}O_{11} + 12O_2 \longrightarrow 12CO_2 + 11H_2O$

| | | |
|---|---|---|
| C: | 12 | 12 |
| H: | 22 | 22 |
| O: | 11+24=35 | 24+11=35. |

QUESTION #4 (Answer: a)

unbalanced: $(NH_4)_2SO_4 + Ca(OH)_2 \longrightarrow NH_3 + H_2O + CaSO_4$
Note: Treat $SO_4^{-2}$ as a group in this case.
$SO_4^{-2}$ and Ca are already balanced
balance N: $(NH_4)_2SO_4 + Ca(OH)_2 \longrightarrow 2NH_3 + H_2O + CaSO_4$
balance O: $(NH_4)_2SO_4 + Ca(OH)_2 \longrightarrow 2NH_3 + 2H_2O + CaSO_4$
(note that the O's in the $SO_4^{-2}$s balance themselves and do not have to be accounted for in this balancing of the O's)
balance H: already balanced.

check: $(NH_4)_2SO_4 + Ca(OH)_2 \longrightarrow 2NH_3 + 2 H_2O + CaSO_4$

| | | |
|---|---|---|
| N: | 2 | 2 |
| H: | 8+2=10 | 6+4=10 |
| S: | 1 | 1 |
| O: | 4+2=6 | 2+4=6. |

QUESTION #5 (Answer: d)

unbalanced: $CuO + H_3PO_4 \longrightarrow Cu_3(PO_4)_2 + 2H_2O$
Note: the $PO_4^{-3}$ can be treated as a group since it is not changed in the reaction.
can select Cu, $PO_4^{-3}$ or H to balance first, the H's appear the most complicated so do them first.
balance H: $CuO + 2H_3PO_4 \longrightarrow Cu_3(PO_4)_2 + 3 H_2O$
balance $PO_4$: already balanced
balance Cu's: $3CuO + 2H_3PO_4 \longrightarrow Cu_3(PO_4)_2 + 3 H_2O$
balance O: already balanced (note again that the O's on the $PO_4^{-3}$'s were balanced by balancing the $PO_4^{-3}$'s)

check:
$$3CuO + 2H_3PO_4 \longrightarrow Cu_3(PO_4)_2 + 3H_2O$$

| | | |
|---|---|---|
| Cu: | 3 | 3 |
| O: | 3+8=11 | 8+3=11 |
| H: | 6 | 6 |
| P: | 2 | 2 |

QUESTION #6   (Answer:  c)

unbalanced:  $Na_2O_2 + H_2O \longrightarrow NaOH + O_2$
balance Na:  $Na_2O_2 + H_2O \longrightarrow 2NaOH + O_2$
balance H:   already balanced
balance O:   $Na_2O_2 + H_2O \longrightarrow 2NaOH + \frac{1}{2}O_2$
remove fractions by multiplying through by 2:

check:
$$2Na_2O_2 + 2H_2O \longrightarrow 4NaOH + O_2$$

| | | |
|---|---|---|
| Na: | 4 | 4 |
| O: | 4+2=6 | 4+2=6 |
| H: | 4 | 4 |

QUESTION #7   (Answer:  d)

unbalanced:  $N_2H_4 + N_2O_4 \longrightarrow N_2 + H_2O$
balance O:   $N_2H_4 + N_2O_4 \longrightarrow N_2 + 4H_2O$
balance H:   $2N_2H_4 + N_2O_4 \longrightarrow N_2 + 4H_2O$
balance N:   $2N_2H_4 + N_2O_4 \longrightarrow 3N_2 + 4H_2O$

check:
$$2N_2H_4 + N_2O_4 \longrightarrow 3N_2 + 4H_2O$$

| | | |
|---|---|---|
| N: | 4+2=6 | 6 |
| H: | 8 | 8 |
| O: | 4 | 4 |

QUESTION #8   (Answer:  c)  These types of problems are solved by using the known ratios of the moles of the compounds from the balanced equation.

Known ratios from equation

$$\frac{x \text{ moles } N_2}{3 \text{ moles } N_2H_4} = \frac{3 \text{ moles } N_2}{2 \text{ moles } N_2H_4}$$

$$x = (3/2)(3) = 9/2 = 4\frac{1}{2}.$$

QUESTION #9   (Answer:  b)  First convert weights to moles:

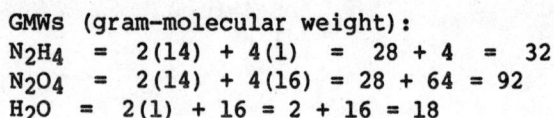

GMWs (gram-molecular weight):
$N_2H_4$ = 2(14) + 4(1)  = 28 + 4  = 32
$N_2O_4$ = 2(14) + 4(16) = 28 + 64 = 92
$H_2O$  = 2(1) + 16 = 2 + 16 = 18

$$\text{moles} = \frac{\text{weight}}{\text{GMW}}$$

$$\text{moles of } N_2H_4 = \frac{8}{32} = \frac{1}{4}$$

$$\text{moles of } N_2O_4 = \frac{92}{92} = 1$$

Then determine if one of these is in limiting amount by using the ratios of the compounds in the balanced equation:

if all of the $N_2H_4$ were used up, then:

$$\frac{x \text{ moles } N_2O_4}{\frac{1}{4} \text{ mole } N_2H_4} = \frac{1 \text{ mole } N_2O_4}{2 \text{ moles } N_2H_4}$$

$$\frac{x}{\frac{1}{4}} = \frac{1}{2}$$

$$x = (\tfrac{1}{2})(\tfrac{1}{4}) = \frac{1}{8} \text{ moles of } N_2O_4 \text{ would be required.}$$

if all of the $N_2O_4$ were used up, then:

$$\frac{x \text{ moles of } N_2H_4}{1 \text{ mole of } N_2O_4} = \frac{2 \text{ moles } N_2H_4}{1 \text{ mole } N_2O_4}$$

$$\frac{x}{1} = \frac{2}{1}$$

$$x = \left(\frac{2}{1}\right)(1) = 2 \text{ moles of } N_2H_4 \text{ would be required.}$$

Since only $\frac{1}{4}$ mole of $N_2H_4$ is available, and not 2 moles as would be required to use up all of the $N_2O_4$, the $N_2H_4$ is the limiting reagent. Then, using the moles of the limiting reagent, calculate the expected moles of the desired product.

$$\frac{x \text{ moles of } H_2O}{\frac{1}{4} \text{ mole of } N_2H_4} = \frac{4 \text{ moles } H_2O}{2 \text{ moles } N_2H_4}$$

$$\frac{x}{\frac{1}{4}} = \frac{4}{2}$$

$$x = \left(\frac{4}{2}\right)(\tfrac{1}{4}) = \frac{1}{2} \text{ mole } O_2.$$

Now calculate the grams of $O_2$:

$$\text{moles} = \frac{\text{weight}}{\text{GMW}}$$

$$\text{weight} = (\text{moles})(\text{GMW}) = (\tfrac{1}{2})(18) = 9 \text{ gms.}$$

QUESTION #10 (Answer: c) Again use moles as the intermediary. First need GMWs and moles where they can be determined:

GMWs:

$$H_2O = 2(1) + 16 = 18$$
$$N_2 = 2(14) = 28$$

$$\text{moles} = \frac{\text{weight}}{\text{GMW}}$$

$$\text{moles of } H_2O = \frac{36}{18} = 2$$

Then use equation to find moles of $N_2$:

$$\frac{x \text{ moles of } N_2}{2 \text{ moles of } H_2O} = \frac{3 \text{ moles } N_2}{4 \text{ moles } H_2O}$$

$$\frac{x}{2} = \frac{3}{4}$$

$$x = \left(\frac{3}{4}\right)(2) = 1\tfrac{1}{2} \text{ moles of } N_2$$

Then since at STP and 22.4 liters = 1 mole of gas:

$$\frac{x \text{ liters of } N_2}{3/2 \text{ moles of } N_2} = \frac{22.4 \text{ liters of } N_2}{1 \text{ mole of } N_2}$$

$$\frac{x}{3/2} = \frac{22.4}{1}$$

$$x = (22.4)(3/2) = 33.6 \text{ liters.}$$

## QUESTION #11   (Answer:  d)

| | |
|---|---|
| unbalanced: | $FeS + O_2 + H_2O \longrightarrow Fe_2O_3 + H_2SO_4$ |
| balance H, S: | already balanced |
| balance Fe: | $2FeS + O_2 + H_2O \longrightarrow Fe_2O_3 + H_2SO_4$ |
| rebalance S: | $2FeS + O_2 + H_2O \longrightarrow Fe_2O_3 + 2H_2SO_4$ |
| rebalance H: | $2FeS + O_2 + 2H_2O \longrightarrow Fe_2O_3 + 2H_2SO_4$ |
| balance O: | $2FeS + 9/2\, O_2 + 2H_2O \longrightarrow Fe_2O_3 + 2H_2SO_4$ |
| multiply by 2: | $4FeS + 9O_2 + 4H_2O \longrightarrow 2Fe_2O_3 + 4H_2SO_4$ |

check:     $4FeS + 9O_2 + 4H_2O \longrightarrow 2Fe_2O_3 + 4H_2SO_4$

| | | |
|---|---|---|
| Fe: | 4 | 4 |
| S: | 4 | 4 |
| O: | 18+4=22 | 6+16=22 |
| H: | 8 | 8 |

## QUESTION #12   (Answer:  c)  Again convert to moles:

$$\text{moles of } O_2 : \frac{x \text{ moles } O_2}{22.4 \text{ liters } O_2} = \frac{1 \text{ mole } O_2}{22.4 \text{ liters } O_2}$$

$$\frac{x}{22.4} = \frac{1}{22.4}$$

$$x = \left(\frac{1}{22.4}\right)(22.4) = 1 \text{ mole}$$

moles of FeS:  GMW of FeS = 56+32=88

$$\text{moles of Fe} = \frac{\text{weight}}{\text{GMW}} = \frac{44}{88} = \frac{1}{2}$$

Then determine if either reagent is in limiting amounts;
    if all the $O_2$ is used up

$$\frac{x \text{ moles FeS}}{1 \text{ mole } O_2} = \frac{4 \text{ moles FeS}}{9 \text{ moles } O_2}$$

$$\frac{x}{1} = \frac{4}{9}$$

x = 4/9 mole of FeS would be required

if all the FeS is used up

$$\frac{x \text{ moles } O_2}{\frac{1}{2} \text{ mole FeS}} = \frac{9 \text{ moles } O_2}{4 \text{ moles FeS}}$$

$$\frac{x}{\frac{1}{2}} = \frac{9}{4}$$

$$x = \left(\frac{9}{4}\right)\left(\frac{1}{2}\right) = \frac{9}{8} \text{ moles of } O_2 \text{ would be required}$$

So, the $O_2$ is in limiting amounts because less than 9/8 mole is available. Note that more than 4/9 mole of FeS is available to react with the $O_2$. Then use moles of $O_2$ to determine how much of $H_2SO_4$ will be produced:

$$\frac{x \text{ moles } H_2SO_4}{1 \text{ mole } O_2} = \frac{4 \text{ moles } H_2SO_4}{9 \text{ moles } O_2}$$

$$\frac{x}{1} = \frac{4}{9}$$

$$x = 4/9 \text{ moles } H_2SO_4$$

since moles $= \dfrac{\text{weight}}{\text{GMW}}$ and

GMW of $H_2SO_4 = 2(1)+32+4(16)=2+32+64=98$

then,

weight of $H_2SO_4$ = (moles)(GMW) $= \left(\dfrac{4}{9}\right)(98) \approx (4)(11) = 44$ gms.

## QUESTION #13 (Answer: b)

$$\frac{x \text{ moles of } Fe_2O_3}{5 \text{ moles of FeS}} = \frac{2 \text{ moles } Fe_2O_3}{4 \text{ moles FeS}}$$

$$\frac{x}{5} = \frac{2}{4}$$

$$x = \left(\frac{2}{4}\right)(5) = \frac{5}{2} = 2\tfrac{1}{2} \text{ moles of } Fe_2O_3$$

## QUESTION #14 (Answer: a)

GMWs: $H_2SO_4 = 2(1) + 32 + 4(16) = 2 + 32 + 64 = 98$
$\quad\quad\quad\; O_2 = 2(16) = 32$

moles: moles $H_2SO_4 = \dfrac{98}{98} = 1$ mole

moles of $O_2$ required:

$$\frac{x \text{ moles } O_2}{1 \text{ mole } H_2SO_4} = \frac{9 \text{ moles } O_2}{4 \text{ moles } H_2SO_4}$$

$$\frac{x}{1} = \frac{9}{4}$$

$$x = \left(\frac{9}{4}\right)(1) = \frac{9}{4} = 2\tfrac{1}{4} \text{ moles of } O_2$$

Volume of $O_2$:

$$\frac{x \text{ liters of } O_2}{9/4 \text{ moles of } O_2} = \frac{22.4 \text{ liters of } O_2}{1 \text{ mole of } O_2}$$

$$\frac{x}{9/4} = \frac{22.4}{1}$$

$$x = \left(\frac{22.4}{1}\right)\left(\frac{9}{4}\right) = 50.4 \text{ liters}$$

VOCABULARY CHECKLIST FOR STOICHIOMETRY


None



**3.7.6**     CONCEPTS, PRINCIPLES, ETC. CHECKLIST FOR STOICHIOMETRY


\_\_\_\_  symbolism of chemical equations
\_\_\_\_  balancing of chemical equations
\_\_\_\_  use of chemical equations in solving problems






**3.8**        **Energy Changes in Reactions**



**3.8.1**     REVIEW OF THE ENERGY CHANGES IN REACTIONS


Enthalpy ($\Delta H$) is the energy change (in terms of heat content) in a chemical reaction that occurs at constant pressure. The natural tendency of systems is toward minimum energy--the lower the energy of the system, the more stable the system. This means that a reaction that occurs with loss of energy (or negative energy) is a favorable reaction. The <u>standard enthalpy of formation</u> ($\Delta H_f^O$) is the enthalpy change when one mole of a compound is formed from its elements at $298^O$k. An example is:

$$C + \tfrac{1}{2} O_2 \text{ (g)} \longrightarrow CO \text{(g)} \qquad \Delta H_f^O(CO) = -26.4 \text{ kcal.}$$

The <u>standard enthalpy change of a reaction</u> ($\Delta H^O$) is:

$$\Delta H^O = \ \text{\Large$\Sigma$}\Delta H_f^O \text{ (products)} - \text{\Large$\Sigma$}\Delta H_f^O \text{ (reactants)}$$

That is, the $\Delta H_f^O$'s of all the products are added together and the $\Delta H_f^O$ of all the reactants are subtracted from them. Note: the enthalpy of elements as they exist at $298^O$k is zero. <u>Hess's Law of Constant Heat Summation</u> states that $\Delta H^O$'s of the reactions can be added algebraically to get the overall $\Delta H^O$ for the overall reaction. Note that when the direction of a reaction is reversed, the sign of the $\Delta H^O$ is changed (from $+\longrightarrow-$, or from $-\longrightarrow+$). Also, if the reaction, as written is multiplied (or divided) by a number, the $\Delta H^O$ must also be multiplied (or divided) by the same number. An example:

Q:  Find the enthalpy of formation ($\Delta H_f^O$) of $Ca(OH)_2(s)$ given the following:

$$2H_2(g) + O_2(g) \longrightarrow 2H_2O(l) \qquad \Delta H = -136.6 \text{ kcal}$$
$$CaO(s) + H_2O(l) \longrightarrow Ca(OH)_2(s) \qquad \Delta H = -15.3 \text{ kcal}$$
$$2CaO(s) \longrightarrow 2Ca(s) + O_2(g) \qquad \Delta H = +303.6 \text{ kcal}$$

A:  $\Delta H_f^O$ of $Ca(OH)_2$ means its formation from $Ca(s)$, $H_2(g)$ and $O_2(g)$. The answer by using the principles above is:

$$\tfrac{1}{2}\left[2H_2(g) + O_2(g) \longrightarrow 2H_2O(l)\right] \qquad \Delta H = \tfrac{1}{2}(-136.6 \text{ kcal})$$
$$CaO(s) + H_2O(l) \longrightarrow Ca(OH)_2(s) \qquad \Delta H = -15.3 \text{ kcal}$$
$$\tfrac{1}{2}\left[2Ca(s) + O_2(g) \longrightarrow 2CaO(s)\right] \qquad \Delta H = \tfrac{1}{2}(-303.6 \text{ kcal})$$

rewriting the above,

$$H_2(g) + \tfrac{1}{2}O_2(g) \longrightarrow H_2O(l) \qquad \Delta H = -68.3 \text{ kcal}$$
$$CaO(s) + H_2O(l) \longrightarrow Ca(OH)_2(s) \qquad \Delta H = -15.3 \text{ kcal}$$
$$Ca(s) + \tfrac{1}{2}O_2(g) \longrightarrow CaO(s) \qquad \Delta H = -151.8 \text{ kcal}$$

---

net:

$$Ca(s) + H_2(g) + O_2(g) \longrightarrow Ca(OH)_2(s) \qquad \Delta H = -235.4 \text{ kcal}$$

(Note: The $CaO(s)$ and $H_2O(l)$ cancel because they are on opposite sides of the equation.)

Entropy ($\Delta S$) is another measure of the stability of a system. It represents that part of the total energy not available for useful work. Entropy can be viewed as a measure of the number of microscopic states associated with a given macroscopic state. The more microscopic states a given macroscopic state has, the higher its entropy. This is also the same as saying the more probable (in the sense of probability) a state is, the higher its entropy. This is also the same as saying the more random a state, the higher its entropy. Systems tend toward maximum entropy for the greatest stability.

$\Delta H$ and $\Delta S$ represent two tendencies of systems. These may oppose each other or be in the same direction. Free energy ($\Delta G$) is a measure of the tendency of a system which takes into account $\Delta H$ and $\Delta S$. It gives the net tendency of the system. The formulation of $\Delta G$ is

$$\Delta G = \Delta H - T\Delta S$$
$T$ = absolute temperature.

For chemical reactions, the following conditions hold:

if $\Delta G = 0$, then the reaction is at equilibrium
   $\Delta G < 0$, then a spontaneous reaction (no energy input) is
        possible
   $\Delta G > 0$, then no reaction spontaneously.

The system tends toward a minimal value of $\Delta G$ which is the maximal stability.

The more negative $\Delta G$, the more probable the reaction will go as written. In summary, the $\Delta G$ represents the useful energy the system has to do work.  As before, with $\Delta H$

$$\Delta G^o = \sum \Delta G_f^o \text{ (products)} - \sum \Delta G_f^o \text{ (reactants)}.$$

Bonded molecules have lower energy than separate atoms; therefore, when atoms combine to form molecules, they lose energy (when spontaneous).  The bond dissociation energy (D) is the enthalpy change of the reaction in wnich a specific bond in a gaseous molecule is broken.  The D is positive (i.e., it requires input of energy to break a bond).  The average bond energy (E) is the approximate energy required to break a bond of a particular type (e.g., C-H) in any compound it may occur in.  Note that each C-H in $CH_4$ has a different D, but the E would be the average of all four of these.  The larger the numerical value (all are positive by definition) of the bond energy, the stronger the bond.

Exothermic reactions proceed with a negative $\Delta H$, and endothermic reactions proceed with a positive $\Delta H$.

That is:

exothermic:     reactants $\longrightarrow$ products + heat
endothermic:    heat + reactants $\longrightarrow$ products.


### 3.8.2     QUESTIONS TO REVIEW ENERGY CHANGES IN REACTIONS

(1)    A measure of the heat of a reaction:

    (a) entropy          (b) enthalpy
    (c) free energy     (d) none of these

(2)    The more stable systems with regard to $\Delta H$ are systems that have

    (a) zero $\Delta H$     (b) maximum $\Delta H$     (c) minimum $\Delta H$

(3)    A measure of the total energy not available for useful work is the:

    (a) entropy          (b) enthalpy
    (c) free energy     (d) none of the above

(4)    The more stable systems with regard to entropy  are systems that have

    (a) minimum $\Delta S$          (b) maximum $\Delta S$
    (c) zero $\Delta S$            (d) none of these

(5)    High values of entropy are associated with all of the following except:

    (a) a large number of microscopic states for a given macroscopic state
    (b) high probability of a state
    (c) high randomness of a state
    (d) all of the above are correct

(6)    The net energy available to a system is given by the:

    (a) entropy          (b) enthalpy
    (c) free energy     (d) none of the above

(7) The relationship between free energy ($\Delta G$), enthalpy ($\Delta H$), entropy ($\Delta S$) and absolute temperature (T) is

(a) $\Delta G = \Delta H + \Delta S$        (b)    $\Delta G = \Delta H + T \Delta S$

(c) $\Delta G = \Delta H - T \Delta S$      (d)    $\Delta G = T \Delta H - \Delta S$

(8) If $\Delta G < 0$, then

(a) the reaction is at equilibrium
(b) a spontaneous reaction is possible
(c) no reaction is possible
(d) none of the above

(9) With regard to $\Delta G$ a system is most stable when

(a) $\Delta G$ is a maximum        (b)    $\Delta G$ is a minimum
(c) $\Delta G$ is zero             (d)    none of the above

(10) The larger the numerical value of a bond energy, the

(a) stronger the bond
(b) weaker the bond
(c) no relation to strength of bond

(11) The following reaction is:

$$\text{reactants} \longrightarrow \text{products} \qquad \Delta H = \text{negative}$$

(a) exothermic     (b) endothermic     (c) neither

Use the following information for the remainder of the Questions.

Enthalpies of Formation, $\Delta H_f^o$ (kcals/mole) at $298^o$K

| $H_2O$(g) | -58 | $NO_2$(g) | 8 | $Ca(OH)_2$ | -236 | $CH_3CH_2OH$($\ell$) | -66 |
| $H_2O$($\ell$) | -68 | $NH_3$(g) | -11 | $CaCO_3$(s) | -288 | $C_2H_4$(g) | 13 |
| $SO_3$(g) | -94 | $CO_2$(g) | -94 | $C_2H_6$(g) | -20 | $C_4H_{10}$(g) | -30 |
| $NO$(g) | 19 | $CaO$(s) | -152 | $CH_3OH$($\ell$) | -57 | | |

Bond Energies ($\Delta H$ in kcals/mole)

| H-H | 104 | O-H | 111 | N≡N | 226 | C-Cl | 79 | C≡C | 194 |
| H-Cl | 103 | O=O | 118 | C-C | 83 | C-N | 70 | C=O | 170 |
| C-H | 99 | Cl-Cl | 58 | C-O | 84 | C=C | 147 | | |

(12) Calculate the $\Delta H_f^o$ of $H_2SO_4$($\ell$) given the following equation:

$$H_2O(\ell) + SO_3(g) \longrightarrow H_2SO_4(\ell) \qquad \Delta H^o = -32 \text{ kcals}$$

(a) -6    (b) -58    (c) -162    (d) -194

(13) Calculate the heat ($\Delta H^o$) of reaction for the following reaction:

$$CaO(s) + CO_2(g) \longrightarrow CaCO_3(s)$$

(a) -534    (b) +534    (c) +42    (d) -42

(14) Calculate the heat ($\Delta H^O$) of reaction for the following reaction:

$$C_2H_4(g) + H_2O(l) \longrightarrow CH_3CH_2OH(l)$$

(a) -121  (b) +15  (c) -15  (d) -11

(15) Calculate the heat ($\Delta H^O$) of a reaction for the combustion of n-butane ($C_4H_{10}$)

$$C_4H_{10}(g) + O_2(g) \longrightarrow CO_2(g) + H_2O(l)$$

(unbalanced)

(a) -132  (b) -192  (c) -310  (d) -686

(16) Which of the following steps requires the most energy?

(1)  $C = O \longrightarrow C - O$

(II)  $C = C \longrightarrow C - C$

(neglect other bonds that might be formed)

(a) I          (b) II          (c) both equal

(17) Which of the following steps releases the most energy?

(I)  $H_2 + $ 

(II)  $H_2 + $ 

(a) I          (b) II          (c) neither releases energy

3.8.3    ANSWERS TO QUESTIONS IN SECTION 3.8.2

(1) b  (2) c  (3) a  (4) b  (5) d  (6) c  (7) c
(8) b  (9) b  (10) a  (11) a  (12) d  (13) d  (14) d
(15) d  (16) a  (17) a

3.8.4    DISCUSSION OF ANSWERS TO QUESTIONS IN SECTION 3.8.2

QUESTIONS #1-#11: Adequately discussed in Section.

QUESTION #12 (Answer: d) The $\Delta H_f^O$ is the formation of one mole of the $H_2SO_4(l)$ from its elements:

$$H_2(g) + S(s) + 2O_2(g) \longrightarrow H_2SO_4(l) \quad \Delta H_f^O = ?$$

Now using the information given, a set of equations must be put together that adds up to this net equation. This is done as follows:

210

$$(1) \quad H_2(g) + \tfrac{1}{2}O_2(g) \longrightarrow H_2O(\ell) \qquad \Delta H_f^O = -68$$

$$(2) \quad S(s) + \tfrac{3}{2}O_2(g) \longrightarrow SO_3(g) \qquad \Delta H_f^O = -94$$

Rearrange these to show how they add up to the equation wanted:

$$H_2(g) + \tfrac{1}{2}O_2(g) \longrightarrow H_2O(\ell) \quad \Delta H_f^O = -68 \text{ kcals}$$

$$S(s) + \tfrac{3}{2}O_2(g) \longrightarrow SO_3(g) \quad \Delta H_f^O = -94 \text{ kcals}$$

$$H_2O(\ell) + SO_3(g) \longrightarrow H_2SO_4(\ell) \quad \Delta H_f^O = -32 \text{ kcals}$$

sum: $\quad H_2(g) + 2O_2(g) + S(s) \longrightarrow H_2SO_4(\ell) \quad \Delta H_f^O = -194 \text{ kcals}$

Or, an alternative method:

$$\Delta H^O (\text{product}) - \Delta H^O (\text{reactant}) = \Delta H^O \text{ reaction}$$
$$\Delta H_f^O H_2SO_4 - \{\Delta H_f^O H_2O_{(\ell)} + \Delta H_f^O SO_{3(g)}\} = -32 \text{ kcal}$$
$$\Delta H_f^O H_2SO_4 - (-68 \text{ kcal} - 94 \text{ kcal}) = -32 \text{ kcal}$$
$$\Delta H_f^O H_2SO_4 = -194 \text{ kcal}$$

QUESTION #13 (Answer: d) This is a direct application of Hess' Law.

$$\textstyle\sum \Delta H_f^O \text{ (products)} = -288$$

$$\textstyle\sum \Delta H_f^O \text{ (reactants)} = -94-152 = -246$$

then,

$$\Delta H^O = \textstyle\sum \Delta H_f^O \text{ (products)} - \sum \Delta H_f^O \text{ (reactants)}$$

$$\Delta H^O = -288 - (-246) = -288 + 246 = -42.$$

QUESTION #14 (Answer: d) This is also a direct application of Hess' Law.

$$\textstyle\sum \Delta H_f^O \text{ (products)} = -66$$

$$\textstyle\sum \Delta H_f^O \text{ (reactants)} = -68+13 = -55$$

and,

$$\Delta H = \textstyle\sum \Delta H_f^O \text{ (products)} - \sum \Delta H_f^O \text{ (reactants)}$$

$$= -66 - (-55) = -66 + 55 = -11.$$

QUESTION #15 (Answer: d) First balance the equation (Section 3.7):

| | | |
|---|---|---|
| unbalanced: | $C_4H_{10} + O_2 \longrightarrow CO_2 + H_2O$ | |
| balance H: | $C_4H_{10} + O_2 \longrightarrow CO_2 + 5H_2O$ | |
| balance C: | $C_4H_{10} + O_2 \longrightarrow 4CO_2 + 5H_2O$ | |
| balance O: | $C_4H_{10} + \tfrac{13}{2}O_2 \longrightarrow 4CO_2 + 5H_2O$ | (leave as 1 mole $C_4H_{10}$ because $\Delta H^O$ based on |
| check: C: | 4 $\quad$ 4 | one mole of the |
| H: | 10 $\quad$ 10 | substance) |
| O: | 13/2(2)=13 $\quad$ 13 | |

Now apply Hess' Law:

$$\leqq \Delta H_f^O \text{ (products)} = 4\Delta H_f^O \text{ of } CO_2(g) + 5\Delta H_f^O \text{ of } H_2O(\ell)$$

$$= 4(-94) + 5(-68) = -376 - 340 = -716$$

$$\leqq \Delta H_f^O \text{ (reactants)} = \Delta H_f^O \text{ of } C_4H_{10} + 13/2\,\Delta H_f^O \text{ of } O_2(g)$$

$$= -30 + 13/2(0) = -30$$

and,

$$\leqq \Delta H^O = \Delta H_f^O \text{ (products)} - \Delta H_f^O \text{ (reactants)}$$

$$= -716 - (-30) = -716 + 30 = -686 \text{ kcals.}$$

QUESTION #16  (Answer: a) This is an application of Hess' Law using bond energies:

| | $\Delta H$ |
|---|---|
| $C = O \longrightarrow C + O$ | 170 |
| $C + O \longrightarrow C - O$ | - 84 |
| $C = O \longrightarrow C - O$ | 86 |
| | |
| $C = C \longrightarrow 2C$ | 147 |
| $2C \longrightarrow C - C$ | - 83 |
| $C = C \longrightarrow C - C$ | 64 |

QUESTION #17  (Answer: a) Again apply Hess' Law to each by adding all bond energies in products and reactants:

| | | $\Delta H$ |
|---|---|---|
| I | $H_2 + C_2H_4 \longrightarrow 6H + 2C$ | |
| | $104 + 4(99) + 147$ | |
| | $\text{H-H} \quad \text{4C-H} \quad \text{C=C}$ | 647 kcal |
| | $6H + 2C \longrightarrow C_2H_6$ | |
| | $83 + 6(99)$ | -677 kcal |
| | $\text{C-C} + \text{6CH}$ | |
| net | $H_2 + C_2H_4 \longrightarrow C_2H_6$ | - 30 kcal |
| | | |
| II | $H_2 + CH_2O \longrightarrow 4H + C + O$ | |
| | $104 + 2(99) + 170$ | 472 kcal |
| | $\text{H-H} + \text{CH} \quad \text{C=O}$ | |
| | $4H + C + O \longrightarrow CH_3OH$ | |
| | $3(99) + 84 + 111$ | -492 kcal |
| | $\text{3C-H} + \text{C-O} + \text{OH}$ | |
| net | $H_2 + CH_2O \longrightarrow CH_3OH$ | - 20 kcal |

3.8.5     VOCABULARY CHECKLIST FOR ENERGY CHANGES IN REACTIONS

____ enthalpy
____ standard enthalpy of formation
____ standard enthalpy of a reaction
____ Hess' Law
____ entropy

____ free energy
____ bond energy
____ exothermic
____ endothermic

212

CONCEPTS, PRINCIPLES, ETC. CHECKLIST FOR ENERGY
             CHANGES IN REACTIONS


____ relation between $\triangle H$, $\triangle S$ and $\triangle G$ and meaning of each
____ use of Hess' Law
____ use and meaning of bond energies


## 3.9        Rate Processes in Chemical Reactions--Kinetics & Equilibrium


### 3.9.1    REVIEW OF RATE PROCESSES IN CHEMICAL REACTIONS


#### 3.9.1.1    Kinetics

Kinetics is concerned with the rates (how fast) of chemical
reactions. This means it is concerned with the activation energy
(see below) rather than the $\triangle H$ (enthalpy change) of a reaction as in
thermodynamics (section 3.8.1).

For a chemical reaction to occur, several conditions must be met.
They are:

(1) the molecules must collide (make contact). The more they
    collide, the greater the chance of a reaction.

(2) The molecules must have enough energy to react once they
    have collided. Remember that molecules have a
    distribution of kinetic energies (Boltzman distribution),
    and only some of the molecules will have enough energy to
    react. Note: $KE \propto T$

(3) Given a collision and sufficient energy, a molecule may
    not react unless the orientation is correct. The energy
    requirements and orientation are related in that some
    orientations require less energy for reaction to occur.


The three factors above help determine the activation energy ($E_A$).
The $E_A$ is the energy barrier which must be overcome for a reaction to
occur. The higher the $E_A$, the slower the reaction. A catalyst (a
substance not used up or changed in a reaction) speeds up reactions
by lowering the $E_A$. This is how enzymes work (Section 2.1.1).


Most reactions proceed as a series of steps which are exemplified by
chain reactions. Chain reactions are exemplified by radical
reactions such as halogenation. The steps are as follows:

(1) Initiation - the production of radicals

$$Cl_2 \longrightarrow 2Cl\cdot$$

(2) **Propagation** - the production of radicals by reaction with radicals, this keeps the reaction going:

$$CL \cdot + R_3CH \longrightarrow R_3C \cdot + HCl$$
$$R_3C \cdot + Cl_2 \longrightarrow R_3CCl + Cl \cdot$$

(3) **Termination** - the destruction of radicals by the reactions of two radicals with each other or by the reactions of radicals with the walls of the container:

$$Cl \cdot + R_3C \cdot \longrightarrow R_3CCl$$
$$R_3C \cdot + R_3C \cdot \longrightarrow R_3C-CR_3 \cdot$$

There are many possible overall paths (reaction coordinates) which may be taken by reactants being converted to products. The path taken will be the one with the lowest $E_A$. Each step, i.e., each $E_A$ in an overall path, is called an <u>elementary process</u>. The elementary process with the highest $E_A$ is the <u>slowest step (rate determining step)</u> and determines the overall rate of the reaction. If one molecule is involved in an elementary process, it is said to be <u>unimolecular</u>. If two molecules, it is said to be bimolecular; if three, then <u>termolecular</u>, etc. Given an overall path (with its composite elementary processes), the <u>principle of microscopic reversibility</u> states that the elementary processes of the reverse reaction are the same as the forward reaction (Fig. 3.10).

reaction coordinate (one of many that are possible)

**Fig. 3.10 – A Reaction Coordinate**

EP  = elementary process
AC  = activated complex, a transient species that may be converted to products or reactants, cannot be isolated; also called the <u>transition state complex</u>
I   = intermediates, transient species that may be isolated in some instances; note they are like "rest points" between the EP's
$E_A$  = activation energies
$E_{A_F}$  = overall $E_A$ for forward reaction
$E_{A_R}$  = overall $E_A$ for reverse reaction
$\triangle E$  = energy of the reaction = $E_{A_R} - E_{A_F}$.

The <u>rates of reactions</u> are quantified in terms of <u>rate expressions</u> which relate the change in concentration of one reactant (or product) with time to the concentration of other reactants (or products):

for,

$$aA + bB \longrightarrow cC + dD \qquad \text{(overall reaction)}$$

the rate expression might be,

$$\text{rate} = \frac{\Delta [A]}{\Delta t} = -k [A]^m [B]^n$$

the minus sign (-) is because $[A]$ is decreasing with time,

k = rate constant for the reaction

$[\ ] \equiv$ concentration in moles/liter (molarity).

Note that the exponents of $A^{(m)}$ and $B^{(n)}$ do not, in general, equal the coefficients of A(a) and B(b). This points out that rate expressions cannot be determined from the stoichiometric equations; they must be determined by experiment. The rate of reaction, and hence, the rate expression, varies during the course of the reaction. This is because the net reaction rate is,

net rate = forward rate - reverse rate,

forward rate = $k_f [A]^m [B]^n$

reverse rate = $k_r [C]^x [D]^y$.

The <u>forward rate</u> depends on the concentration of the reactants, and the <u>reverse rate</u> depends on the concentration of the products. Early (initially) in the reaction, there are more reactants and the forward rate dominates. As reactants are converted to products, there accumulates more products and the reverse rate increases until it equals the forward rate. This point is equilibrium (Fig. 3.11).

The rate is $\Delta c / \Delta t$ = slope and this changes going from t = 0 to equilibrium.

**Fig. 3.11 – Course of a Reaction**

For the reason above, most rate expressions are for <u>initial rates</u> (reactants present but no products) and, hence, are <u>forward rates</u> and take the form:

$$\text{rate} = k [A]^m [B]^n$$

The problem then is to determine the values of m and n. This is done by varying the concentration of one reactant while holding other reactants constant and determining how the rate is affected by this. The <u>order</u> of the reaction (contrasted with molecularity) is the sum of the exponents in the experimentally derived rate expression. For example:

given: rate = $k [A]^2 [B]^{1/2}$

215

then:  order of reaction = 2 + ½ = 2½
order of reactant in $\underline{A}$ = 2
order of reactant in $\underline{B}$ = ½

First order kinetics means the order is one, second order is two, etc.  The rate constant can be calculated once the orders in each reactant is known:

$$k = \frac{rate}{[A]^2[B]^{\frac{1}{2}}}$$

From the collision theory of gaseous reactions, the following equation is derived:

$k = Ae^{-Ea/RT}$
k = rate constant
A = a constant which includes collision, orientation, and molecular factors
e = base of natural logs
Ea = activation energy
R = 1.99 cal/mole-$^{\circ}$K
T = absolute temperature

The $E_a$ can be calculated by determining the rate constant at a number of different temperatures and making this plot:

$$\ln k = \ln A - \frac{EA}{R} \cdot \frac{1}{T}$$

$(y = b + m \cdot x)$

## 3.9.1.2    Equilibrium

All chemical reactions proceed toward an equilibrium state.  The equilibrium state exists when the forward rate equals the reverse rate: hence, there is no change in the components of the reaction (see 3.9.1.1).  This points out that the equilibrium state is a dynamic state; i.e., the reactions have not ceased, and reactants are being converted to products and products are being converted to reactants.  At equilibrium, $\triangle G$ (free energy) is zero, $\triangle H$ (enthalpy) is a minimum, and $\triangle S$ (entropy) is a maximum (see section 3.8.1).  This means that there is a minimum energy and maximum randomness in a system at equilibrium.

The equilibrium constant (K) is a quantitative way of describing the interrelationships of the concentrations of components at equilibrium.  It is:

given the reaction:  $aA + bB \underset{k_2}{\overset{k_1}{\rightleftharpoons}} cC + dD$

forward rate = $k_1 [A]^a [B]^b$

backward rate = $k_2 [C]^c [D]^d$

216

then the equilibrium constant is:

forward rate = backward rate

$$K_1 = [A]^a[B]^b = K_2[C]^c[D]^d$$

$$K = \frac{k_1}{K_2} = \frac{[C]^c[D]^d}{[A]^a[B]^b} \quad \text{depends only on temperature}$$

[ ] = concentration in moles/liter (molarity)
[ gases ] = atmospheres
[ pure solids ] = constant and are essentially = 1.

The K is a measure of the capacity of reactants to be converted to products. The larger the K, the more reactants will be converted to products. The expression:

$$\frac{[C]^c[D]^d}{[A]^a[B]^b}$$

can be determined <u>at points other than equilibrium</u>. <u>The direction the reaction must proceed to get to equilibrium</u> can be determined by comparing the values of the expression with the K:

if $\quad \frac{[C]^c[D]^d}{[A]^a[B]^b} < K$

then the reaction proceeds to equilibrium from left to right as written (the numerator, products, must increase and/or the denominator, reactants, must decrease for the expression to equal K);

if $\quad \frac{[C]^c[D]^d}{[A]^a[B]^b} > K$

then the reaction proceeds to equilibrium from right to left as written (the reverse of the above).

Note that the equilibrium constant for the reverse ($K_R$) of a given reaction (K) is:

$$K_R = 1/K.$$

The overall equilibrium constant (K) for a series of reactions that sum to this overall reaction is:

$$K = K_1K_2K_3.....$$

When a reaction is <u>exothermic</u> ($\triangle H$ is negative), the K actually decreases as the temperature increases. The reverse is true for an endothermic reaction (see 3.8.1).

<u>Le Chatelier's Principle</u> is a good way to determine what the effect of a change in condition (e.g. concentration) will do the relative concentrations of reactants/products and other factors (e.g. heat, volume) in a reaction. The Principle is:

Any perturbation (change) to a system initially at equilibrium will cause that system (if left alone) to adjust in such a way as to offset that perturbation.

This means the system will go toward a new equilibrium but with concentrations and other factors appropriately adjusted. A practical way of using Le Chatelier's Principle is:

(1) Write all the components and conditions of the reaction on the appropriate side of the equation. This includes all the reactants, products, heat and volume. The heat is the heat of the reaction. If positive, it is a reactant; if negative, it is a product (see 3.8.1). Remember that an increase in temperature is like increasing the energy (heat) and vice versa. The volume can be related to the moles (in the balanced equation) of gases in the reaction. Put the volume on the side with the fewer moles of gas ("balances" out the volume). Remember that as pressure increases, the volume decreases and vice versa.

(2) Apply these rules (from Le Chatelier's) to determine how the equilibrium will shift:

   (a) if a component or condition increases, the reaction is shifted to the opposite side; i.e., components/conditions on the other side will increase and those on the same side will decrease;

   (b) if a component/condition decreases, the reaction is shifted to its side, the other components/conditions on that side increase and the components/conditions on the opposite decrease.

An example is:

given the reaction,

$$M_2(g) + 3 E_2(g) \rightleftharpoons 2 ME_3(g) \qquad \triangle H = +10 \text{ kcals}$$

Rewrite using the rules above.

$$\text{heat} + M_2(g) + 3E_2(g) \rightleftharpoons 2ME_3(g) + \text{volume}$$

Examples of effects of perturbations are:

   if   $\uparrow M_2$,
       reaction shifts to right

   if   $\downarrow E_2$,
       reaction shifts to left

   if   $\uparrow$ pressure,
       this causes volume to decrease
       reaction shifts to right

   if   $\downarrow$ temperature,
       same as decreasing heat and decreasing volume
       reaction shift is indeterminate

   if   add a catalyst
       no shift in equilibrium by a catalyst,
       catalyst only affects rate of reaction.

(1)     All of the following conditions must be met in order for a chemical reaction to occur except:

(a) collisions between molecules
(b) sufficient energy per molecule to react
(c) appropriate orientation of colliding molecules
(d) all of the above are necessary


(2)     The energy that must be overcome for a chemical reaction to occur is called the

(a) enthalpy                    (b)  activation energy
(c) entropy                     (d)  free energy

(3)     The steps in a chain reaction include all except

(a) initiation                  (b)  propagation
(c) acceleration                (d)  termination

(4)     The step in which radicals already present are used to generate new radicals is called

(a) initiation                  (b)  propagation
(c) acceleration                (d)  none of the above

Use the following diagram to answer Questions #5 through #7.

(5)     The activation energy of the forward reaction is given by:

(a) II       (b) III      (c) IV       (d) V

(6)     The heat of the reaction is given by:

(a) II       (b) III      (c) IV       (d) V

(7)     The activated complex would be located at:

(a) I       (b) II       (c) III       (d) none of the above

(8)     The rate determining step of a reaction with a series of steps is characterized by:

(a) the lowest energy of activation
(b) the highest energy of activation
(c) the highest enthalpy
(d) none of the above

(9)   The role of a catalyst is to:

(a) shift the equilibrium of the reaction in favor of products
(b) speed up the reaction by raising the activation energy
(c) speed up the reaction by lowering the activation energy
(d) none of the above


(10)   At equilibrium:

(a) the forward reaction continues
(b) the reverse reaction continues
(c) there is minimum energy and maximum randomness
(d) all of the above

(11)   As the value of K (the equilibrium constant) becomes larger:

(a) more products will be present at equilibrium
(b) less products will be present at equilibrium
(c) the faster the reaction will proceed
(d) the slower the reaction will proceed

(12)   Given a reaction symbolized as:

$$A \underset{\longleftarrow}{\overset{K}{\longrightarrow}} B$$

if          $\frac{[B]}{[A]} = 2 \times 10^{-5}$   and it is known that

$K = 5 \times 10^{-4}$ from other experiments, in what direction must the
reaction proceed to reach equilibrium?

(a) $\begin{bmatrix} B \end{bmatrix}$ must increase and/or $\begin{bmatrix} A \end{bmatrix}$ decrease

(b) $\begin{bmatrix} B \end{bmatrix}$ must decrease and/or $\begin{bmatrix} A \end{bmatrix}$ decrease

(c) cannot be determined from the information given

(13)   For the reaction:

$$A + 2B \underset{\longleftarrow}{\overset{K}{\longrightarrow}} 2C$$

the concentrations, in moles/liters, of the components at
equilibrium are:

$\begin{bmatrix} A \end{bmatrix} = 1 \times 10^{-2} M$, $\begin{bmatrix} B \end{bmatrix} = 2 \times 10^{-3} M$, $\begin{bmatrix} C \end{bmatrix} = 5 \times 10^{-6} M$.

What is the equilibrium constant (K) of the reaction?

(a) 6.25 x 10$^{-4}$          (b)   0.225
(c) 25                              (d)   none of the above

Use the following information for Questions #14 through #17.

$C_2H_5OH(\ell) + 3O_2(g) \rightleftharpoons 2CO_2(g) + 3H_2O(\ell)$    $\Delta H^o = -327$ kcals

(14)   If the temperature is increased, the equilibrium:

(a) shifts to the left
(b) shifts to the right
(c) is unchanged

(15)  If the pressure is increased, the equilibrium:

      (a) shifts to the left
      (b) shifts to the right
      (c) is unchanged

(16)  If $O_2$(g) is added, the equilibrium:

      (a) shifts to the left
      (b) shifts to the right
      (c) is unchanged

(17)  A chemical is added which absorbs $CO_2$(g).  This will cause the
      equilibrium to be:

      (a) shifted to the left
      (b) shifted to the right
      (c) unchanged

Use the following information for Questions #18 through #21.

$$CH_4(g) + H_2O(\ell) \rightleftharpoons CH_3OH(\ell) + H_2(g) \qquad \Delta H = +29 \text{ kcal}$$

(18)  If the $H_2$(g) formed is allowed to escape from the reaction; the
      equilibrium will be:

      (a) shifted to the left
      (b) shifted to the right
      (c) unchanged

(19)  If the pressure is doubled, the equilibrium:

      (a) shifts to the left
      (b) shifts to the right
      (c) is unchanged

(20)  Suppose $Co^{+2}$ catalyzes this reaction.  If it is added, the
      equilibrium:

      (a) shifts to the left
      (b) shifts to the right
      (c) is unchanged

(21)  The temperature is decreased, this causes the equilibrium to:

      (a) shift to the left
      (b) shift to the right
      (c) be unchanged

3.9.3      ANSWERS TO QUESTIONS IN SECTION 3.9.2

( 1)  d   (2)  b   (3)  c   (4)  b   (5)  d   (6)  c   (7)  b
( 8)  b   (9)  c  (10)  d  (11)  a  (12)  a  (13)  a  (14)  a
(15)  b  (16)  b  (17)  b  (18)  b  (19)  c  (20)  c  (21)  a

QUESTIONS #1-#11:  Adequately discussed in the text.

QUESTION #12  (Answer:  a)  In this case $[B]/[A] < K$ because 2 x $10^{-5} < 5$ x $10^{-4}$.  Then for $[B]/[A]$ to become equal to K, the $[B]$ must increase and the $[A]$ must decrease.

QUESTION #13  (Answer:  a)  The equilibrium constant (K) is,

$$K = \frac{[C]}{[A][B]^2} = \frac{[5 \times 10^{-6}]^2}{[1\times10^{-2}][2\times10^{-3}]^2} = \frac{25 \times 10^{-12}}{(10^{-2})(4\times10^{-6})}$$

$$K = \frac{25 \times 10^{-12}}{4 \times 10^{-8}} = \frac{25}{4} \times 10^{-12+8} = 6.25 \times 10^{-4}.$$

QUESTION #14  (Answer:  a)  The complete equation is

$$C_2H_5OH(\ell) + 3O_2(g) \rightleftharpoons 2CO_2(g) + 3H_2O(\ell) + vol. + heat.$$

Volume goes on the right side because there are fewer moles of gas on that side.  Heat goes on the right because the reaction is exothermic, i.e., heat is a product.  Then an increase in temperature causes an increase in heat which shifts the reaction to the opposite side (the left).  Increased temperature also increases the volume (Charles' Law).  This also shifts the reaction to the left.

QUESTION #15  (Answer:  b)  See #14.  An increase in pressure causes a decrease in volume.  A decrease in volume pulls a reaction to its side (the right).

QUESTION #16  (Answer:  b)  The added $O_2$ shifts the reaction to the opposite side (the right).  Increased temperature also increases the volume (Charles' Law).  This also shifts the reaction to the left.

QUESTION #17  (Answer:  b)  The $CO_2$(g) decreases and this pulls the reaction to its side (the right).

QUESTION #18  (Answer:  b)  The overall equation is:

$$heat + CH_4(g) + H_2O(\ell) \rightleftharpoons CH_3OH(\ell) + H_2(g).$$

The heat is on the left because the reaction is endothermic which means heat is used as a reactant.  There is no volume factor because there is an equal number of moles of gases on both sides.  Since the $H_2$ is being removed, the reaction is pulled to its side (the right).

QUESTION #19  (Answer:  c)  See #18.  There is no volume factor so the pressure has no effect.

QUESTION #20  (Answer:  c)  Catalysts do not affect the equilibrium of a reaction.

QUESTION #21  (Answer:  a)  A decrease in temperature is like decreasing the heat which shifts the reaction to that side (the left).

## 3.9.5    VOCABULARY CHECKLIST FOR KINETICS & EQUILIBRIUM

| | | | |
|---|---|---|---|
| ✗ | kinetics | ⟋ | transition states |
| ⟋ | Le Chatelier's Principle | ⟋ | catalyst |
| ⟋ | activation energy | ⟋ | chain reactions |
| ⟋ | equilibrium constant | ⟋ | initiation |
| ⟋ | propagation | ⟋ | termination |
| ⟋ | intermediates | | |

## 3.9.6    CONCEPTS, PRINCIPLES, ETC. CHECKLIST FOR KINETICS AND EQUILIBRIUM

____ requirements for a chemical reaction to occur
____ steps in chain reactions
____ meaning of equilibrium and the equilibrium constant
____ use of Le Chatelier's Principle

## 3.10    Solubility

## 3.10.1    REVIEW OF SOLUBILITY

### 3.10.1.1    Concentration Units

A liquid solution is a homogenous, continuous liquid of variable composition over a limited range consisting of two or more components.  Note that a solution may also be gaseous or solid.

Given a two component solution, the solvent is the component in greater amount (herein, usually a pure liquid), and the solute is the component in lesser amount (herein, usually a solid or second liquid).  Note that solids, gases or other liquids can be dissolved in a given pure liquid to make a solution.

There are many possible ways of measuring the composition of solutions.  The common ones are:

(1)  Percent composition can be weight/volume, weight/weight, volume/volume, etc.  It must be designated as to the type and the units of mass and volume used.

$$\% = \frac{\text{amt. of solute}}{\text{total amt. of solution}} \times 100 \text{ (usual form)}.$$

(2)  Density ($\rho$)

$$\rho = \frac{\text{mass of solution}}{\text{total volume of solution}}$$

(3)  Mole Fraction (X)

$$x_1 = \frac{\text{moles of one component}}{\text{moles of all components}} = \frac{n}{\sum\limits_{i=1}^{i=m} n_i}$$

$n_1$ = moles of component #1.

$\sum\limits_{i=1}^{i=m} n_i$ = sum over moles of all m components.

$(i=1,2,\ldots,m)$.

This is useful when emphasizing the relation between concentration-dependent properties of solutions and the relative amounts of the components (see below).

(4)  Molarity (M)

$$M = \frac{\text{moles of solute}}{\text{liter of solution}}$$

Varies with the temperature.

(5)  Molality (m)

$$m = \frac{\text{moles of solute}}{\text{kilogram of solvent}}$$

Does not vary with temperature.

(6)  Formality (F)

$$F = \frac{\text{moles of solute}}{\text{liter of solution}}$$

Essentially the same as M.  Technically more correct for substances that do not exist as molecules, and the formula is used to calculate the gram-formula weight (e.g., NaCl is the formula for "salt" which has no discrete molecules).

The following concept is important for solving problems dealing with solutions and concentrations.  Most problems can be solved by realizing there is usually a conservation of mass.  This means:

given: C = concentration unit = $\dfrac{\text{amt. of solute}}{\text{volume of solution}}$

(all of the above are like this except for molality; just substitute kilograms for volume and solvent for solution)

V = volume of solution

then:  (C)(V) = amount of solute
amount = gms, moles, equivalents, etc., depending on the concentration unit (C) used

then:  this amount of solute is conserved

(1) as solutions are diluted,
$C_1 V_1 = C_2 V_2$ = amount
e.g., $M_1 V_1 = M_2 V_2$ = moles
$(\%_1)(V_1) = (\%_2)(V_2)$ = grams if % is (W/V).

(2) as solutions are made from solid and liquids,
CV = amount of solute used to make the solution, e.g.,

$(M)(V)$ = moles = $\dfrac{\text{weight}}{\text{gram-molecular weight}}$

$(\%)(V)$ = grams (% is w/v here).

Then the correct combination of formulas is chosen depending upon the problem.

224

Electrolytes are substances that dissociate into positive and negative ions when dissolved in solvent. The ions are positive (cations) and negative (anions) and are surrounded by solvent molecules in solution (a process called solvation; when the solvent is $H_2O$, this is hydration). Our discussion will refer to water as a solvent.

Some substances are only partially soluble in water. The ion product is a means of quantifying the solubility:

$$M_mA_a + H_2O \longrightarrow mM^{+a}(aq) + aA^{-m}(aq)$$

(aq) = dissolved in water

$$\text{ion product} \equiv [M^{+a}]^m[A^{-m}]^a$$

$[\;\;]$ = concentration in moles/liter, i.e. molarity.

The ion product can be calculated for any solution. The solubility product ($K_{sp}$) is the ion product for a saturated solution (as much as possible of the solute has been dissolved at a given temperature):

$$K_{sp} = [M^{+a}]^m[A^{-m}]^a$$

for a saturated solution. The smaller the $K_{sp}$, the less soluble is a solid. The $K_{sp}$ is larger than the ion product except at saturation where they are equal. As long as the ion product is less than the $K_{sp}$, more solute can be dissolved.

The common ion effect on solubility can be understood in terms of LeChatelier's Principle (Section 3.9.1.2). Explanation of the effect is based on analysis of the following equation:

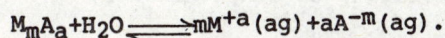

$$M_mA_a + H_2O \rightleftharpoons mM^{+a}(ag) + aA^{-m}(ag).$$

The common ions would be $M^{+a}$ or $A^{-m}$. These are increased by adding compounds that dissociate into them and add them to solution, and they are decreased by adding species that react with them and remove them from solution. If $M^{+a}$ or $A^{-m}$ are increased, the reaction shifts to the left and less of $M_mA_a$ dissolves. If $M^{+a}$ or $A^{-m}$ are decreased, the reaction shifts to the right and more of the $M_mA_a$ dissolves. Note that $K_{sp}$ is not affected--the ion not changed compensates (by increasing or decreasing) for the ion changed (the common ion). For example:

for $CaSO_4$     $K_{sp} = 2.4 \times 10^{-5}$

$$CaSO_4(s) + H_2O \longrightarrow Ca^{+2}(aq) + SO_4^{-2}(aq)$$

if, given $NaSO_4$ which gives $SO_4^{-2}$, the reaction shifts to the left and more solid $CaSO_4$ forms, this leaves less $Ca^{+2}(aq)$ in solution.

if, given $Na_3PO_4$, the $PO_4^{-3}$ reacts with $Ca^{+2}(aq)$ to form $Ca_3(PO_4)_2$ which has a $K_{sp} = 1.3 \times 10^{-32}$ and is very insoluble, this removes $Ca^{+2}(aq)$ from the solution which causes the reaction to shift to the right, this causes more of the $CaSO_4$(s) to dissolve and this results in more $SO_4^{-2}$(aq) in solution.

## 3.10.2    QUESTIONS TO REVIEW SOLUBILITY

(1)  Fifty grams of sugar are dissolved in enough water (approximately 168 ml) to make 200 ml of solution. The percent composition of sugar in solution in terms of gms/ml is:

(a) 40%    (b) 0.25%    (c) 2.5%    (d) 25%

(2)  The density of the sugar solution in question #1 in gms/ml (assume water weighs 1 gm/ml) is:

(a) 0.8    (b) 1.00    (c) 1.05    (d) 1.09

(3)  What weight of salt is in 50 mls of solution with a density of 1.05 gms/ml? Assume the volume is due mostly to water and water weighs 1 gm/ml.

(a) 1.05    (b) 2.5    (c) 3.25    (d) 5.0

(4)  A gas mixture contains 84g of $N_2$ (N=14), 64g of $O_2$ (O=16), and 10g of $H_2$ (H=1). What is the mole fraction of $O_2$ in this mixture?

(a) 0.4    (b) 0.3    (c) 0.2    (d) need more information

(5)  A solution is made by dissolving 23g of ethyl alcohol ($C_2H_5OH$; C = 12, O = 16, H = 1) in 500 mls of water. Water has a density of 1 gm/ml. What is the molality of ethyl alcohol?

(a) 0.25    (b) 0.5    (c) 1.0    (d) none of the above

(6)  Seventy-five grams of $Na_2CO_3$ (Na = 23), C = 12, O = 16) are dissolved in enough water to make 1 liter of solution. What is the molarity of the solution?

(a) 1.1    (b) 1.0    (c) 0.71    (d) none of the above

(7)  One-hundred milliliters of a 2M solution of $H_2SO_4$ contains how many moles of $H_2SO_4$?

(a) 0.2    (b) 2    (c) 200    (d) none of the above

(8)  A 3M solution of $H_3PO_4$ (all H's react) contains how many equivalents of $H_3PO_4$ in 500 mls?

(a) 1    (b) 2    (c) 6    (d) none of the above

(9)  What weight of NaCl (Na = 23, Cl = 35) would be required to make 2 liters of a 1.5F solution?

(a) 174    (b) 116    (c) 58    (d) none of above

226

(10) How many mls will need to be added to 500 mls of a 1.5M solution in order to make a 1.0M solution:

(a) 100 mls
(c) 5000 mls

(b) 250 mls
(d) none of the above

$\frac{x}{500} = 1.5$

$x = 750$

(11) Given the following data:

| Ion | Radius (A) | Charge |
|-----|-----------|--------|
| Li | 0.68 | +1 |
| K | 1.33 | +1 |
| Cs | 1.67 | +1 |

Which ion would <u>most likely</u> have the largest hydration shell in solution?

(a) $Li^+$    (b) $K^+$    (c) $Cs^+$    (d) cannot be predicted

Use the following information for Questions #16 through #19. (The numbers are $K_{sp}$'s)

$BaSO_4...1 \times 10^{-10}$
$PbS.....7 \times 10^{-29}$
$PbCO_3...2 \times 10^{-13}$
$Ag_2S....1 \times 10^{-51}$
$HgS.....3 \times 10^{-53}$

$BaF_2....2 \times 10^{-6}$
$PbSO_4...1 \times 10^{-8}$
$AgCl....3 \times 10^{-10}$
$FeS.....1 \times 10^{-19}$

(12) If a saturated solution of $Cu(OH)_2$ contains $[Cu^{+2}] = 3.4 \times 10^{-7}$ and $[OH^-] = 6.8 \times 10^{-7}$ the $K_{sp}$ is:

(a) $8.2 \times 10^{-21}$
(c) $4.6 \times 10^{-13}$

(b) $1.6 \times 10^{-19}$
(d) none of the above

$[3.4 \times 10^{-7}][6.8 \times 10^{-7}]^2$

$\begin{matrix} 68 \\ \underline{68} \\ 544 \\ 408 \\ \hline 46.24 \end{matrix}$

$\begin{matrix} 14+7 \\ \end{matrix}$

$\begin{matrix} 3.4 \\ \underline{\times 10} \\ 13.8 \times 10 \end{matrix}$ 79

(13) A saturated solution of $Cu(IO_3)_2$ is $3.0 \times 10^{-3}$ moles/liter (m). The $K_{sp}$ is:

$[3.0 \times 10^{-3}][6 \times 10^{-3}]^2$

(a) $6 \times 10^{-6}$
(c) $9 \times 10^{-9}$

$\begin{matrix} 36 \\ \underline{3} \\ 108 \end{matrix}$

(b) $2.7 \times 10^{-8}$
(d) none of the above

(14) A saturated solution of $BaSO_4$ contains what concentration of $Ba^{+2}$?

(a) $2 \times 10^{-10}$
(c) $0.5 \times 10^{-10}$

(b) $1 \times 10^{-5}$
(d) none of the above

(15) If enough $Na_2SO_4$ is added to a saturated solution of $PbSO_4$ to make the total $[SO_4^{-2}] = 2 \times 10^{-2}M$, how much $[Pb^{+2}]$ is in solution?

$[Pb][SO_4] = \frac{1 \times 10^{-8}}{2 \times 10^{-2}}$  0.5

(a) $2 \times 10^{-16}$
(c) $5 \times 10^{-7}$

(b) $1 \times 10^{-4}$
(d) none of the above

3.10.3    <u>ANSWERS TO QUESTIONS IN SECTION 3.10.2</u>

(1 ) d    (2) d    (3) b    (4) c    (5) c    (6) c    (7) a
(8 ) d    (9) a    (10) b    (11) a    (12) b    (13) d    (14) b
(15) c

QUESTION #1    (Answer:   d)

$$\% = \frac{\text{weight of solute}}{\text{volume of solution}} \times 100 = \frac{50}{200} \times 100 = \frac{50}{2} = 25\%.$$

QUESTION #2    (Answer:   d)

$$\text{density} = \frac{\text{total mass of solution}}{\text{total volume of solution}} = \frac{\text{weight of sugar + weight of water}}{\text{total volume of solution}}$$

$$= \frac{50+168}{200} = \frac{218}{200} = \frac{25}{20} = \frac{5}{4} = 1.09 \text{ gms./ml.}$$

QUESTION #3    (Answer:   b)

$$\text{density (d)} = \frac{\text{total weight (w)}}{\text{total volume (v)}}$$

$$d = \frac{w}{v}$$

w = (v)(d) = (50 mls)(1.05 gm/ml) = 52.5 gms total
w = total weight = weight of salt + weight of water
    weight of water = (1gm/ml)(50 mls) = 50 gms
    52.5 = weight of salt + 50
    weight of salt = 2.5 gms.

QUESTION #4    (Answer:   c)

$$X_{O_2} = \frac{n_{O_2}}{n_{O_2}+n_{N_2}+n_{H_2}} = \frac{2}{2+3+5} = \frac{2}{10} = 0.2$$

$$n_{O_2} = \frac{\text{weight}}{\text{GMW}} = \frac{64}{32} = 2; \; n_H = \frac{10}{2} = 5; \; n_H = \frac{84}{28} = 3$$

QUESTION #5    (Answer:   c)

$$m = \frac{\text{moles of solute}}{\text{kg's of solvent}} = \frac{\frac{1}{2}}{\frac{1}{2}} = 1.0$$

$$\text{moles of } C_2H_5OH = \frac{\text{weight}}{\text{GMW}} = \frac{23}{46} = \frac{1}{2}$$

$$\text{GMW} = C_2H_5OH = 2(12) + 5(1) + 16 + 1 = 24 + 5 + 17 = 46$$

$$\text{kg's of water} = (500 \text{ mls})\left(\frac{1 \text{ gm}}{1 \text{ ml}}\right)\left(\frac{1 \text{ kg}}{1000 \text{gm}}\right) = \frac{500}{1000}\text{kg} = \frac{1}{2} \text{ kg}$$

QUESTION #6    (Answer: c)

$$m = \frac{\text{moles of solvent}}{\text{liters of solution}} = \frac{.71}{1} = 0.71$$

$$\frac{\text{moles of}}{Na_2CO_3} = \frac{\text{weight}}{\text{GMW}} = \frac{75}{106} = .71$$

$$\text{GMW of } CaCO_3 = 2(23)+12+3(16) = 52+48 = 106$$

QUESTION #7    (Answer: a)

$$\text{moles} = (M)(V) = (2)(0.1) = 0.2$$

$$V = (100\text{mls})\left(\frac{1 \text{ }\ell}{1000 \text{ mls}}\right) = \frac{100}{1000} = \frac{1}{10} = 0.1$$

QUESTION #8    (Answer:  d)

$$equivalents = (N)(V) = (9)(\tfrac{1}{2}) = 9/2 = 4.5$$
$$N = nM = (3)(3) = 9$$
$$V = (500\ mls)\left(\frac{1\ell}{1000\ mls}\right) = \frac{500}{1000} = 1/2$$

QUESTION #9    (Answer:  a) First find the number of moles that are required, then find the weight from this:

$$moles = (F)(V) = (1.5)(2) = 3$$

$$since\ moles = \frac{weight}{GMW}$$

$$weight = (GMW)(moles) = (58)(3) = 174$$
$$GMW\ of\ NaCl = 23+35=58$$

QUESTION #10    (Answer:  b)

$$M_2V_2 = M_1V_1$$

$$V_2 = \frac{M_1V_1}{M_2} = \frac{(1.5)(500)}{1.0} = 750\ mls\ is\ the\ total\ volume.$$

Then 750 - 500 = 250 mls for the added volume (pure water, e.g.).

QUESTION #11    (Answer:  a)  In general, the ion with the highest charge to volume (or radius) will be the most hydrated.  Since all the charges are the same, the ion with the smallest radius will be the most densely charged and have the greatest hydration--this is Lithium.

QUESTION #12    (Answer:  b)

$$Cu(OH)_2 \rightleftharpoons Cu^{+2}+2OH^-$$

$$Ksp = \left[Cu^{+2}\right]\left[OH^-\right]^2 = (3.4 \times 10^{-7})(6.8 \times 10^{-7})^2$$

$$\approx (3 \times 10^{-7})(7 \times 10^{-7})^2 \quad \approx (3 \times 10^{-7})(49 \times 10^{-14})$$
$$\approx (3 \times 10^{-7})(50 \times 10^{-14}) \quad \approx 150 \times 10^{-21} \approx 1.5 \times 10^{-19}$$

Note that estimation works well here.

QUESTION #13    (Answer:  d)

$$Cu(IO_3)_2 \rightleftharpoons Cu^{+2}+2IO_3^-$$

$$Ksp = \left[Cu^{+2}\right]\left[IO_3^-\right]^2$$

$$\left[Cu^{+2}\right] = amt\ dissolved = 3 \times 10^{-3}$$

$$\left[IO_3^-\right] = twice\ the\ amount\ dissolved = 2(3 \times 10^{-3}) = 6 \times 10^{-3}$$

$$Ksp = (3 \times 10^{-3})(6 \times 10^{-3})^2 = (3 \times 10^{-3})(36 \times 10^{-6}) = 108 \times 10^{-9}$$
$$= 1.08 \times 10^{-7}.$$

Notice that the options are very nearly equal and estimation might prove hazardous.

QUESTION #14    (Answer:  b)

$$BaSO_4 \rightleftharpoons Ba^{+2}+SO_4^{-2}$$

$$Ksp = \left[Ba^{+2}\right]\left[SO_4^{-2}\right]$$

$$\left[ Ba^{+2} \right] = \left[ SO_4^{-2} \right]$$

$$Ksp = 1 \times 10^{-10} = \left[ Ba^{+2} \right] \left[ Ba^{+2} \right] = \left[ Ba^{+2} \right]^2$$

$$\left[ Ba^{+2} \right] = (1 \times 10^{-10})^{\frac{1}{2}} = 1 \times 10^{-5}$$

QUESTION #15 (Answer: c)

$$PbSO_4 \rightleftharpoons Pb^{+2} + SO_4^{-2}$$

$$K_{sp} = \left[ Pb^{+2} \right] \left[ SO_4^{-2} \right] = 1 \times 10^{-8}$$

$$\left[ Pb^{+2} \right] \left[ 2 \times 10^{-2} \right] = 1 \times 10^{-8}$$

$$\left[ Pb^{+2} \right] = \frac{1 \times 10^{-8}}{2 \times 10^{-2}} = 0.5 \times 10^{-6} = 5 \times 10^{-7}$$

Note that since each $PbSO_4$ gives only one $Pb^{+2}$ per molecule, the $\left[ Pb^{+2} \right]$ in solution is the same as the amount of $PbSO_4$ that dissolves in the solution. The above is an example of the common ion in effect.

3.10.5     VOCABULARY CHECKLIST FOR SOLUBILITY

____ solvent                ____ molarity
____ solute                 ____ formality
____ solubility product     ____ ion product
____ density                ____ percent composition
____ mole fraction          ____ common ion effect
____ molality

3.10.6     CONCEPTS, PRINCIPLES, ETC. CHECKLIST FOR SOLUBILITY

____ concentration units and their use in solving problems
____ ions in solution
____ common ion effect

## 3.11    Acids and Bases


### 3.11.1    REVIEW OF ACIDS AND BASES


### 3.11.1.1    Acids and Bases

There are three common definitions of acids and bases:

(1)    Arrhenius

Substances that can dissociate into $H^+$ are acids.  Substances that can dissociate into $OH^-$ are bases.

(2)    Bronsted-Lowry

An acid is a substance that can donate $H^+$.  A base is a substance that can accept $H^+$.

(3)    Lewis

An acid is an electron pair acceptor, so it needs a vacant orbital.  A base is an electron pair donator, so it needs a free pair of electrons.

Certain acids or bases fall under one classification; others may fall under more than one.  The Bronsted-Lowry concept is stressed herein.

The strength of an acid (protic, esp.) is determined by its ability to donate protons ($H^+$).  The strength of a base is determined by its ability to accept protons.  This strength is measured by the acid (or base) dissociation constant:

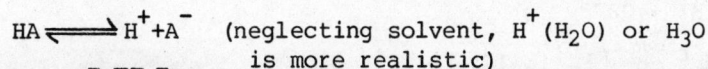

Acid
$$HA \rightleftharpoons H^+ + A^- \quad \text{(neglecting solvent, } H^+(H_2O) \text{ or } H_3O \text{ is more realistic)}$$
$$K_A = \frac{[H^+][A^-]}{[HA]} \quad \text{at equilibrium}$$

Base
$$MOH \rightleftharpoons M^+ + OH^-. \quad \text{(for hydroxy bases)}$$
$$K_B = \frac{[M^+][OH^-]}{[MOH]} \quad \text{at equilibrium}$$

The larger the $K_A$ ($K_B$), the stronger the acid (base).  The smaller the $pK_A$ ($pK_B$), the stronger the acid (base)--see below for pH.  If an acid is strong its conjugate base is weak and vice versa.  The same is true for bases and their conjugate acids.  This terminology is:

$$\underset{\text{acid}_1}{H_A} + \underset{\text{base}_2}{B} \rightleftharpoons \underset{\substack{\text{conjugate} \\ \text{base}_1}}{A^-} \quad \underset{\substack{\text{conjugate} \\ \text{acid}_2}}{HB^+}$$

A strong acid is one that dissociates completely.  A weak acid is one that dissociates incompletely.  The conjugate base (acid) of a weak acid (base) is also weak.

Salts of strong acids (bases) are neutral. Salts of weak acids or bases are basic·and acidic, respectively. This is because they hydrolyze in water; the process is hydrolysis:

a salt of a weak acid is basic

$CH_3CO_2H$ (acetic acid) is a weak acid
$CH_3CO_2^-Na^+$ (sodium acetate) is the salt
$CH_3CO_2^-Na^+ + HOH \rightleftharpoons CH_3CO_2H + Na^+ + OH^-$
        solution is basic

a salt of a weak base is acidic

$NH_4OH$ is a weak base
$NH_4Cl$ is the salt
$NH_4Cl + HOH \rightleftharpoons NH_4OH + H^+ + Cl^-$
        solution is acidic

Examples of strong acids are $H_2SO_4$, HCl, $HNO_3$, HI, HBr, $HClO_4$. Examples of weak acids are $H_2CO_3$, $H_3PO_4$ and $CH_3CO_2H$. Examples of strong bases are NaOH, KOH, LiOH and $Ca(OH)_2$. The important weak base is $NH_3$ (ammonia) or $NH_4OH$. Organic acids (Section 4.10.1) and some phenols (Section 4.9.1) may be strong or weak acids. The organic bases are amines (Section 4.11.1) and are weak.

The pH is defined as follows:

$$pH = -\log \left[ H^+ \right] = \log (1/\left[ H^+ \right])$$

$\left[ H^+ \right]$ = hydrogen ion concentration in moles/liter as molarity or normality (both are the same in this case).

The $pK_A$ and pOH are similarly defined. The pH of water solutions at 25°C range from pH = 1 to pH = 14. A pH = 7 is neutral, a pH < 7 is acid and a pH > 7 is basic. The dissociation of water is:

$$H_2O \rightleftharpoons H^+ + OH^-$$

$$K_w = \left[ H^+ \right] \left[ OH^- \right] = 10^{-14}$$

Note that $K_w$ is not the equilibrium constant. This results in this relationship:

$$pH + pOH = 14.$$

The $H^+$ of a strong acid or the $OH^-$ of a strong base can be calculated from the normality (discussed in Section 3.10.1) of the acid or base. The $H^+$ ($OH^-$) from a weak acid (base) cannot be calculated from the normality of the acid (base) because they are only partially dissociated. These problems are rigorously solved by using the equations below:

(1) $K_A = \dfrac{[H^+] [A^-]}{[HA]}$

(2) $K_w = [H^+] [OH^-]$

232

Equation (1) can be simplified if $K_A \ll [HA_o]$ (original concentration of acid), then:

$$[H^+] \approx \sqrt{K_A[HA_o]}$$

The $[H^+]$ can also be arrived at as follows:

$$HA \rightleftharpoons H^+ + A^-$$

original:          $[HA_o]$     0     0
at equililbrium:  $[HA_o]-x$    x     x    (assume negligible $H^+$
                                              from $H_2O$)

then:  $K_A = \dfrac{[H^+][A^-]}{[HA]} = \dfrac{(x)(x)}{[HA_o]-x}$

x = amount of HA that dissociates in moles/liter = $[H^+]$

The equation can be solved using the quadratic formula, or if the x is small relative to $[HA_o]$, then neglect x in the expression $[HA_o]-x$, and solve to get

$$[H^+] \approx \sqrt{K_A[HA_o]}$$

as before.

Neutralization reactions are solved using the following equation:

$N_A V_A$   $= N_B V_B$
N       = normality (see Section 3.10.1.1)
V       = volume in liters
A       = acid
B       = base.

A neutralization reaction is one in which the number of equivalents of acid is exactly neutralized by an equal number of equivalents of base.

A titration reaction is one in which a given amount of acid (base) is neutralized by a base (acid) which is added step-wise. A titration reaction may be done as follows:

   f = fraction of acid neutralized = equivalents of base added/$n_o$
   $n_o$ = original equivalents of acid
   V = original volume of acid
   v = volume of base added
   $[H^+]$(from acid and water) $= [OH^-]$ at the equivalence point

then,

$[H^+] = (n_o)(1-f)/(V+v)$ + contribution from the $H_2O$ (usually neglect
       = acid concentration at  any given point during the titration
         up to neutralization by base (f = 1.0)

     note that $(n_o)(1-f)/(V+v)$ = amount of  acid not neutralized
        by added base.

Titration reactions can be used to calculate the normality of unknown acid (base) solutions, the equivalent weights of an unknown base or acid  or the $pK_A$'s ($pk_B$'s). Examples of titration curves are in Fig. 3.12.

Fig. 3.12 – Titration Curves

Note that the curve differs for strong and weak acids, and that the $pK_A$ = pH where the acid is half neutralized.

### 3.11.1.2    Buffers

A buffer solution resists changes in pH.  This means a buffer solution is able to hold the pH of a solution relatively constant when an acid or base is added to that solution.  Buffers are mixtures of weak acids or bases and their salts.  For example:

(1)    acetic acid            sodium acetate
       $CH_3CO_2H$            $CH_3CO_2^-Na^+$

(2)    carbonic acid          sodium bicarbonate
       $H_2CO_3$              $NaHCO_3$

(3)    ammonium hydroxide   ammonium chloride
       $NH_4OH$              $NH_4Cl$

Most strong acids or bases and their salts do not make good buffers because they cannot hold the pH constant (see below).

A buffer works by having an acid component to neutralize added bases and a basic component to neutralize added acids.  This can be accomplished by using weak acids or bases and their salts.  For example:

for acetic acid-acetate buffer

$CH_3CO_2H$ combines with added base
$CH_3CO_2H + OH^- \rightleftharpoons CH_3CO_2^- + H_2O$
$CH_3CO_2^-$ combines with added acid
$CH_3CO_2^- + H^+ \rightleftharpoons CH_3CO_2H$

Hence the pH (depends on free $H^+$ or $OH^-$) is held nearly constant.

It may be obvious that it is the ratio of salt and weak acid or base that is important.

The <u>Henderson-Haselbach</u> relation points out the importance of the ratio:

$$HA + H_2O \underset{K_A}{\rightleftharpoons} H_3O^+ + A^-$$

$$K_A = \frac{[H_3O^+][A^-]}{[HA]}$$

(HA = acid and $A^-$ = salt of the acid)

solving for $[H_3O^+]$

(1) $[H_3O^+] = \left(\frac{[HA]}{[A^-]}\right)\left(K_A\right)$ OR,

(2) $pH = pK_A + \log\frac{[A^-]}{[HA]}$

(1) and (2) are equivalent expressions of the Henderson-Haselbach relation.

The <u>effectiveness of a buffer</u> can be understood in terms of this relation. The key points are:

(1)   buffers are most effective when the desired pH (of the solution) is near the $pK_A$,

(2)   ratios ($[A^-]/[HA]$) in the range of 0.1 to 10 are where buffers are effective. Note that this is because the ratio changes slowly and, thus, the pH changes slowly when the ratio

= 1 (i.e., $[A^-]$ = $[HA]$).

Important buffers in the body are:

(1) phosphates - inorganic and organic (least important)
(2) carbonic acid - bicarbonate (most important)
(3) proteins - moderate importance.

3.11.2       <u>QUESTIONS TO REVIEW ACIDS, BASES AND BUFFERS</u>

(1)   An acid is a substance that can donate hydrogen ion ($H^+$); this is a definition of acids given by:

(a) Lewis                        (b)   Arrhenius
(c) Bronsted-Lowry               (d)   none of the above

(2)   A base is an electron pair donor; this is a definition of bases given by:

(a) Arrhenius                    (b)   Bronsted-Lowry
(c) Lewis                        (d)   none of the above

(3)   The conjugate base of a weak acid (one that dissociates incompletely) is:

(a) strong          (b) weak

(4)   Given the reaction of acid (HA) and base (B) below:

$$HA + B \rightleftharpoons A^- + HB^+$$

   (a) $A^-$ is the conjugate acid of HA
   (b) $A^-$ is the conjugate base of B
   (c) $HB^+$ is the conjugate acid of B
   (d) $HB^+$ is the conjugate base of HA

(5)   The salt of a strong acid is:

   (a) basic            (b)   neutral            (c)   acidic

(6)   The salt of a weak acid is:

   (a) basic            (b)   neutral            (c)   acidic

(7)   The salt of a weak base is:

   (a) basic            (b)   neutral            (c)   acidic

(8)   Select the weak acid:

   (a) HCl       (b)   $HNO_3$       (c)   $H_2SO_4$       (d)   $CH_3CO_2H$

(9)   Select the strongest acid:

   (a) $CH_3CO_2H$       (b)   $H_3PO_4$       (c)   $H_2CO_3$       (d)   $H_2SO_4$

(10)   Select the weak base:

   (a) NaOH       (b)   KOH       (c)   $NH_3$       (d)   $Ca(OH)_2$

(11)   All of the following are important buffer systems of the body except:

   (a) carbonic acid-bicarbonate       (b)   phosphates
   (c) proteins                        (d)   nucleic acids

(12)   A buffer solution is most effective when

   (a) a strong acid or base and its salt are used;
   (b) the desired pH is near the pK of the acid or base;
   (c) the ratio of salt to acid (base) is less than 1/10 or
       greater than 10
   (d) all of the above

(13)   A buffer solution

   (a) is made of strong acids and their salts;
   (b) is made of strong bases and their salts;
   (c) resists changes in pH when acids or bases are added;
   (d) all of the above.

(14) Borane,

H
|
H—B—H

with boron having an atomic number of five and B-H bonds being relatively strong covalent bonds, is a(n):

(a) acid by Bronsted-Lowry      (b)  acid by Lewis
(c) acid by Arrhenius            (d)  base by Lewis

(15) Ammonia,

H—N—H
|
H

is a(n):

(a) acid by Bronsted-Lowry      (b)  base by Bronsted-Lowry
(c) base by Lewis               (d)  both (b) and (c)

(16) Pyruvic acid is a weak acid. Sodium hydroxide is a strong base. These are combined to form water and sodium pyruvate (a salt). If this salt is placed in water, the solution will be:

(a) basic        (b)  neutral        (c)  acidic

(17) Given the acid HA that dissociates into $H^+$ and $A^-$, the acid dissociation constant ($K_A$) is:

(a) $K_A = \dfrac{[H^+][A^-]}{[HA]}$     (b) $K_A = \dfrac{[HA]}{[H^+][A^-]}$

(c) $K_A = [HA][H^+][A^-]$     (d) $K_A = \dfrac{[HA][H^+]}{[A^-]}$

(18) Acid #1 has an acid dissociation constant ($K_{A_1}$) of $5 \times 10^{-5}$. Acid #2 has a $K_{A_2} = 9 \times 10^{-7}$:

(a) acid #1 is a weaker acid than acid #2
(b) the conjugate base of acid #1 is a weaker base than the conjugate base of acid #2
(c) both (a) and (b)
(d) neither (a) or (b)

(19) Fifty mls of a 2M solution of HCl contains how many milliequivalents of acid?

(a) 100      (b)  10      (c)  1      (d)  0.1

(20) What volume of an 0.1M acid would be required to neutralize 50 mls of an 0.3M base?

(a) about 17 mls      (b)  150 mls
(c) 300 mls           (d)  450 mls

(21) If 100 mls of a 2M solution of acid neutralizes 25 mls of a solution of base, the normality of the base is:

(a) 0.5M   (b) 2M   (c) 4M   (d) 8M

(22) Select the incorrect expression of pH ($[H^+]$ = hydrogen ion concentration):

(a) $pH = -\log [H^+]$     (b) $pH = \log [H^+]^{-1}$
(c) $pH = 1/\log [H^+]$    (d) $pH = \log(1/[H^+])$

(23) A solution has a hydroxide ion concentration of $10^{-8}$, the pH is

(a) 0   (b) 1   (c) 6   (d) 8

(24) A solution has a hydrogen ion concentration ($[H^+]$) of $2 \times 10^{-6}$; the pH is (log 2 = 0.30):

(a) 4.3   (b) 5.7   (c) 6.3   (d) 12.3

(25) A solution has a pH = 9.3. The hydrogen ion concentration is: (antilog 0.30 = 2, antilog 0.70 = 5):

(a) $5 \times 10^{-9}$   (b) $2 \times 10^{-9}$   (c) $5 \times 10^{-10}$   (d) $2 \times 10^{-10}$

(26) A solution has a pOH = 9, the hydrogen ion concentration is:

(a) $10^{-9}$   (b) $10^9$   (c) $10^5$   (d) $10^{-5}$

(27) The pH of a 0.01M solution of HCl (strong acid) is:

(a) 1   (b) 2   (c) -1   (d)  need more information

(28) Calculate the pH of a 0.001M solution of NaOH (strong base):

(a) 11   (b) 4   (c) 1   (d) 3

(29) A 0.10M solution of a monoprotic weak acid is 10% ionized, the pH is:

(a) 0.01   (b) 0.1   (c) 1   (d) 2

(30) If the $K_A$ is much less than the original concentration $HA_0$ of a _weak_ acid in solution, and $H^+$ = hydrogen ion concentration, then:

(a) $K_A \not\approx [H^+] + [HA_0]$     (b) $[H^+] \approx \sqrt{K_A [HA_0]}$
(c) $K_A \approx [H^+] / [HA_0]$     (d) $[H^+] \approx \sqrt{K_A / [HA_0]}$

(31) The acid dissociation constant ($K_A$) of a weak monoprotic acid is $4 \times 10^{-5}$. The $[H^+]$ of a 0.1M solution is:

(a) $4 \times 10^{-6}$   (b) $4 \times 10^{-5}$   (c) $2 \times 10^{-4}$   (d) $2 \times 10^{-3}$

(32) Which point (or line) on the graph below showing the titration of a weak monoprotic acid by a base represents the $pK_A$ of the acid?

fraction of acid neutralized (f)

(a) A     (b) B     (c) C     (d) D

(33) All of the following could be used to make a buffer solution except:

(a) $H_2CO_3$     (b) $H_2SO_4$     (c) $NH_4OH$     (d) $CH_3CO_2H$

(34) A buffer solution that is 0.1M in an acid (with a $pK_A=5$) and its salt which is 1.0M would have a pH of:

(a) 5.1     (b) 6     (c) 6.1     (d) 7

(35) A buffer solution with a pH = 3.3 is desired. An acid (with a $pK_A=4.3$) and its salt are available. What ratio of salt to acid is required?

(a) 10     (b) 1     (c) 1/10     (d) 1/100

3.11.3     ANSWERS TO QUESTIONS IN SECTION 3.11.2

| (1) c | (2) c | (3) b | (4) c | (5) b | (6) a | (7) c |
|---|---|---|---|---|---|---|
| (8) d | (9) d | (10) c | (11) d | (12) b | (13) c | (14) b |
| (15) d | (16) a | (17) a | (18) b | (19) a | (20) b | (21) d |
| (22) c | (23) c | (24) b | (25) c | (26) d | (27) b | (28) a |
| (29) d | (30) b | (31) d | (32) b | (33) b | (34) b | (35) c |

3.11.4     DISCUSSION OF ANSWERS TO QUESTIONS IN SECTION 3.11.2

QUESTIONS #1-#13: Adequately discussed in Section.

QUESTION #14 (Answer: b) Since the atomic number is five, the electron configuration is $1s^2\ 2s^2\ 2p^1$. Then there are only 3 bonding electrons ($2s^2\ 2p^1$) to fill the four possible bonding orbitals ($2s$, $2p_x$, $2p_y$, $2p_z$). This means there is one vacant orbital that can accept an electron pair. Lewis' definition of an acid is an electron pair acceptor. The information about the covalent bond is to suggest that the H's do not dissociate, and, therefore, the Arrhenius and Bronsted-Lowry definitions do not hold.

239

QUESTION #15 (Answer: d) Ammonia is a base by Bronsted-Lowry because it is a proton acceptor. It is also a base by Lewis because it is an electron pair donator.

QUESTION #16 (Answer: a) The reaction is,

$$pyruvic\ acid + NaOH \longrightarrow H_2O + Na\ pyruvate$$
$$Na\ pyruvate + HOH \rightleftharpoons pyruvic\ acid + Na^+ + OH^-$$

It is the free $OH^-$ in solution that makes the solution basic. Undissociated acid (e.g., pyruvic acid) has no effect on the acidity or basicity of the solution.

QUESTION #17 (Answer: a) The $K_A$ is defined as the equilibrium constant of this reaction:

$$HA \rightleftharpoons H^+ + A^-\ at\ equilibrium$$

This is given as:

$$K_A = \frac{[H^+][A^-]}{[HA]}$$

QUESTION #18 (Answer: b) The larger the $K_A$, the stronger the acid. Also, stronger acids have weaker conjugate bases (see Section for terminology). Note that $10^{-5} > 10^{-7}$, this means acid #1 is stronger than acid #2 and its conjugate base is weaker.

QUESTION #19 (Answer: a)

MV = moles                     if V = liters, M = moles/liter
MV = millimoles (mm)           if V = mls, M = mm/ml
(2mm/ml) (50 mls) = 100 mm.

QUESTION #20 (Answer: b)

$$M_A V_A = M_B V_B$$

$$V_A = \frac{M_B V_B}{M_A} = \frac{(0.3)(50)}{(0.1)} = (3)(50) = 150\ mls.$$

QUESTION #21 (Answer: d)

$$M_A V_A = M_B V_B$$

$$M_B = \frac{M_A V_A}{V_B} = \frac{(2)(100)}{(25)} = (2)(4) = 8M$$

QUESTION #22 (Answer: c) Recall that,

$$-\log x = \log x^{-1} = \log\left(\frac{1}{x}\right).$$

QUESTION #23 (Answer: c) Since,

$$K_W = [H^+][OH^-] = 10^{-14}$$

$$[H^+] = \frac{10^{-14}}{[OH^-]} = \frac{10^{-14}}{10^{-8}} = 10^{-6}$$

then:

$$pH = -\log[H^+] = -\log 10^{-6} = -(-6) = +6$$

$(\log 10^{-6} = -6$ the log of any power of 10 is the exponent).

Or:

$$pOH = -\log[OH^-] = -\log 10^{-8} = -(-8) = 8$$
$$pH + pOH = 14$$
$$pH = 14 - pOH = 14 - 8 = 6$$

QUESTION #24   (Answer:  b)

$$pH = -\log[H^+] = -\log 2 \times 10^{-6} = -(\log 2 + \log 10^{-6})$$
$$= -(0.30 - 6) = -(-5.7) = 5.7$$

Note carefully the signs above.

QUESTION #25   (Answer:  c)

$$pH = -\log[H^+]$$
$$9.3 = -\log[H^+] = \log[H^+]^{-1}$$
$$10^{9.3} = 10^{\log[H^+]^{-1}} = [H^+]^{-1} = 1/[H^+]$$
$$[H^+] = 1/10^{9.3} = 10^{-9.3} = 10^{-10+0.7} = 10^{0.7} \times 10^{-10} =$$
$$= 5 \times 10^{-10}$$

(antilog of $0.7 = 5$ or $10^{0.7} = 5$).

Study the steps carefully.  Several important log relationships are shown.

QUESTION #26   (Answer:  d)  First method:

Step (a):  $pH + pOH = 14$
$$pH = 14 - pOH = 14 - 9 = 5$$

Step (b):
$$pH = -\log[H^+]$$
$$5 = -\log[H^+]$$
$$-5 = \log[H^+]$$
$$10^{-5} = [H^+]$$

Second method,

Step (a):  $pOH = -\log[OH^-]$
$$9 = -\log[OH^-]$$
$$-9 = \log[OH^-]$$
$$10^{-9} = [OH^-]$$
Step (b):  $[H^+][OH^-] = 10^{-14}$
$$[H^+] + 10^{-14}/[OH^-] = 10^{-14}/10^{-9} = 10^{-5}$$

QUESTION #27  (Answer:  b)  The $[H^+]$ of a strong acid is the normality of the acid.  For HCl, the molarity and normality are equal.  Then:

(a)  $[H^+] = 0.01 = 1 \times 10^{-2}$

(b)  $pH = -\log[H^+] = -\log(10^{-2}) = -(-2) = 2$

QUESTION #28   (Answer:  a)  The hydroxide concentration of a strong base is its normality.  The molarity (M) is the same as normality (N) for NaOH.  Then:

(a)  $[OH^-] = 0.001 = 1 \times 10^{-3} = 10^{-3}$

(b) $[H^+][OH^-] = 10^{-14}$
$[H^+] = 10^{-14}/[OH^-] = 10^{-14}/10^{-3} = 10^{-11}$.

(c) $pH = -\log[H^+] = -\log 10^{-11} = -(-11) = 11$.

Or, the problem may be solved by:

(a) $pOH = -\log[OH^-] = -\log(10^{-3}) = -(-3) = 3$

(b) $pH + pOH = 14$
$pH = 14 - pOH = 14-3 = 11$.

<u>QUESTION #29</u>   (Answer:  d)   For the reaction given:

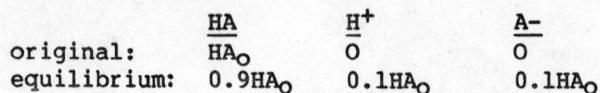

|  | HA | H$^+$ | A$^-$ |
|---|---|---|---|
| original: | $HA_O$ | O | O |
| equilibrium: | $0.9HA_O$ | $0.1HA_O$ | $0.1HA_O$ |

Then:

$$[H^+] = (0.1)(0.1) = 0.01 = 10^{-2}$$

Then:

$$pH = -\log[H^+]$$
$$= -\log(10^{-2}) = -(-2) = 2.$$

<u>QUESTION #30</u>   (Answer:  b)   This serves to point out a formula that can be used in the often met situation described in this question. It is discussed in the Section.

<u>QUESTION #31</u>   (Answer:  d)  The $[H^+]$ of a weak acid must be calculated from $K_A$.  Since $0.1 >> 4 \times 10^{-5}$,    use the formula:

$$[H^+] = \sqrt{K_A[HA_O]} = \sqrt{(4 \times 10^{-5})(10^{-1})} = \sqrt{4 \times 10^{-6}}$$
$$= \sqrt{4} \times \sqrt{10^{-6}} = 2 \times 10^{-3}$$

and:

$2 \times 10^{-3} << 10^{-1} (0.002 << 0.1)$ so the assumption is correct.  An alternative method to solve the problem is:

$$HA \rightleftharpoons H^+ + A^-$$

start:          0.1     0     0
equilibrium     0.1-x   x     x

$$K_A = \frac{[H^+][A^-]}{[HA]} = \frac{[x][x]}{[0.1-x]} = \frac{x^2}{0.1-x} = \frac{x^2}{0.1} \quad \text{(assume } x << 0.1)$$
$$4 \times 10^{-5} = x^2/10^{-1}$$
$$x^2 = (10^{-1})(4 \times 10^{-5}) = 4 \times 10^{-6}$$
$$x = \sqrt{4 \times 10^{-6}} = \sqrt{4} \times \sqrt{10^{-6}} = 2 \times 10^{-3}$$

<u>QUESTION #32</u>   (Answer:  b)   This is shown in the Section.  The $pK_A$ of an acid is the pH at which it can be half neutralized or f = 0.5.

<u>QUESTION #33</u>   (Answer:  b)  $H_2SO_4$ is a strong acid.  Strong acids or bases do not make good buffers.

242

<u>QUESTION #34</u>  (Answer:  b)   Use Henderson-Haselbach relation:

$$pH = pK_A + \log\frac{[A^-]}{[HA]} = 5 + \log\frac{1.0}{0.1} = 5 + \log 10 = 5 + 1 = 6$$

<u>QUESTION #35</u>  (Answer:  c)   Use the Henderson-Haselbach relation,

$$pH = pK_A + \log\frac{[A^-]}{[HA]}$$

$$3.3 = 4.3 + \log\frac{[A^-]}{[HA]}$$

$$-1 = \log\frac{[A^-]}{[HA]}$$

$$10^{-1} = [A^-]/[HA]$$

$$\frac{1}{10} = \frac{[A^-]}{[HA]}.$$

**3.11.5**       <u>VOCABULARY CHECKLIST FOR ACIDS AND BASES</u>

____  Arrhenius                    ____  neutralization
____  Bronsted-Lowry               ____  buffers
____  Lewis                        ____  Henderson-Haselbach
____  conjugate base              ____  titration
____  conjugate acid              ____  pH

**3.11.6**       <u>CONCEPTS, PRINCIPLES, ETC. CHECKLIST FOR ACIDS AND BASES</u>

____  definitions of acids and bases
____  strengths of acids/bases and their salts
____  definition and calculations using pH
____  titrations
____  neutralizations
____  buffer solutions and calculations

**3.12**       **Electrochemistry**

**3.12.1**       <u>REVIEW OF ELECTROCHEMISTRY</u>

Electrochemistry is the study of chemical reactions in which the reactants undergo a change in oxidation state (i.e., there is a transfer of electrons between atoms).  The <u>oxidation state</u> (OS) of an atom is a convenient bookkeeping device for keeping track of the electrons in a reaction.  The atoms do not actually possess the charge (when in a molecule) designated by the OS.  The following rules (general with exceptions) are useful for determining the OS:

(1)    all elements have an OS = 0 in the elemental form, e.g., $O_2$, Fe, Na (these can exist as ions but then they are not in the elemental form);

243

(2)   hydrogen is +1  except when combined with metals as hydrides
      (-1);

(3)   oxygen is -2 except when combined with fluorine, then it is +2,
      or in peroxides (-1), or in superoxides (-½);

(4)   Fluorine is always = -1;

(5)   Group I metals (Li, Na, K, etc.) are +1;

(6)   Group II metals (Mg, Ca, Sr, Ba) are +2;

(7)   Halogens (Cl, Br, I) are -1 unless combined with F or O;

(8)   Al = +3;

(9)   charges (not O.S.) of some common complex ions:

| | | | |
|---|---|---|---|
| $SO_4^{-2}$ | sulfate | $CO_3^{-2}$ | carbonate |
| $NO_3^{-1}$ | nitrate | $CH_3CO_2^-$ | acetate |
| $PO_4^{-3}$ | phosphate | $ClO_4^-$ | perchlorate |
| $OH^-$ | hydroxide | | |

In an oxidation-reduction reaction, one (or more) atom(s) is always
oxidized, and one (or more) atoms is always reduced. Oxidation is
the loss of electrons (or equivalently the loss of hydrogen in
organic chemistry), and reduction is the gain of electrons (or
equivalently the gain of hydrogen in organic chemistry). An
oxidizing agent is a substance that can take electrons from other
atoms and is reduced. A reducing agent is a substance that can give
electrons to other atoms and is oxidized. The overall reaction can
be divided into the oxidation half-reaction and the reduction half-
reaction, for example:

overall reaction:            $Zn + Cu^{+2} \rightleftharpoons Zn^{+2} + Cu$

oxidation half-reaction:     $Zn \rightleftharpoons Zn^{+2} + 2e$

reduction half-reaction:     $Cu^{+2} + 2e \rightleftharpoons Cu$

Note:

(1) the $e^-$ (electrons) in the oxidation (loss) half-reaction
    are on the right side (of the arrow), and for the reduction
    (gain) half-reaction they are on the left;

(2) the sum of the electrons in the balanced half-reactions
    must cancel out when added (algebraically) to get the
    overall reaction.

These half-reactions may occur at electrodes (a substance, a metal
or carbon, at which electrons may be exchanged). An anode is an
electrode that attracts the "negative" (relatively) substance, is
positive itself and is where reduction of electrode occurs and
oxidation of the solution occurs. A cathode is an electrode that
attracts the "positive" (relative to less positive) substance, is
negative itself, and is where oxidation of electrode and reduction
of the solution occurs. That is, electrons enter the anode by the
oxidation of some substance and move to the cathode where they exit
by reducing some substance. To get from the anode to the cathode
there must be a conducting connector, e.g., a wire or a salt bridge.

The capacity of one substance to give or take electrons from another substance is complex. Suffice it to say that electron affinities, ionization potentials, concentrations, pressures and temperature are all important. Fortunately, the relative ability of a substance to give or take electrons can be quantified in one number symbolized by E. E is the potential difference (or voltage, Section 5.7) that is generated when two substances are connected. This potential, when standardized, is called the <u>standard half-cell potential</u> (E°) as follows:

(1) a <u>reference half-reaction</u> is established and its $E^o = 0$,
$$2H^+(1M) + 2e^- \longrightarrow H_2(1 \text{ atm})$$
atm = atmosphere and M = molar,

(2) all other half-reactions are compared to this and the $E^o$ for each of them is determined,

(3) to be $E^o$, these standard conditions must hold:
concentration of all solutes is 1M (one molar),
pressure of all gases is 1 atm,
temperature is 25°C (298°K).

The <u>standard half-cell potential</u> ($E^o$) can be written as an oxidation half-reaction,

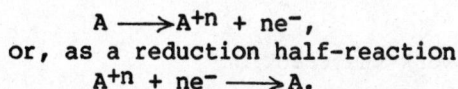

$$A \longrightarrow A^{+n} + ne^-,$$
or, as a reduction half-reaction
$$A^{+n} + ne^- \longrightarrow A.$$

The first is called an <u>oxidation cell potential</u>; the second is called a <u>reduction cell potential</u>. Usually the reduction cell potentials are used. Regardless of which one is used, the <u>interpretation</u> of $E^o$ is the same. The more positive the $E^o$, the more likely the reaction to proceed to the right as written. Please note:

(1) if the direction of the equation is reversed, the sign of $E^o$ changes to the opposite $(+ \longrightarrow -)$ or $(- \longrightarrow +)$,

(2) the value of $E^o$ <u>is not</u> affected by the stoichiometry of the reaction.

To determine the <u>potential for a reaction</u>, call it $\triangle E^o$, the appropriate $E^o$ for the half-cell reactions must be looked up, given the correct sign, and then added up. For example, given the reaction,

$$2A + B^{+2} \longrightarrow 2A^{+1} + B$$

the oxidation half-reaction (O) is,

$$(O): \quad 2A \longrightarrow 2A^{+1} + 2e^-$$

the reduction half (R) is,

$$(R): \quad B^{+2} + 2e^- \longrightarrow B.$$

Then if a table of reduction potentials is available, one will find these (in the table)

$$A^{+1} + e^- \longrightarrow A \qquad\qquad E^o = -1.10V$$
$$B^{+2} + 2e \longrightarrow B \qquad\qquad E^o = +0.50V$$

These half-reactions from the reduction potential table are rewritten as they occur (the direction) in the given reaction:

$$\text{(O):} \quad 2A \longrightarrow 2A^{+1} + 2e^- \qquad E^O = +1.10V$$
$$\text{(R):} \quad 2e^- + B^{+2} \longrightarrow B \qquad E^O = +0.50V$$

_____

$$\text{overall:} \qquad 2A + B^{+2} \longrightarrow 2A^{+1} + B \qquad \triangle E^O = +1.60V$$

Note: (1) when balancing the half-reaction, the $E^O$, is not affected as for the (O) above,

(2) when reversing the equation as found in the table, the sign of $E^O$ (from the table) is reversed as for the (R),

(3) if the overall $\triangle E^O$ is positive, then the reaction proceeds from left to right as written,

(4) if the overall $\triangle E^O$ is negative, then the reaction proceeds in the reverse direction and it should be rewritten as such.

The value of $\triangle E^O$ determines the maximal amount of work the reaction can perform. The relation is:

$$\text{work (Joules)} = (\triangle E)(q) = (\triangle E)(I)(\triangle t)$$
$$\triangle E = \text{volts} \qquad q = \text{charge in Coulombs}$$
$$I = \text{current in amperes (Coulombs/sec)}$$
$$t = \text{time in seconds.}$$

The equation is valid for electrolysis (below).

Galvanic cells produce a current and voltage internally by a chemical reaction. For example, a lead storage battery. The size of the potential, $\triangle E^O$, is as calculated by the methods above.

Concentration cells can produce a current and voltage by differences in concentrations of the same substance. The larger the concentration difference, the larger the potential produced by the cell.

Electrolysis is the process whereby electrons are pushed into a system by an external voltage, and a reaction can be forced to go in a direction it could not go spontaneously. This is one way metals may be recovered from their salts. Also, gold or silver electroplating is done this way. The key relations are:

1F (Faraday) = 96,500 Coulombs = 1 mole of electrons
(Faraday's Relation)
1 ampere of current = 1 Coulomb/sec.

These relations are used to determine how much of a metal can be plated out by a given current acting over a certain time, or they can be used to calculate the reverse.

The suggested sequence of steps to balance oxidation-reduction equations is:

(1)     identify which substance(s) is(are) oxidized and reduced in the net ionic equation,

(2)     write half-reactions for each substance oxidized and reduced,

(3)     balance each half-reaction,

(4)     add half-reactions and the electrons should cancel out (multiply each half-reaction by a small whole number as necessary),

(5)     check by counting elements on each side,

(6)     Note: for each half—reaction and the overall reaction, the charges should be equal on each side of the equation as should the mass (number of each element on each side); often $H^+$, $OH^-$, or $H_2O$ can be added as needed depending on the pH of the solution.


3.12.2          QUESTIONS TO REVIEW ELECTROCHEMISTRY

(1)     The oxidation state of an element in its elemental form is:

        (a)  +1                           (b)  O
        (c)  -1                           (d)  need electron
                                               configuration

(2)     All of the following generally have an oxidation state of +1 except:

        (a)  F      (b)  Na      (c)  H      (d)  K

(3)     All of the following generally have an oxidation state of +2 except:

        (a)  Al      (b)  Ca      (c)  Ba      (d)  Mg

(4)     Which complex ion below has a charge of -2?

        (a)  $NO_3^{-?}$                   (b)  $PO_4^{-?}$
        (c)  $ClO_4^{-?}$                  (d)  $SO_4^{-?}$

(5)     Oxidation of a molecule

        (a)  results in a gain of electrons;
        (b)  results in a more negative oxidation state;
        (c)  may be viewed as the loss of hydrogen in some cases;
        (d)  all of the above.

(6)     An oxidizing agent is a species that

        (a)  goes to a more negative oxidation state;
        (b)  gains electrons;
        (c)  is reduced;
        (d)  all of the above.

(7) In the reduction half-reaction, the electrons appear on the _____ of the equation.

    (a) right side    (b) left side    (c) either side

(8) When the oxidation and reduction half-reactions are added, the sum of the electrons is:

    (a) positive            (b) negative
    (c) zero              (d) any of the above

(9) Oxidation of the solution (or solute) occurs at the:

    (a) anode    (b) cathode    (c) neither    (d) both

(10) "Positive" substances are attracted to the:

    (a) anode    (b) cathode    (c) neither    (d) both

(11) The direction of electron flow is:

    (a) from anode to cathode
    (b) from cathode to anode
    (c) either way

(12) All the half-cell potentials ($\triangle E$) use the _____ as the reference.

    (a) hydrogen ($H_2$) half-cell
    (b) oxygen ($O_2$) half-cell
    (c) carbon (C) half-cell
    (d) arbitrarily set zero point

(13) The $\triangle E^O$ depends on all the following variables except:

    (a) temperature         (b) concentrations
    (c) pressures of gases    (d) all of the above

(14) Half-cell potentials are usually written as:

    (a) oxidation half-reactions
    (b) reduction half-reactions

(15) The more negative the value of $\triangle E^O$,

    (a) the more likely the reaction is to proceed left to right (as written);
    (b) the more likely the reaction is to proceed right to left (the reverse of the way it is written);
    (c) either of the above.

(16) If the coefficients in a half-reaction are doubled, the $\triangle E^O$ is:

    (a) doubled    (b) halved    (c) not affected

(17) If $\triangle E$ = electrical potential, I = current and $\triangle t$ = time the current is flowing, then the work (or energy) = W generated is:

    (a) $W = \dfrac{(\Delta E)(I)}{\Delta t}$         (b) $W = \dfrac{\Delta E}{(I)(\Delta t)}$

    (c) $W = (\Delta E)(I)(\Delta t)$        (d) none of the above

(18) If the potential created by a chemical reaction is used to move a current, the **cell** created is called a:

(a) concentration **cell**       (b) galvanic cell

(c) electrolytic cell       (d) none of the above

(19) One Faraday corresponds to

(a) one volt of cell potential;

(b) 96,487 amperes;

(c) one mole of electrons;

(d) all of the above.

(20) What is the oxidation state of Pt in $PtCl_4^{-2}$ ?

(a) +2     (b) -2     (c) +4     (d) -4

(21) The oxidation state of Co in $Co_3(PO_4)_2$ is:

(a) +2     (b) +3     (c) -2     (d) -3

(22) The oxidation state of Cr in $K_2Cr_2O_7$ is:

(a) +3     (b) +6     (c) +12     (d) -12

(23) The oxidation state of Fe in $FeCl_2$ is:

(a) -4     (b) -2     (c) +4     (d) +2

(24) Which of the following would be considered a reduction half-reaction?

(a) $A^{+2} + 2e^- \longrightarrow A$      (b) $A \longrightarrow A^{+2} + 2e^-$

(c) both      (d) neither

(25) The reduction half-reaction of the following reaction is:

$$A^{+2} + 2B \longrightarrow A + 2B^{+1}$$

(a) $2B \longrightarrow 2B^{+1} + 2e^-$      (b) $A \longrightarrow A^{+2} + 2e^-$

(c) $A^{+2} + 2e^- \longrightarrow A$      (d) $2B^{+1} + 2e^- \longrightarrow 2B$

(26) Suppose A and $B^{+2}$ are placed in the same solution. Will there be a spontaneous reaction? If so, what is the balanced equation? Below are the pertinent reduction potentials:

$$A^{+1} + e^- \longrightarrow A \qquad E^o = -1.50 \text{ volts}$$

$$B^{+2} + 2e^- \longrightarrow B \qquad E^o = -1.00 \text{ volts}$$

(a) no, because the $\triangle E^o$ of the reaction is negative

(b) yes, $A + B^{+2} \longrightarrow A^{+1} + B$

(c) yes, $2A + B^{+2} \longrightarrow 2A^{+1} + B$

(d) yes, $2A + B \longrightarrow 2A^{+1} + B^{+2}$

Use the following data for the remainder of the problems.

## Standard Reduction Potentials at 25°C

### Acid Solutions

| Half-Reaction | $E^O$ (volts) |
|---|---|
| $Ca^{+2} + 2e^- \longrightarrow Ca$ | -2.9 |
| $Na^+ + e^- \longrightarrow Na$ | -2.7 |
| $Al^{+3} + 3e^- \longrightarrow Al$ | -1.7 |
| $Mn^{+2} + 2e^- \longrightarrow Mn$ | -1.2 |
| $Zn^{+2} + 2e^- \longrightarrow Zn$ | -0.8 |
| $Cu^{+2} + 2e^- \longrightarrow Cu$ | +0.3 |
| $I_2(s) + 2e^- \longrightarrow 2I^-$ | +0.5 |
| $PtCl_4^{-2} + 2e^- \rightarrow Pt + 4Cl^-$ | +0.7 |
| $Ag^+ + e^- \longrightarrow Ag$ | +0.8 |
| $O_2 + 4H^+ + 4e^- \rightarrow 2H_2O(\ell)$ | +1.23 |
| $Cr_2O_7^{-2} + 6e^- \rightarrow Cr^{+3}$ | +1.33 |
| $Cl_2 + 2e^- \longrightarrow 2Cl^-$ | +1.36 |
| $MnO_4^- + 5e^- \longrightarrow Mn^{+2}$ | +1.51 |

### Equations

$$\Delta E = \Delta E^O - \frac{0.059}{n} \log \frac{[C]^c[D]^d}{[A]^a[B]^b} = \Delta E^O - \frac{0.059}{n} \log K \text{ at } 25^OC$$

(the Nernst Equation)
for $aA + bB \longrightarrow cC + dD$

note $[$ solids $] = 1$, $[$ gases $] =$ atmospheres

$\Delta E^O$ = standard cell potential
$\Delta E$ = cell potential at new set of concentrations
n = number of electrons exchanged in the reaction as written
K = equilibrium constant

$$\Delta G^O = -nF\Delta E^O \quad \text{or} \quad \Delta G = -nF\Delta E$$

F = Faraday = 23,000 cals/volt (= 96,500 Coulombs)
n = number of electrons exchanged in reaction as written
$\Delta E$ = cell potential
$\Delta G$ = free energy of reaction = cals

(27) The sum of all the coefficients in the following equation when balanced (the solution is acidic and aqueous) is:

$$Ag + NO_3^- \longrightarrow Ag^+ + NO$$

(a) 9     (b) 14     (c) 15     (d) 18

(28) The sum of all the coefficients in the following equation when balanced (solution is basic and aqueous) is:

$$N_2H_4 + Cu(OH)_2 \longrightarrow N_2 + Cu$$

(a) 8     (b) 10     (c) 12     (d) 14

(29)  The sum of all the coefficients in the following equation when balanced (solution is basic and aqueous) is:

$$ClO_2 + OH^- \longrightarrow ClO_2^- + ClO_3^-$$

(a) 5        (b) 7        (c) 9        (d) 10

Use the following information for Questions #30 to #39.

both solutions are acidic

(30)  Which substances are the reactants in the above cell assuming concentrations are all standard (1M)?

(a) $Al + Ag$                    (b) $Al^{+3} + Ag^+$
(c) $Al + Ag^+$                  (d) $Ag + Al^{+3}$

(31)  Write the balanced oxidation half-reaction of the above cell:

(a) $Ag^+ + e^- \longrightarrow Ag$          (b) $Al^{+3} + 3e^- \longrightarrow Al$
(c) $Ag \longrightarrow Ag^+ + e^-$          (d) $Al \longrightarrow Al^{+3} + 3e^-$

(32)  Reduction of the solution is occurring at the _____ electrode.

(a) Al      (b) Ag      (c) neither      (d) both

(33)  The Al electrode is _____ and is called the _____.

(a) positive, anode              (b) positive, cathode
(c) negative, anode              (d) negative, cathode

(34)  The flow of electrons is from the _____ electrode to the _____ electrode.

(a) Al, Ag                              (b) Ag, Al

(35)  The sum of coefficients in the balanced equation for the reaction is:

(a) 4        (b) 6        (c) 8        (d) 10

251

(36) The <u>standard</u> cell potential ($\Delta E^o$) for the reaction is _____ volts.

(a) −0.9    (b) 0.9    (c) 2.5    (d) 4.1

(37) Using the Nernst equation, the cell potential ($\Delta E$), in volts, at 25°C as written in #37 for $[Al^{+3}] = 0.1m$ and $[Ag^+] = 0.1m$ is:

(a) −1.14    (b) 1.14    (c) 2.46    (d) 2.10

(38) The free energy ($\Delta G$) of the reaction for the conditions, given in calories, is:

(a) +169,740                    (b) −169,740
(c) +56,580                     (d) −56,580

(39) This type of cell may be <u>best</u> considered a(n):

(a) concentration cell          (b)  galvanic cell
(c) electrolytic cell           (d)  none of these

(40) Which of the following substances will oxidize Mn?

(a) $Al^{+3}$                    (b)  Na
(c) $Zn^{+2}$                    (d)  $Ca^{+2}$

(41) Which of the following substances will reduce $I_2(s)$?

(a) Pt      (b) $Ag^+$      (c) $Cl^-$      (d) Zn

(42) Which of the following is a stronger oxidizing agent than $Cr_2O_7^{-2}$?

(a) $Cl^-$    (b) $MnO_4^-$    (c) $O_2$    (d) $Ag^+$

(43) Which of the following is a stronger reducing agent than Zn?

(a) $Cu^{+2}$    (b) $Na^+$    (c) Al    (d) Pt

(44) A current of 10 amps is passed through a solution of $Ag^+$ for one hour.  What weight of Ag (GAW = 108) will be plated out?

(a) 40.3g      (b) 22.4g      (c) 5.6g      (d) 1.2g

3.12.3      ANSWERS TO QUESTIONS IN SECTION 3.12.2

( 1)  b  ( 2)  a  ( 3)  a  ( 4)  d  ( 5)  c  ( 6)  d  ( 7)  b
( 8)  c  ( 9)  a  (10)  b  (11)  a  (12)  a  (13)  d  (14)  b
(15)  b  (16)  c  (17)  c  (18)  b  (19)  c  (20)  a  (21)  a
(22)  b  (23)  d  (24)  a  (25)  c  (26)  c  (27)  b  (28)  b
(29)  b  (30)  c  (31)  d  (32)  b  (33)  a  (34)  a  (35)  c
(36)  c  (37)  c  (38)  b  (39)  b  (40)  c  (41)  d  (42)  b
(43)  c  (44)  a

QUESTIONS #1-#19:  Adequately explained in Section.

QUESTION #20   (Answer:  a)  An equation is:

$$Pt + 4Cl = -2 \qquad (Cl = -1 \text{ from rules in section})$$
$$Pt + 4(-1) = -2$$
$$Pt - 4 = -2$$
$$Pt = +2.$$

QUESTION #21   (Answer:  a)  An equation is:

$$3\,Co + 2\,PO_4 = 0 \qquad (PO_4 = -3 \text{ from Section})$$
$$3\,Co + 2(-3) = 0$$
$$3\,Co - 6 = 0$$
$$3\,Co = +6$$
$$Co = +2$$

QUESTION #22   (Answer:  b)  An equation is:

$$2K + 2Cr + 70 = 0$$
$$2(+1) + 2Cr + 7(-2) = 0$$
$$2\,Cr - 12 = 0$$
$$2\,Cr = +12$$
$$Cr = +6$$

QUESTION #23   (Answer:  d)  The equation is:

$$Fe + 2Cl = 0$$
$$Fe + 2(-1) = 0$$
$$Fe - 2 = 0$$
$$Fe = +2.$$

QUESTION #24   (Answer:  a)  A reduction half—reaction has the electrons on the left side (so that there is a gain) as in (a).

QUESTION #25   (Answer:  c)  In the reaction as written, the $A^{+2}$ is being reduced to A:  i.e., $A^{+2} \longrightarrow A$ is a change to a more negative (less positive) oxidation state which is reduction.

QUESTION #26   (Answer:  c)  The half-reactions would be:

$$A \longrightarrow A^{+1} + e^- \qquad E^O = +1.50V \text{ (because reversed)}$$
$$B^{+2} + 2e^- \longrightarrow B \qquad E^O = -1.00V,$$

This is because A and $B^{+2}$ are the reactants given.  Then balance electrons (by multiplying half-reactions as necessary) so they sum to zero:

$$2A \longrightarrow 2A^{+1} + 2e^- \qquad E^O = +1.50V \text{ (note } E^O \text{ does not change)}$$
$$B^{+2} + 2e^- \longrightarrow B \qquad E^O = -1.0V$$

---

Sum:  $2A + B^{+2} \longrightarrow 2A^{+1} + B \quad \triangle E^O = +0.50V$

Since, the $\triangle E^O$ is positive, the reaction will occur spontaneously as written.

QUESTION #27    (Answer:  b)   Follow the scheme given in the Section:

(1)    Ag is oxidized; the N in $NO_3^-$ is reduced

$$Ag + NO_3^- \longrightarrow Ag^+ + NO$$

oxidation
states:              0      +5,-2      +1      +2,-2

(2)    (a) oxidation half–reaction

$$Ag \longrightarrow Ag^+ + e^-$$

       (b) reduction half–reaction

$$3e^- + NO_3^- \longrightarrow NO$$

(3)    (a) $Ag \longrightarrow Ag^+ + e^-$                already balanced
       (b) $NO_3^- + 3e^- \longrightarrow NO$           N's are balanced
           $4H^+ + NO_3^- + 3e^- \longrightarrow NO$     Add $H^+$ to left to balance
                                                  charge on <u>both</u> sides
           $4H^+ + NO_3^- + 3e^- \longrightarrow NO + 2H_2O$  Add $H_2O$ to right to
                                                  balance H's and O's

(4)            $3\ Ag \longrightarrow 3\ Ag^+ + 3e^-$
        $\underline{4H^+ + NO_3^- + 3e^- \longrightarrow NO + 2H_2O}$
        $4H^+ + 3Ag + NO_3^- \longrightarrow 3Ag^+ + NO + 2H_2O$
        sum of coefficients = 4 + 3 + 1 + 3 + 1 + 2 = 14

(5)    everything checks

Note that for acidic or basic solutions the $H^+$ or $OH^-$, respectively,
are usually on the left side of the equation.  Also, the balancing of
charge does not have to make the overall charge neutral but must make
the net charge on one side equal the net charge on the other.


QUESTION #28    (Answer:  b)   As in #28,

(1)    N is oxidized, Cu is reduced
       $$N_2H_4 + Cu(OH)_2 \longrightarrow N_2 + Cu$$
oxidation
states:    -2,+1    -2,-2,+1      0      0

(2)    (a) oxidation half–reaction
           $$N_2H_4 \longrightarrow N_2 + 4e^-$$             (each  N  loses  two
                                                  electrons)

       (b) reduction half–reaction
           $$2e^- + Cu(OH)_2 \longrightarrow Cu$$

(3)    balance each half–reaction

       (a) $N_2H_4 \longrightarrow N_2 + 4e^-$             N's are already balanced
           $4\ OH^- + N_2H_4 \longrightarrow N_2 + 4e^-$   Add $OH^-$ to left to
                                                  balance charge
           $4\ OH^- + N_2H_4 \longrightarrow N_2 + 4e^- + 4\ H_2O$  Add $H_2O$ to right to
                                                  balance the O's (and
                                                  H's)

(b)  $2e^- + Cu(OH)_2 \longrightarrow Cu$
      $2e^- + Cu(OH)_2 \longrightarrow Cu + 2OH^-$

Cu's are balanced balance charge by adding $OH^-$ to the right side, H's and O's are then balanced

(4)    $4OH^- + N_2H_4 \longrightarrow N_2 + 4H_2O + 4e^-$
    $4e^- + 2Cu(OH)_2 \longrightarrow 2Cu + 4OH^-$    (multiply by 2)

$N_2H_4 + 2Cu(OH)_2 \longrightarrow N_2 + 2Cu + 4H_2O$
sum of coefficients = 1 + 2 + 1 + 2 + 4 = 10.

(5)    everything checks out


QUESTION #29  (Answer: b)  Follow steps as in #27:

(1)    Cl is oxidized, Cl is reduced

        $ClO_2 + OH^- \longrightarrow ClO_2^- + ClO_3^-$

oxidation
states:    +4,−2  −2,+1    +3,−2    +5,−2

(2)    (a) oxidation half−reaction

        $ClO_2 \longrightarrow ClO_3^- + e^-$

    (b) reduction half−reaction

        $e^- + ClO_2 \longrightarrow ClO_2^-$

(3)    balance each half−reaction

    (a) $ClO_2 \longrightarrow ClO_3^- + e^-$

Cls already balanced, add $OH^-$ to left to balance charge

        $2 OH^- + ClO_2 \longrightarrow ClO_3^- + e^-$
        $2 OH^- + ClO_2 \longrightarrow ClO_3^- + H_2O + e^-$

Add $H_2O$ to right to balance O and H

    (b) $e^- + ClO_2 \longrightarrow ClO_2^-$

Cl's, O and charge are already balanced

(4)    $2 OH^- + ClO_2 \longrightarrow ClO_3^- + H_2O + e^-$
    $e^- + ClO_2 \longrightarrow ClO_2^-$

    $2OH^- + 2ClO_2 \longrightarrow ClO_2^- + ClO_3^- + H_2O$
    sum of coefficients = 2 + 2 + 1 + 1 + 1 = 7


QUESTION #30  (Answer: c)  There are four possible substances for reactants Al, $Al^{+3}$, Ag and $Ag^+$; only two can be reactants.  One will be oxidized and one will be reduced.  The candidates for oxidation are Al and Ag; the candidates for reduction are $Al^{+3}$ and $Ag^{+1}$.  Since the $\Delta E^O$ for $Al \longrightarrow Al^{+3} + 3e^-$ (+1.7) is larger than the $\Delta E^O$ for $Ag \longrightarrow Ag^+ + e^-$ (+0.8) which is larger than the $\Delta E^O$ for $Al^{+3} + 3e \longrightarrow Al$ (−1.7), the Al must be oxidized and the $Ag^+$ reduced.


QUESTION #31  (Answer: d)  From #30, the Al is oxidized to get:
        $Al \longrightarrow Al^{+3} + 3e^-$.

QUESTION #32   (Answer: b)   From #30, the Ag$^+$ is being reduced so reduction must be occurring at the Ag electrode.

QUESTION #33   (Answer: a) Oxidation is occurring at the Al electrode from #32. Oxidation occurs at the anode which is positive.

QUESTION #34   (Answer: a)  The Al electrode is losing electrons (Al$\longrightarrow$Al$^{+3}$ + 3e$^-$) which travel through the wire to the Ag electrode where they are used (Ag$^+$ + e$^- \longrightarrow$Ag).

QUESTION #35   (Answer: c)  Following the steps in the Section for balancing equations:

(1)   Al is oxidized, Ag$^+$ is reduced
$$Al + Ag^+ \longrightarrow Al^{+3} + Ag$$
oxidation
states:   0   +1      +3      0

(2)   (a) oxidation half-reaction

$$Al \longrightarrow Al^{+3} + 3e^-$$

(b) reduction half-reaction

$$e^- + Ag^+ \longrightarrow Ag$$

(3)   both are already balanced

(4)   Al $\longrightarrow$ Al$^{+3}$ + 3e$^-$
3e$^-$ + 3Ag$^+ \longrightarrow$ 3Ag      (multiplied by 3)
Al + 3Ag$^+ \longrightarrow$ Al$^{+3}$ + 3Ag
sum of coefficients = 1 + 3 + 1 + 3 = 8

(5)   everything checks

QUESTION #36   (Answer: c)  Using the balanced half-reactions from #37 and the E$^o$ from the table:

Al$\longrightarrow$Al$^{+3}$ + 3e$^-$            E$^o$ = +1.7 (sign reversed)
3e$^-$ + 3Ag$^+ \longrightarrow$ 3Ag          E$^o$ = +0.8
Sum:  Al + 3Ag$^+ \longrightarrow$ Al$^{+3}$ + 3Ag      $\triangle$E$^o$ = +2.5 volts

QUESTION #37   (Answer: c)  The Nernst equation for the balanced reaction is:

$$\Delta E = \Delta E^o - \frac{0.059}{n} \log \frac{[Al^{+3}]}{[Ag^+]^3} \approx 2.5 - \frac{0.06}{3} \log \frac{0.1}{(0.1)^3} \approx 2.5 - 0.02 \log \frac{10^{-1}}{(10^{-1})^3}$$

$$\approx 2.5 - 0.02 \log \frac{10^{-1}}{10^{-3}} \approx 2.5 - 0.02 \log 10^2$$

$$\approx 2.5 - 0.02(2) \approx 2.5 - 0.04 \approx 2.46 \text{ volts.}$$

QUESTION #38   (Answer: b)  The equation for $\triangle$G is,

$$\triangle G = -nF\triangle E = -(3)(23,000)(2.46) \approx (-3)(2.5)(23,000) \approx -(7.5)(23,000)$$
$$\approx -(7)(23,000) - (\tfrac{1}{2})(23,000) \approx -161,000 - 11,500 = -172,500 \text{ cals}$$
$$= -172.5 \text{ kcals}$$

Exact answer by calculator = -169,740 cals.

256

QUESTION #39  (Answer: b)  The voltage in this cell is generated by a chemical reaction.  The 'difference in concentrations reflect that the conditions are not standard.  The classic concentration cell would have either $Al^{+3}/Al$ or $Ag^+/Ag$ in both beakers but in different concentrations in each.

QUESTION #40  (Answer: c)  If a substance (X) oxidizes Mn, it must take electrons from it and be reduced.  The half—reactions are

$$\text{oxidation:} \qquad Mn \longrightarrow Mn^{+2} + 2e^- \qquad E^O = +1.2$$
$$\text{reduction:} \qquad X^{+n} + ne \longrightarrow X.$$

Therefore any substance will oxidize Mn if its reduction potential is greater than -1.2 volts (more positive than).  Since the reduction potentials for $Ca^{+2}$ (-2.9) and $Al^{+3}$ (-1.7) are too negative and Na cannot be reduced normally, $Zn^{+2}$ (-0.8) is the best answer.  Or any substance on the left side of the arrows below Mn will oxidize Mn.

QUESTION #41  (Answer: d)  If a substance (X) reduces $I_2(s)$, it must be oxidized in the process.  The half—reactions are:

$$\text{reduction:} \qquad I_2(s) + 2e^- \longrightarrow 2I \quad E^O = +0.5$$
$$\text{oxidation:} \qquad X \longrightarrow X^{+n} + ne^-.$$

Therefore, any substance will reduce $I_2(s)$ if its oxidation potential (reverse of that found in table) is more positive than -0.5 volts.  This makes Zn, with an oxidation potential = +0.8 volts, the only possibility given.

QUESTION #42  (Answer: b)  Since oxidizing agents are reduced, another way of asking the problem is which substance has a more positive reduction potential.  Referring to the table, $MnO_4^-$ is the only possibility.

QUESTION #43  (Answer: c)  This question can be rephrased to ask which substance has a more positive oxidation potential than Zn. This is because reducing agents are oxidized.  Remembering that the signs of the $\triangle E^O$ and the directions of the equations are reversed to get oxidation potentials, the table shows that Al is the only possibility.

QUESTION #44  (Answer: a)  This is an electrolysis problem. First, moles of electrons are determined:

$$\text{moles of electrons} = \frac{\text{charge passed}}{96,500 \text{ coulombs/mole of elec.}} = \frac{36,000}{96,500} = \frac{360}{965}$$

$$\text{charge passed} = (\text{current})(\text{time in secs}) = \text{coulombs}$$
$$= (10)(60 \times 60) = (10)(3600) = 36,000$$

Since $Ag^+ + e^+ \longrightarrow Ag$, the moles of electrons correspond to the moles of Ag plated out.  (If, e.g., one had $Ni^{+2} + 2e^- \longrightarrow Ni$, then each mole of electrons would plate out only ½ mole of Ni).  Then,

$$\text{moles of electrons} = \text{moles of AG} = \text{weight of AG/GAW of Ag}$$

and,

$$\text{weight of Ag} = (\text{moles of Ag})(\text{GAW of Ag})$$
$$= (360/965)(108) \approx (360/970)(110) \approx (3/8)(110)$$
$$\approx (3/4)(55) \approx 165/4 \approx 41.25.$$

Exact answer by calculator = 40.29.

____ reduction half-cell potential          ____ oxidation state
____ oxidation                              ____ Galvanic cells
____ reduction                              ____ concentration cells
____ oxidizing agent                        ____ electrolysis
____ reducing agent                         ____ Faraday
____ half-reactions                         ____ Coulomb
____ anode                                  ____ amperes
____ cathode                                ____ current
____ reference half-reaction                ____ standard half-cell
                                                 potential


3.12.6    CONCEPTS, PRINCIPLES, ETC. CHECKLIST FOR ELECTROCHEMISTRY

____ terminology of electrochemistry
____ writing and balancing half-reactions and electrochemical
     equations
____ determination of cell potentials
____ reactions at electrodes
____ Faraday's relation and its application


## 3.13    References for Review of General Chemistry

Mahan, B.  University Chemistry.  (Addison-Wesley Publishing Co., Inc.)

   Excellent introductory general chemistry text, but which goes
   beyond what is required for the MCAT.

Masterson, W. L., and Slowinski, E. J.  Chemical Principles.  (W. B.
   Saunders Company.)

   A good introductory text with very good problems.  Might be one
   of the best texts for review, especially in problem solving,
   for the MCAT.

Murphy, D. B., and Rousseau, V.  Foundations of College Chemistry.
   (The Ronald Press Company.)

   A very good introductory text.  More commensurate with the
   expectations of the MCAT.

# CHAPTER 4:

## REVIEW

## OF

## ORGANIC CHEMISTRY

### 4.1.1    REVIEW OF COVALENT BONDING

The major elements involved in organic compounds are carbon (C),
hydrogen (H), oxygen (O), nitrogen (N) and the halides (fluorine-F,
chlorine-Cl, bromine-Br, iodine-I).  Sulfur (S) and phosphorus (P)
are also in many organic compounds.  Carbon forms 4 bonds, N forms 3
and has one unshared pair of electrons, O forms 2 and has 2 unshared
pairs of electrons.  H forms one bond and each halogen forms one bond
and has 3 unshared pairs of electrons—all of the above are assumed
to be neutral.  The possible bonds are single bonds (SB, one shared
pair of electrons), double bonds (DB, two shared pairs of electrons)
and triple bonds (TB, three shared pairs of electrons).  C and N form
all three types, O forms DB and SB and H and the halides (in organic
compounds) form SB's only.

The C atom has one s orbital and three p orbitals in its outer
bonding electron shells.   (See Section 3.1.1).    In organic
molecules, these original atomic orbitals are recombined into hybrid
orbitals made of part s and part p.  If one s and three p's are mixed,
there result four hybrid sp³ orbitals (each consisting of one part s
and three parts p) on  the carbon  atom.   If one s orbital and two
p orbitals mix, there result three sp² orbitals  and  one  original
p orbital on each carbon atom.  If one s and one p mix, there result
two sp orbitals and two original p orbitals on each carbon.   The
geometry of each of the orbitals is: sp³-tetrahedral, sp²-triangular
and sp-linear (Fig.  4.1).

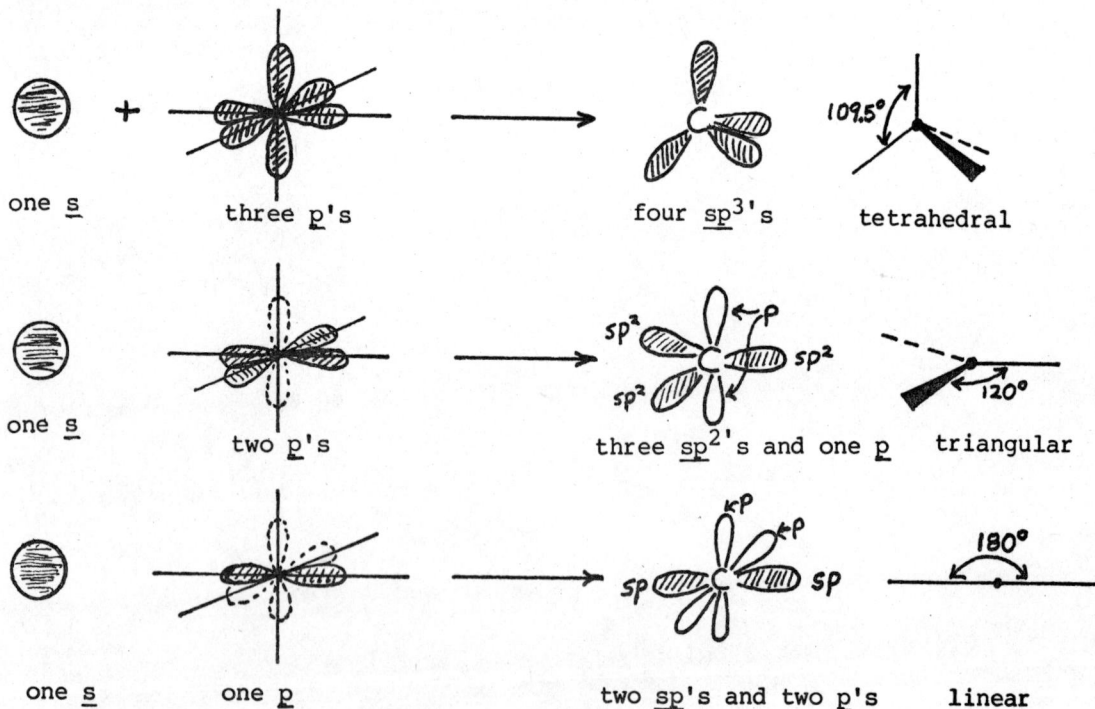

**Fig. 4.1 – Hybrid Bonding Orbitals**

<u>Sigma (σ) bonds</u> have electron density between the nuclei. Sigma bonds are formed when hybrid orbitals (sp, sp$^2$, sp$^3$) overlap directly. <u>Pi (π) bonds</u> have electron density (overlap) above and below the axis (and plane) of the atoms. They are formed by "sideways" overlap of the p orbitals. <u>Single bonds</u> are σ bonds. <u>Double bonds</u> are made of one σ bond and one π bond, <u>triple bonds</u> include one σ and two π bonds. Note that σ bonds are symmetric about the axis and can rotate freely. <u>Multiple bonds</u> (DB, TB), with π components, are not symmetric about the axis and are not free to rotate about it (Fig. 4.2).

single atoms are sp$^2$ hybridized                double bond formed

Note: the sp$^2$'s overlap between the nuclei to form the σ bond

the p's overlap above and below the axis between the C's to form a π bond

**Fig. 4.2 – Sigma and Pi Bonds**

When adjacent atoms are sp$^2$ or sp hybridized, there is the possibility of side to side overlap of the leftover p orbitals over all of these atoms. This is called delocalization of the electrons in the π bonds of the molecule. Two ways of depicting these molecules are by the molecular orbital (MO) or the valence bond (resonance) approach. The MO aproach takes a linear combination of atomic orbitals (LCAO) to form molecular orbitals which electrons go into to form bonds. These molecular orbitals cover the whole molecule, and, hence, the delocalization of electrons is depicted. In the <u>valence bond (resonance) approach</u>, there is a linear combination of different structures with localized π bonds (and unpaired electrons), which together depict the true molecule (the resonance hybrid). There is no one structure that is representative of the molecule (Fig. 4.3, on the following page).

electron density of the MO

$C_4H_6$
butadiene

MO

The atomic orbitals are rearranged to form a set of
MO's--one is shown above. Note that the MO is over
the whole molecule and π bonds and p orbitals do not
exist as such.

valence
bond

Note that no one structure represents the molecule which
is a composite of all of them. The π bonds and p orbitals
do exist in each structure above.

### Fig. 4.3 - Comparison of MO and Valence Bond Approaches

It is the valence electrons (outer shell electrons) that enter into
the formation of chemical bonds.  (See sections 3.1.1 and 3.2.1).
Electron dot structures are a means  of illustrating the valence
electrons and how they enter into bond formation.  They are used in
conjunction with the octet rule that states that a maximum of eight
electrons is possible in the outermost shell of atoms.  This rule
holds only for the second row elements (C,N,O,F).  Third row elements
(Si,P,S,Cl) can use d orbitals and, hence, can have more.  Examples
of the use of electron dot formulas:

(1) $CO_2$

C-4 valence electrons  ·Ç·
O-6 valence electrons    :Ö:
combine single electrons (may have to make double or triple
bonds)   Ö::C::Ö

(2) $CO_3^{-2}$   (an example of resonance)
C-4 valence electrons
O-6 valence electrons
-2 means two extra electrons to place on the atoms

Each element, in the final structure, counts one half the electrons
in a bond as its own and counts all unpaired electrons as its own.
The sum of these two numbers should equal the number of valence
electrons the element began with.

When atoms of differing electronegativity form the chemical bond, a
situation of charge separation exists.  For example,

electron
density

262

There is a slight pulling of electron density by the oxygen (the more electronegative) from the carbon (the less electronegative) as shown. This results in the C-O bond having <u>partial ionic character</u>. The separation of charge also causes an electrical dipole to be set up in the direction of the arrow as shown. A dipole has a positive end (the C above) and a negative end (the O above). A dipole will line up in an electric field (see Section 5.7.1). The most electronegative elements are: fluorine (4.0) > oxygen (3.5) > nitrogen (3.0) = chlorine (3.0). These are often combined with hydrogen (2.1) and carbon (2.5) and, hence result in bonds with partial ionic character. The numbers in parenthesis show electronegativities. The <u>dipole moment</u> is a measure of the charge separation and, hence, the electronegativities of the elements that make up the bond. The larger the dipole moment, the larger the charge separation.

See Section 3.11.1.1 for a discussion of Lewis acids and bases.

### 4.1.2     <u>QUESTIONS TO REVIEW COVALENT BONDING</u>

(1)    Which type of bond has electron density directly between the nuclei?

     (a) pi ($\pi$)    (b) sigma ($\sigma$)    (c) both    (d) neither

(2)    Which type of bond is formed by overlap of p orbitals perpendicular to the 2 nuclei?

     (a) pi ($\pi$)    (b) sigma ($\sigma$)    (c) both    (d) neither

(3)    Single bonds are composed of _____ bonds.

     (a) pi ($\pi$)    (b) sigma ($\sigma$)    (c) both    (d) neither

(4)    Double bonds are composed of _____ bonds.

     (a) pi ($\pi$)    (b) sigma ($\sigma$)    (c) both    (d) neither

(5)    Rotation about the bonding axis can occur with:

     (a) pi ($\pi$) bonds          (b) double bonds
     (c) both                  (d) neither

(6)    Delocalization of electrons (i.e., resonance) occurs over

     (a) sigma bonds between separated atoms;
     (b) sigma bonds on adjacent atoms;
     (c) pi bonds on adjacent atoms;
     (d) pi bonds between separated atoms.

(7)    The resonance approach implies that

     (a) one structure cannot be drawn which accurately depicts the electrons in the true molecule;

     (b) one structure can be drawn which accurately depicts the electrons in the true molecule.

(8)   The octet rule does not have to hold for which of the following elements?

(a) C      (b) O      (c) F      (d) P

(9)   An acceptable resonance form of the following ion is:

$$H-\overset{H}{\underset{H}{\overset{|}{\underset{|}{C}}}}_5-\overset{H}{\underset{H}{\overset{|}{\underset{|}{C}}}}_4-\overset{H}{\underset{3}{\overset{|}{C}}}=\overset{H}{\underset{2}{\overset{|}{C}}}-\overset{\oplus}{\underset{1}{C}}\diagdown^{H}_{H}$$

(a) $H-\overset{H}{\underset{H}{\overset{|}{\underset{|}{C}}}}_5-\overset{H}{\underset{H}{\overset{|}{\underset{|}{C}}}}_4-\overset{H}{\underset{3}{\overset{|}{C}}}=\overset{}{\underset{2}{C}}=\overset{}{\underset{1}{C}}\diagdown^{H}_{H}$

(b) $H-\overset{H}{\underset{H}{\overset{|}{\underset{|}{C}}}}_5-\overset{H}{\underset{H}{\overset{|}{\underset{|}{C}}}}_4-\overset{H}{\underset{3}{\overset{|}{C}}}=\overset{H}{\underset{2}{\overset{|}{C}}}-\overset{H\oplus}{\underset{1}{C}}\diagdown_{H}$

(c) $H-\overset{H}{\underset{H}{\overset{|}{\underset{|}{C}}}}_5-\overset{}{\underset{4}{C}}=\overset{H}{\underset{3}{\overset{|}{C}}}-\overset{H}{\underset{2}{\overset{|}{C}}}=\overset{}{\underset{1}{C}}\diagdown^{H}_{H}$

(d) $H-\overset{H}{\underset{H}{\overset{|}{\underset{|}{C}}}}_5-\overset{H}{\underset{4}{\overset{|}{C}}}-\overset{\oplus}{\underset{3}{C}}-\overset{H}{\underset{2}{\overset{|}{C}}}=\overset{}{\underset{1}{C}}\diagdown^{H}_{H}$

(10)   All of the following are acceptable resonance forms of the following ion except:

(11)   What is the electron dot formula of $H_2O$?
(Atomic numbers:  H = 1, O = 8)

(a) H:H:Ö:      (b) H:Ö:H      (c) ·H:Ö:H·      (d) Ḣ:Ḣ:Ö:

(12)   What is the electron dot formula for $SO_4^{-2}$?
(Atomic numbers:  O = 8, S = 16)

(a) :S̈:Ö:Ö:Ö:Ö:$^{-2}$

(b) Ö::S̈::Ö$^{-2}$ (with :O: above and :O: below)

(c) ⁻:Ö:Ö::S̈::Ö:Ö:⁻

(d) Ö::S̈::Ö (with :Ö:⁻ above and :Ö:⁻ below)

For the following questions use the electronegativities given in the section.

(13)   In which compound does the starred carbon have the largest partial positive charge?

(a) $H-\overset{H}{\underset{H}{\overset{|}{\underset{|}{C}}}}*-\overset{H}{\underset{H}{\overset{|}{\underset{|}{C}}}}-F$

(b) $H-\overset{H}{\underset{H}{\overset{|}{\underset{|}{C}}}}*-Cl$

(c) $H-\overset{H}{\underset{H}{\overset{|}{\underset{|}{C}}}}*-F$

(d) $H-\overset{H}{\underset{H}{\overset{|}{\underset{|}{C}}}}*-O-H$

(14) Select the following compound with the largest dipole moment:

(a) $CH_3-CH_2-CH_3$                    (b) $CH_3-CH_2-Cl$
(c) $CH_3-CH_2-OH$                      (d) $CH_3-CH_2-H$

(15) Select the compound with the largest dipole moment:

(a) $CCl_4$                             (b)
                                        Cl
                                        ⬡
                                        Cl

(c)  H       Cl                         (d)  Cl      Cl
      \C=C /                                  \C=C /
     Cl      H                              H      H

## 4.1.3    ANSWERS TO QUESTIONS IN SECTION 4.1.2

( 1) b   (2) a   (3) b   (4) c   (5) d   (6) c   (7) **a**
( 8) d   (9) d   (10) b  (11) b  (12) d  (13) c  (14) c
(15) d

## 4.1.4    DISCUSSION OF ANSWERS TO QUESTIONS IN SECTION 4.1.2

QUESTIONS #1-8:  Adequately discussed in the Section.

QUESTION #9  (Answer:  d)  Pi ($\pi$) electrons can be delocalized over charges (+ or -) and over radicals.  So, view the plus charge as if it were an adjacent p orbital ready for overlap.  Option (a) is not acceptable because an atom is displaced (the H)--resonance forms are of the same molecule, so no atoms can move.  This is also true of option (c).  Option (c) also places a p orbital on C where none existed.  Hydrogens have no p orbitals and can form only one bond so option (b) is incorrect.  Option (d) is correct which shows a simple 'shift' of the bond from $C_3-C_2$ to $C_2-C_1$.

QUESTION #10  (Answer:  b)  Options (a), (c) and (d) are arrived at by simple 'shifts' of the $\pi$ bonds around the ring.  There is no way to get the structure in option (b)--also, one carbon has five bonds.

QUESTION #11  (Answer:  b)  Oxygen has an electron configuration of $1s^2 2s^2 2p^4$, so there are 6 valence electrons (see sections 3.1.1 and 3.2.1).  The hydrogen's is $1s^1$, and it has one valence electron.  These are symbolized and combined as:

$$H\bullet + \bullet\ddot{O}\bullet + \bullet H \longrightarrow H:\ddot{O}:H.$$

Note: (1) that the single element is usually the central element, (2) single electrons are paired up, (3) the octet rule is followed for oxygen, and (4) the number of electrons that belong to each element is the same as the number of valence electrons it started with (see section discussion).

QUESTION #12  (Answer:  d)  If you thought that none of the structures accurately depicts the true $SO_4^{-2}$ ion, you are correct because resonance is possible with this structure.  The electron configurations are:

$$O = 1s^2\ 2s^2\ 2p^4 \qquad S = 1s^2\ 2s^2\ 2p^6\ 3s^2\ 3p^4.$$

The valence electrons (in the outer shell only) are:

$$O = 6 \qquad \text{and } S = 6 \text{ plus two electrons for charge } (-2).$$

The electron dot formula is:

Note: (1) The electron "pairs" on S (I⟶II) broken up to accommodate the free electron pairs of O (esp. #1 and #3). Hence, sulfur does not follow the octet rule (II, III). (2) The O's in II (i.e., #2 and #4) have one unpaired electron each; these are paired with the two extra electrons (II⟶III) to make the O's follow the octet rule. (3) An equivalent structure is,

(4) In counting up the valence electrons for each atom, remember the two extra electrons are spread out among the O's (actually the O's and the S). See Question #11 for other points.

QUESTION #13 (Answer: c) The element with the highest electronegativity is F, so this pulls the most electron density away from the C making it slightly positive. The F is more effective when attached directly to the C as in (c) than when another atom (the other C) intervenes as in (a).

QUESTION #14 (Answer: c) The reasoning is the same as in #13. The O is the most electronegative and causes the largest charge separation,

$$\underset{\delta^+ \qquad\ \delta^-}{C \longrightarrow O}$$

and, hence, the largest dipole moment.

QUESTION #15 (Answer: d) This is to point out that dipole moments are vectors (directions and magnitude) and are additive as such. The molecules in (a), (b) and (c) are all symmetric and the dipoles are opposite and equal and, hence, cancel. This is not true for (d):

no net dipole          no net dipole          no net dipole

____ sigma bonds
____ pi bonds
____ resonance
____ dipole moment

____ electron dot
structures
____ partial ionic
character

## 4.2     Stereochemistry

## 4.2.1     REVIEW OF STEREOCHEMISTRY

If two molecules have the same number and type of atoms, they are called isomers. Structural isomers have different atoms and/or bonding patterns in relation to each other. Stereoisomers differ by virtue of different spatial orientations of isomers even though the same atoms are attached to each other and the bonding patterns (i.e., location and number of single bonds, double bonds, etc, and to the same atoms) are the same. Geometric isomers are stereoisomers that differ by virtue of orientation about a double bond or ring, i.e., cis or trans isomers. Optical isomers are stereoisomers that differ by different spatial orientations about an asymmetric carbon atom (all four substituents are different) (Fig. 4.4).

STRUCTURAL ISOMERS

OPTICAL ISOMERS

GEOMETRIC ISOMERS

Fig. 4.4(a) - Isomers

and

STRUCTURAL ISOMERS

and

OPTICAL ISOMERS

and

GEOMETRIC ISOMERS

trans

cis

**Fig. 4.4(b) - Isomers**

Cis-Trans isomers can be distinguished by differences in dipole moments, melting and boiling points, chemical reactivity and spectra (UV, NMR). The number of possible geometric isomers in a molecule is $2^n$, where n = 1, 2, 3, etc., and is the number of double bonds in a molecule.

Structural and geometric isomers in general, differ in most chemical and physical properties. Optical isomers differ from each other only in the rotation of plane polarized light. Light travels as waves in all planes. Certain substances can select out one of these planes to yield plane polarized light. When this polarized light passes through an optical isomer it will be rotated in a given direction. If it is rotated clockwise, the direction is called dextrorotatory and symbolized by a d or a +. When rotation is counterclockwise, it is called levorotatory and is symbolized by an l or a -. Equal amounts of d and l together is a racemic mixture, the rotation is zero degrees. The specific rotation ($\propto$) is:

$$\propto = \frac{observed \ rotation \ in \ degrees}{(length \ of \ sample \ in \ decimeters)(concentration \ in \ gm/ml)}$$

Since the rotation depends upon the temperature, the wavelength of light used, concentration of substance, the solvent and the structure (d or l) of the molecule, these should all be specified.

Optical isomers are called enantiomers when they are non-superimposable mirror images of each other. This occurs when the absolute configuration at each asymmetric carbon is the inverse of the other. Optical isomers which are not mirror images (at one or more asymmetric carbons) are called diastereomers. The maximum number of possible optical isomers in a compound is given by,

268

$2^n$ where n = 1,2,3 = the number of asymmetric carbons (Fig. 4.5)

$$
\begin{array}{c}
CH_3 \\
H-C^*-OH \\
H_3C-C^*-OH \\
CH_2CH_3
\end{array}
$$

*the starred carbons are asymmetric
there are $2^2$ = 4 optical isomers

**Fig. 4.5(a) - Stereoisomers**

enantiomers: A & B; C & D
diastereomers: (A) & (D); (A) & (C); (B) & (C); (B) & (D).

**Fig. 4.5(b) - Stereoisomers**

A racemic mixture contains both d and l forms of an enantiomer. Since these differ only in rotation of light, it is impossible to separate them unchanged. One way of separating enantiomers is by reacting them with a second optically active compound. For example,

       A(d) and A(l) are original enantiomers
        react with B(d) to get
         A(d)-B(d) and A(l)-B(d)
       now the compounds A(d)-B(d) and A(l)-B(d) are no
       longer optical isomers and can be separated by
       chemical or physical means.

(1)    Stereoisomers, in contrast to structural isomers, have

    (a) the same number and types of atoms;
    (b) different numbers of single, double and triple bonds;
    (c) the same atoms bonded to each other;
    (d) none of the above.

(2)    Asymmetric carbons are key features of:

    (a) optical isomers        (b)  geometric isomers
    (c) structural isomers      (d)  all of the above

(3)    Cis-trans isomers can be distinguished by:

    (a) dipole moments       (b)  chemical reactivity
    (c) melting points       (d)  all of the above

(4)    Optical isomers can be best distinguished from each other by:

    (a) chemical reactivity
    (b) rotation of polarized light
    (c) melting points
    (d) all of the above

(5)    A symbol of + or _____ indicates that a molecule causes _____ rotation of polarized light.

    (a) d, counterclockwise    (b)  d, clockwise
    (c) l, counterclockwise    (c)  l, clockwise

(6)    The specific rotation of light by a substance depends upon all the following except:

    (a) concentration of substance
    (b) length of sample
    (c) wavelength of light used
    (d) refractive index of substance

(7)    Enantiomers are:

    (a) geometric isomers
    (b) racemic
    (c) optically inactive
    (d) nonsuperimposable mirror images

(8)    If n is the number of asymmetric carbons in a compound, the number of optical isomers possible is:

    (a) $n^2$    (b) $2^n$    (c) 2n    (d) 4n

(9)    A racemic mixture

    (a) is composed of geometric isomers;
    (b) rotates plane polarized light;
    (c) contains equal amounts of enantiomers;
    (d) contains equal amounts of diastereomers.

(10) The components of a racemic mixture may be separated (resolved) by:

(a) precipitation        (b) distillation
(c) hydrolysis         (d) none of the above

(11) How many structural isomers does $C_5H_{12}$ have?

(a) 1    (b) 2    (c) 3    (d) 4

(12) Select the structural isomer of the following compound:

$$CH_3-CH_2-\overset{\overset{\displaystyle O}{\|}}{C}-CH_3$$

(a) H₃C / C=C / CH₂-OH (with H substituents)

(b) cyclic: O bridging CH₂ CH₂ over HC=CH

(c) $CH_3-CH_2-CH_2-O-CH_3$

(d) $CH_3-\underset{OH}{CH}-\underset{OH}{CH}_2-CH_3$ (OH OH on CH₃-CH₂-CH₂-CH₃)

(13) Select the geometric isomer of the following compound:

H₃C-CH₂ and CH₂-Cl on one carbon; C=C; CH₃ and Cl

(a) H₃C-CH₂ / C=C \ Cl ; CH₃ / \ CH₂-Cl

(b) H₃C-CH₂ / C=C \ CH₂Cl ; Cl / \ CH₃

(c) H₃C-CH₂ / C=C \ Cl ; ClCH₂ / \ CH₃

(d) CH₃ / C=C \ Cl ; CH₃-CH₂ / \ CH₂Cl

(14) Select the geometric isomer of the following compound:

(a)  (ring structure with O, OH, OH)

(b) HO— ... —OH (ring structure with O)

(c) (ring structure with OH, OH)

(d) (ring structure with OH, O)

(15) In #14 select the compound(s) that is(are) optical isomer(s) of the given compound:

(a)      (b)      (c)      (d)

(16) In #14 select the compound(s) that is(are) structural isomer(s) of the given compound:

(a)      (b)      (c)      (d)

271

(17) Ten gms of a compound are placed in 2 mls of $H_2O$ in a sample cylinder 10 cms long. The observed rotation of light is -15°, the specific rotation (for Na light and 25°C) is:

    (a) -3°     (b) -0.3°    (c) +5°    (d) none of these

(18) The substance in #17 is:

    (a) dextrorotatory               (b) levorotatory

(19) Which of the labeled carbon(s) in the following compound is(are) asymmetric?

    (a) 1,5     (b) 2,4    (c) 2,3,4    (d) 3 only

(20) How many optical isomers does the compound in #19 have?

    (a) 2    (b) 4    (c) 6    (d) 8

(21) An enantiomer of the following compound is

valine (an amino acid)

(d) none of the above

4.2.3       ANSWERS TO QUESTIONS IN SECTION 4.2.2

( 1) c  (2) a  (3) d  (4) b  (5) b  (6) d  (7) d
( 8) b  (9) c (10) d (11) c (12) a (13) a (14) b
(15) d (16) a,c (17) a (18) b (19) b (20) b (21) c

QUESTIONS #1-#10:  Adequately discussed in Section.

QUESTION #11  (Answer:  c)  The H's can be neglected and use only the carbon skeleton.  Work systematically, starting with $C_5$ then $C_4$ then $C_3$ and place the extra carbons onto these systematically:

$C_5$:        C—C—C—C—C            only possible one

$C_4$:        C—C—C—C            only possible one
              1  2  3  4

      note that the last C cannot go on $C_1$ or $C_4$ (the <u>end</u> carbons) because this gives $C_5$ again.
      and $C_2 \equiv C_3$ so only one compound is possible.

$C_3$:    ～

      C—C—C
      1  2  3

      the extra carbons can be C,C or C-C, but C-C will give either $C_4$ or $C_5$ and just duplicate prior structures.
      the C,C cannot go on $C_1$ or $C_3$.

Since the formula was $C_5H_{12}$, which is a $C_nH_{2n+2}$, there were no double bonds or rings (see Sections 4.3.1 and 4.4.1).

QUESTION #12  (Answer:  a)  The other options (b, c and d) either contain too few or too many H's or O's.

QUESTION #13  (Answer:  a)  Options (b) and (c) have atoms or groups of atoms bonded to different atoms.  Option (d) is just the original compound flipped over.  Note: (b) and (c) are structural isomers of the original compound.

QUESTION #14  (Answer:  b)  Option (b) is the CIS isomer of the compound.

QUESTION #15  (Answer:  d)  Option (d) is the mirror image of the compound:

QUESTION #16  (Answer:  a,c)  Both (a) and (c) have atoms which are attached to different atoms in contrast to (b) and (d) which are stereoisomers.

QUESTION #17  (Answer:  a)

$$\text{specific rotation} = \frac{-15^\circ}{(1)(5)} = \frac{-15^\circ}{5} = -3^\circ/dm \cdot gm/ml$$

observed rotation = $-15^\circ$

$$\text{length of sample in decimeters (dm)} = (10 \text{ cms})\left(\frac{1 \text{ dm}}{10 \text{ cms}}\right) = 1 \text{ dm}$$

$$\text{conc. in gms/ml} = \frac{10 \text{ gms}}{2 \text{ mls}} = 5 \text{ gms/ml}$$

QUESTION #18   (Answer:   b)   Negative   observed   rotation   is levorotatory.

QUESTION #19   (Answer:   b)   Only (2) and (4) are asymmetric, (1) and (5) have 3 hydrogens each; (3) has two identical groups attached:

$$H - \overset{\displaystyle OH}{\underset{\displaystyle CH_3}{C}} - OH$$

QUESTION #20   (Answer:   b)   $2^n = 2^2 = 4$.

QUESTION #21   (Answer:   c)   Only the carbon containing the $-NH_2$ is asymmetric, the rest are not asymmetric.   Then,

Mirror image = option (C)

Options (a) and (b) are rotations about the bond labelled (1) above.


4.2.5          VOCABULARY, CONCEPTS, ETC.   CHECKLIST FOR STEREOCHEMISTRY

____ isomers                           ____ dextrorotatory
____ structural isomers                ____ levorotatory
____ stereoisomers                     ____ specific rotation
____ geometric isomers                 ____ enantiomers
____ optical isomers                   ____ diastereomers
____ cis-trans isomers                 ____ racemic mixtures
____ polarized light                   ____ separation of
                                            racemers


4.3        Alkanes


4.3.1        REVIEW OF ALKANES

The basic ideas of nomenclature for alkanes will hold for more complex molecules also.   Alkanes are simple because they contain only carbon and hydrogen (also called hydrocarbons) and contain no aromatic rings.   The longest straight carbon chain is determined and is named depending upon the number of carbons:

$C_1$—meth-, $C_2$—eth-, $C_3$—prop-, $C_4$—but(a), $C_5$—pent(a), $C_6$—hex(a), $C_7$—hept(a) $C_8$—oct(a), $C_9$—non(a), $C_{10}$—dec(a).

If these carbons contain only C and H the suffix -yl is added:

$CH_3$- = methyl, $CH_3CH_2$- = ethyl, $CH_3CH_2CH_2$- = propyl, etc.

There are special names for some branched chain alkanes:

Once the longest chain is determined, the groups attached to it are numbered such that the lowest set of numbers is obtained. The side groups are placed in the molecule name in alphabetical order or in order of increasing size. The prefixes di-(two), tri-(three), tetra-(four), etc., are used when a particular group is present more than once. The suffix indicating alkanes is -ane. For example:

2,5,5,6-Tetra methyl-4-ethyl-6-isopropyl octane or 2,5,5,6,7-Pentamethyl-4,6-diethyl octane.

Alkanes (if no rings, $C_nH_{2n+2}$; and lose 2 hydrogens for each ring) may be open chains or rings. The rings are named for the number of carbons that make them up:

cyclo-propane

ethylcyclopropane

cis-1,Methyl-2-ethyl cyclopropane

cyclobutane

cyclopentane

cyclohexane

The main chemical features are the lack of functional groupings (e.g., -OH, Br) and full saturation (no double or triple bonds). These factors cause them to be chemically unreactive except when induced by heat or light.

Physical properties of alkanes are fairly straightforward. Because they are nonpolar and have weak intermolecular forces, they have low boiling points and are not soluble in water. Branching makes the molecules more symmetrical and this lowers the boiling points even more, which is true for other classes of compounds as well. With increasing molecular weights, the intermolecular forces increase and the boiling point increases; this is also observed in other classes of molecules. Melting points increase as molecular weights increase. Solubility is in nonpolar solvents and not in aqueous solvents.

The main reactions of alkanes are combustion and substitution (radical) reactions:

(1)    Combustion

$$C_nH_{2n+2}+O_2 \text{ (excess)} \xrightarrow{\text{flame}} nCO_2+(n+1)H_2O$$

(2)    Substitution (radical)

$$CH_3CH_3+Cl_2 \xrightarrow{\text{light}} CH_3CH_2Cl+HCl$$

also get di, tri, etc. substitutions.

The mechanism is:

(a) initiation - production of radicals de novo, e.g. from heat or ultraviolet light
$Cl_2 \longrightarrow 2Cl\cdot$

(b) propagation - generation of radicals by radicals
$Cl\cdot +CH_3-CH_3 \longrightarrow CH_3-CH_2\cdot +HCl$
$CH_3-CH_2\cdot +Cl_2 \longrightarrow CH_3-CH_2Cl+Cl\cdot$

(c) termination - reaction of radicals with radicals
$Cl\cdot +CH_3-CH_2\cdot \longrightarrow CH_3-CH_2-Cl$
$CH_3-CH_2\cdot +CH_3-CH_2\cdot \longrightarrow CH_3-CH_2-CH_2-CH_3$

Chain reactions will result when one intermediate adds to a molecule producing another radical which can react further, and then this repeats itself:

$CH_3-CH_2 + H_2C{=}CH_2 \rightarrow CH_3-CH_2-CH_2-CH_2 + H_2C{=}CH_2 \rightarrow CH_3-CH_2-CH_2-CH_2-CH_2-CH_2$, etc.

Radicals result from homolytic cleavage of chemical bonds:

$$X-Y \longrightarrow X\cdot + Y\cdot$$

Note that each species is neutral (if begun neutral), and that each has a free unpaired electron. Because of the free unpaired electron, radicals are paramagnetic. Most radicals are very unstable and react rapidly. The stability of radicals depends on the ability to delocalize the free electron. Remember that benzene rings and allylic double bonds can delocalize electrons readily:

benzyl    allylic    tertiary($3^0$) secondary($2^0$) primary($1^0$) methyl.

The smaller the number of carbons in a ring, the less stable the ring is. This is due to <u>ring strain</u> of the bonding orbitals. The usual angle between bonds is $109.5^0$ in the $sp^3$ hybridized carbon. The expected bond angles in the following ring compounds are:

cyclopropane    cyclobutane    cyclopentane    cyclohexane    chair
                                                normal angles

The ring strain is very high in cyclopropane. This makes cyclopropane as reactive with $H_2, Br_2$ as alkenes are (see 4.4.1). Cyclobutane relieves some of the ring strain by assuming a bent conformation,

Cyclopentane is puckered to relieve the strain,

Cyclohexane has no strain in the chair form as shown. Cyclobutane is fairly reactive, but cyclopentane or cyclohexane are not.

4.3.2    QUESTIONS TO REVIEW ALKANES

(1) Alkanes tend to have _____ boiling points because they are _____ and, hence, have _____ intermolecular forces.

   (a) low, nonpolar , weak    (b) high, polar, strong
   (c) low, polar, weak        (d) high, nonpolar , strong

(2) Alkanes are _____ in water because they are _____.

   (a) soluble, polar          (b) insoluble, polar
   (c) soluble, nonpolar       (d) insoluble, nonpolar

277

(3) Branching tends to make an alkane more _____ and this _____ the boiling point.

(a) symmetric, lowers      (b) symmetric, raises
(c) asymmetric, lowers      (d) asymmetric, raises

(4) The step in which radicals react with radicals is:

(a) termination      (b) propagation
(c) initiation      (d) none of these

(5) Of the following radicals, in general, the most stable is:

(a) allylic      (b) primary
(c) secondary      (d) tertiary

(6) Which ring has the greatest ring strain?

(a) cyclohexane      (b) cyclopentane
(c) cyclobutane      (d) cyclopropane

(7) Which of the following rings has no ring strain?

(a) cyclohexane      (b) cyclobutane
(c) cyclopropane      (d) none of the above

(8) Name the following compound:

(a) 2-Isopropyl pentane      (b) 2,3 Dimethylpentane
(c) 3,4-Dimethyl pentane      (d) none of the above

(9) Name the following compound:

(a) 2,4,8-Trimethyl-2-ethyl-5-isopropylnonane    (b) diisoprene
(c) 3,3,5,9-Tetramethyl-6-isopropyldecane    (d) none of the above

(10) Give the structure of 2,6-Dimethyl-4-ethyloctane:

278

(11) Name the following compound:

(a) cis-1-Methyl-2-ethylcyclopropane   (b) 2,3-Methylpentane
(c) trans-Dimethylcyclopropane   (d) none of the above

(12) What is the structure of trans-1-Ethyl-4-t-butylcyclohexane?

(a)

(b)

(c)

(d) none of the above

(13) Which compound probably has the higher boiling point?

$$CH_3-CH_2-CH_2-CH_2-CH_3$$
(I)

$$CH_3-CH(CH_3)-CH_2-CH_3$$
(II)

(a) I   (b) II   (c) both equal

(14) Which compound probably has the higher boiling point?

$$CH_3-CH_2-CH_3$$
(I)

$$CH_3-CH_2-CH_2-CH_2-CH_3$$
(II)

(a) I   (b) II   (c) both equal

(15) How many $CO_2$'s are produced by the complete combustion of 3,3-Diethylhexane?

6 + 2 + 2

(a) 10   (b) 8   (c) 6   (d) 4

(16) Which of the following radicals is the most stable?

(a)

(b) $CH_3-C(CH_3)(CH_3)\cdot$

(c) $CH_3-CH(CH_3)$

(d) $CH_3$

(17) The removal of which H will result in the most stable radical in the following compound?

$$CH_3 - \underset{\underset{\text{(II)}}{H}}{\overset{\overset{CH_2-H \text{ (I)}}{|}}{C}} - \underset{\underset{\text{(III)}}{H}}{\overset{CH_3}{\overset{|}{CH}}} - CH_2-H \text{ (IV)}$$

(a)   I      (b)   II      (c)   III      (d)   IV

(18)   The formula for an <u>alkane</u> is $C_4H_8$. Therefore, this compound:

        (a)  is a straight chain        (b)  is branched
        (c)  contains a ring           (d)  none of these

## 4.3.3      ANSWERS TO QUESTIONS IN SECTION 4.3.2

( 1)  a   (2)  d   (3)  a   (4)  a   (5)  a   (6)  d   (7)  a
( 8)  b   (9)  c  (10)  b  (11)  d  (12)  b  (13)  a  (14)  b
(15)  a  (16)  a  (17)  b  (18)  c

## 4.3.4      DISCUSSION OF ANSWERS TO QUESTIONS IN SECTION 4.3.2

<u>QUESTIONS #1-#7</u>:  Adequately discussed in Section.

<u>QUESTION #8</u>   (Answer:  b)   The numbering is:

$$C_1 - \underset{\underset{C}{|}}{\overset{\overset{C}{|}}{C_2}} - C_3 - C_4 - C_5$$

<u>QUESTION #9</u>   (Answer:  c)   The numbering is,

<u>QUESTION #10</u>   (Answer:  b)   Study answer and options given.

<u>QUESTION #11</u>   (Answer:  d)   The correct answer is trans-1-Methyl-2-ethylcyclopropane.

<u>QUESTION #12</u>   (Answer:  b)   Study the answer and options given.

<u>QUESTION #13</u>   (Answer:  a)   Compound (II) is more branched than (I) and has a lower predicted boiling point.

<u>QUESTION #14</u>   (Answer:  b)   Compound (II) has the higher molecular weight and the higher predicted boiling point.

QUESTION #15 (Answer: a) The structure is,

$$CH_3-CH_2-\underset{\underset{CH_2CH_3}{|}}{\overset{\overset{CH_2-CH_3}{|}}{C}}-CH_2-CH_3$$

The formula is: $C_{10}H_{22}$.

The equation is: $C_{10}H_{22} + \frac{31}{2} O_2 \longrightarrow 10\ CO_2 + 11\ H_2O$

QUESTION #16 (Answer: a) Given in Section.

QUESTION #17 (Answer: b) The resulting radicals would be:

$$CH_3-\underset{\underset{H}{|}}{\overset{\overset{\bullet CH_2}{|}}{C}}-CH_2-CH_3 \quad (1^O)$$
(I)

$$CH_3-\overset{\overset{CH_3}{|}}{\underset{\underset{\bullet}{|}}{C}}-CH_2-CH_3 \quad (3^O)$$
(II)

$$CH_3-\overset{\overset{CH_3}{|}}{CH}-\underset{\bullet}{CH}-CH_3 \quad (2^O)$$
(III)

$$CH_3-\overset{\overset{CH_3}{|}}{CH}-CH_2-\overset{\bullet}{CH_2} \quad (1^O)$$
(IV)

Then the $3^O$ radical (II) is the most stable.

QUESTION #18 (Answer: c) Since the compound is an alkane, there are no double or triple bonds. One would expect $C_4H_{10}$ for a fully saturated alkane without rings. The two missing H's ($C_4H_8$) suggest the presence of one ring.

4.3.5    VOCABULARY, CONCEPTS, ETC.    CHECKLIST FOR ALKANES

____ nomenclature of alkanes
____ meth-, methyl
____ eth-, ethyl
____ prop-, propyl
____ but(a)-, butyl
____ pent(a)-, pentyl
____ hex(a)-, hexyl
____ hept(a)-, heptyl
____ oct(a)-, octyl
____ non(a)-, nonyl
____ dec(a)-, decyl
____ stability of radicals

____ isobutyl
____ sec-butyl
____ tert-butyl
____ cyclopropane
____ cyclobutane
____ cyclopentane
____ cyclohexane
____ combustion reactions
____ physical properties
      of alkanes
____ radical reactions
____ isopropyl
____ ring strain

4.4.1     REVIEW OF ALKENES

See Section 4.2.1 for cis-trans isomerism.  See Section 4.3.1 for basic points on nomenclature.  See Section 4.1.1 for composition of the double bond.

Alkenes (if no ring, $C_nH_{2n}$) have the double bond as the functional group.  For each double bond, the molecule loses two hydrogens from the alkane formula of $C_nH_{2n+2}$.  The only addition to the nomenclature as discussed in 4.3.1 is that the double bond(s) is(are) numbered in the molecule.  Again try to get the smallest possible number(s) for the double bonds:

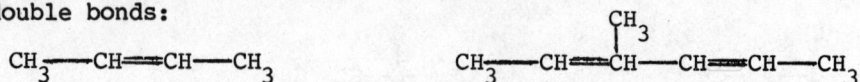

$$CH_3\!\!-\!\!CH\!\!=\!\!CH\!\!-\!\!CH_3 \qquad\qquad CH_3\!\!-\!\!CH\!\!=\!\!\overset{\overset{\textstyle CH_3}{|}}{C}\!\!-\!\!CH\!\!=\!\!CH\!\!-\!\!CH_3$$

  2-Butene                              3-Methyl-2,4-hexadiene

Nearly all of the chemistry of alkenes can be understood in terms of the double bond and its key feature of attack by electrophiles (partial or complete positively charged substances seeking out electron rich substances) with the resulting carbonium ions (positive charges on carbon):

(I)

E = electrophile       carbonium        Nu = nucleophile
                          ion              (see below)

The other key feature of the double bond is its ability to stabilize carbonium ions, or radicals which are on adjacent carbons:

(II)
   carbonium ion

   carbanion

   radical

   All are resonance stabilized (Section 4.1.1)

The stability of the intermediate carbonium ion as shown in (I) above depends on the groups (G) attached which can stabilize or destabilize it.  In general, groups which can share electrons by $\pi$ orbital overlap (resonance) stabilize the carbonium ion (as the double bond in (II) above).  In general, groups which place a positive (partial or total) charge adjacent to the carbonium ion withdraw electrons inductively (by sigma bonds) to destabilize it (see electronegativity in Section 4.1.1).  (Fig. 4.6).

$$G-\overset{|}{\underset{|}{C}}\oplus$$

G = stabilizes = O, N, benzyl, allyl, $CH_3$- or alkyls
benzyl ~ allyl>$3^O$>$2^O$>$1^O$ in terms of stability

benzyl

allyl

$$CH_3-\overset{CH_3}{\underset{CH_3}{\overset{|}{\underset{|}{C}}}}\oplus \qquad 3^O$$

$$CH_3-\overset{H}{\underset{CH_3}{\overset{|}{\underset{|}{C}}}}\oplus \qquad 2^O$$

$$CH_3-\overset{H}{\underset{H}{\overset{|}{\underset{|}{C}}}}\oplus \qquad 1^O$$

G = destabilizes = carbonyl, alkyl halide

carbonyl

alkyl halide

### Fig. 4.6 – Stability of Carbonium Ions

The above points are useful in predicting which carbon (1 or 2 in (I) above) will become the carbonium ion and which one the E and Nu will bond to. The intermediate carbonium ion formed must be the most stable. Markownikoff's rule is a sequel to this: the nucleophile (a molecule with a free pair of electrons and sometimes a negative charge that seeks out partially or completely positive charge species) will be bonded to the most substituted carbon (fewest hydrogens attached) in the product, or equivalently, the electrophile will be bonded to the least substituted (most hydrogens attached) carbon in the product. An example:

$H^+$ = electrophile      $Br^-$= nucleophile
$C_1$ = most substituted C,   $C_2$ = least substituted C
$C_1$ forms the most stable carbonium ion.

The _physical properties_ of alkenes are similar to the alkanes (Section 4.3.1). One difference is that alkenes may be polar due to cis-trans isomers and to the nature of the double bond itself (an electron withdrawer):

has a small
dipole moment

has no dipole
moment

small dipole
moment

no dipole
moment

Also trans compounds tend to have higher melting points (due to better symmetry) but lower boiling points (due to less polarity) than the corresponding cis compounds (see Sections 3.4.1 and 3.5).

(1)    The general formula for an alkene with one double bond and no rings is:

(a) $C_nH_{2n-2}$     (b) $C_nH_{2n+2}$     (c) $C_nH_n$     (d) $C_nH_{2n}$

(2)    Select the most stable carbonium ion:

(3)    Select the most unstable carbonium ion:

(4)    Although alkanes and alkenes are both composed of carbon and hydrogen, alkenes may show _____ due to _____.

(a) hydrogen bonding, the double bond
(b) less reactivity, double bond
(c) polarity, cis-trans isomerism
(d) none of the above

(5)    Name the following compound:

(a) 2-Ethyl-trans-6-octene     (b) 6-Ethyl-trans-2-octene
(c) 2-Ethyl-cis-6-octene       (d) 6-Ethyl-cis-2-octene

(6) Give the structure for 3,4 Dimethyl—cis—2—trans-4-heptadiene:

(d) none of the above

284

(7) A double bond can stabilize an adjacent carbonium ion by
_____ (of) the positive charge with its ____-bond.

(a) neutralizing, $\pi$       (b) neutralizing, $\sigma$
(c) delocalization, $\pi$      (d) delocalization, $\sigma$

(8) The reaction of $H^+$ with the following compound will form which carbonium ion:

(a)                (b)

(c)                (d) none of these

(9) The product of the following reaction is:

(a)                (b)

(c)                (d)

(10) Which compound has the higher boiling point?

(I)                (II)

(a) I      (b) II      (c) both equal

(11) Which compound has the higher dipole moment?

(I)                (II)

(a) I      (b) II      (c) both equal

**4.4.3**   ANSWERS TO QUESTIONS IN SECTION 4.4.2

( 1)  d   (2)  c   (3)  a   (4)  c   (5)  b   (6)  b   (7)  c
( 8)  b   (9)  d   (10)  b  (11)  a


**4.4.4**   DISCUSSION OF ANSWERS TO QUESTIONS IN SECTION 4.4.2

QUESTIONS #1 to #4, #7:  Adequately discussed in Section.

QUESTION #5   (Answer:  b)  The numbering is,

QUESTION #6   (Answer:  b)  Study correct answer vs. other options.

QUESTION #8   (Answer:  b)  The only possible cations from this double bond are (a) which is $2^O$ and (b) which is $3^O$.  Tertiary ($3^O$) is more stable than secondary ($2^O$).

QUESTION #9   (Answer:  d)  The mechanism is,

This carbonium ion is more stable than the alternate because of the adjacent brominated carbons,

QUESTION #10   (Answer:  b) Cis-compounds tend to have higher boiling points because of higher polarity than the corresponding trans compound.

QUESTION #11   (Answer:  a)  See #10 and discussion in Section.


**4.4.5**   VOCABULARY, CONCEPTS ETC.   CHECKLIST FOR ALKENES


____  carbonium ions
____  stability of carbonium ions
____  dipole moments of alkenes
____  nomenclature of alkenes
____  physical properties of alkenes

## 4.5    Benzene

### 4.5.1    REVIEW OF BENZENE

Many monosubstituted benzenes have special names or they can be named by the substituent attached:

Benzene    Phenol    Toluene    Aniline    Nitrobenzene    Benzoic Acid

Disubstituted benzenes can be named as a derivative of the primary substituent with numbers or the o-p-m system:

o=ortho
m=meta
p=para

o-Nitrotoulene    m-Dinitrobenzene

2-methyl-4-Hydroxybenzoic acid     m-Methylaniline, or m-Aminotoluene     2,4,6-Trinitro-toluene

Tri and higher substituted benzenes require the numbering system as above.

The benzene ring is a set-up for resonance delocalization of charges (Section 4.1.1):

The key reaction of the benzene ring is the addition and eventual substitution of an electrophile ($E^+$, see Section 4.4.1) for a hydrogen (H) which requires stabilization of the intermediate positive charge:

This stabilization of the intermediate positive charge is affected

greatly by the substituents attached to the ring.   Two types of
substituents are identified.   One group directs substituents to the
ortho-para positions (o-p directors), and the other type directs
substituents to the meta positions (meta directors):

<u>o-p directors</u> (e.g., -OH, -NH$_2$, -OR, -NR$_2$, alkyls)

--note the electron density is at the o-p positions so the E$^+$
   favors attack at o-p positions,
--with a substituent (E$^+$) at ortho or para get good
   stabilization:

--with a substituent at meta:

the -OH can no longer help delocalize the positive charge so
the o-p is favored over the meta.

<u>meta directors</u>  (e.g. -NO$_2$, -SO$_2$-, -CN)

--without a substituent:

notice that + charge is put at the o-p positions so the E$^+$
favors attack at meta position

--with a substituent at meta positions:

--with a substituent at o-p position:

resonance form III is useless because of the adjacent positive charge; analogous situations exist with the other meta directors also; so, meta substitution is favored.

### 4.5.2     QUESTIONS TO REVIEW BENZENE

(1)  Name the following compound:

    (a) o-Chlorotoluene           (b) p-Chloromethylbenzene
    (c) l-Methyl-2-chlorobenzene   (d) none of the above

(2)  Name the following compound:

    (a) p-Dichlorobenzene       (b) m-Dichlorobenzene
    (c) 1,3-Dichlorobenzene      (d) none of the above

(3)  Give the structure of 2-Chloro-4-Iodonitrobenzene:

(a)

(b)

(c)

(d) none of the above

(4)  Given the following compound, give the positions which will have the most electron density due to delocalization:

   (a) 1,3,5     (b) 3,4,5     (c) 2,5     (d) none of these

(5)    Given the following compound, give the positions which will
       have the most electron density due to delocalization:

       (a) 3,5      (b) 2,4,6      (c) 3,4,5      (d) none of these

(6)    If $Br^+$ is an electrophile (e.g., from $Br_2$ + $AlCl_3$), the most
       likely product of its reaction with the following compound is:

       (a)          (b)          (c)          (d) none of these

(7)    Assume the $Br^+$ from #6 reacts with the following compound, the
       most likely product is:

       (a)          (b)          (c)          (d) none of these

4.5.3      ANSWERS TO QUESTIONS IN SECTION 4.5.2

(1)  d   (2)  a   (3)  c   (4)  d   (5)  a   (6)  c   (7)  c

4.5.4      DISCUSSION OF ANSWERS TO QUESTIONS IN SECTION 4.5.2

QUESTION #1  (Answer: d)  The  correct  name  is  m-Chlorotoluene
(others also possible).

QUESTIONS #2 - #5:  Are adequately discussed in the Section.

QUESTION #6 (Answer: c) The -O-CH₃ is an o-p director. Of the products given (c) is the most likely. This para-product is also favored over the ortho product because of steric (bulk) considerations.

QUESTION #7 (Answer: c) The -NO₂ is a meta director.


## 4.5.5 VOCABULARY, CONCEPTS, ETC.: CHECKLIST FOR BENZENE

✓ nomenclature of benzene
✓ resonance of benzene
✓ reactions of benzene


## 4.6 Alcohols


## 4.6.1 REVIEW OF ALCOHOLS

See Section 4.3.1 for the basics of nomenclature. Alcohols are named by replacing the -e of the corresponding alkane with -ol for simple alcohols:

| | | | |
|---|---|---|---|
| $CH_4$ | $CH_3OH$ | $CH_3CH_2CH_3$ | $CH_3CH_2CH_2OH$ |
| methane | methanol | propane | propanol |
| | (methyl alcohol) | | (propyl alcohol) |

The use of sec-, iso-, and tert- are also appropriate:

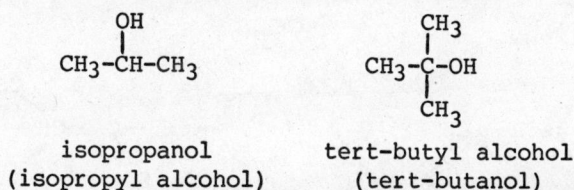

$$CH_3-\underset{\overset{|}{OH}}{CH}-CH_3$$

$$CH_3-\underset{\overset{|}{CH_3}}{\overset{\overset{CH_3}{|}}{C}}-OH$$

isopropanol                tert-butyl alcohol
(isopropyl alcohol)         (tert-butanol)

For more complex alcohols, the numbering system is used and the carbon with the -OH should, in general, have the lowest number (if the compound is named as an alcohol):

$$CH_3-CH_2-CH_2-\underset{\overset{|}{CH_3}}{CH}-CH_2-\underset{\overset{|}{OH}}{CH}-CH_2-C\begin{smallmatrix}CH_3\\CH_3\end{smallmatrix}$$

2,6-Dimethyl-4-nonanol

$$CH_3CH_2\underset{\overset{|}{OH}}{CH}CH_2CH_3$$

3-Pentanol

Alcohols are acidic because of the -OH group:

$$\underset{\delta^-}{\overset{|}{C}}-\underset{\delta^+}{O-H} \rightleftharpoons -\overset{|}{C}-O^{\ominus} + H^{\oplus}$$

They are very weakly acidic, being less strong than water. As the number

291

of carbon groups attached to the C increases, the acidity decreases:

$$CH_3OH > CH_3CH_2OH \quad \text{in acidity}$$

CH_3CH_2OH > CH_3—CH(H)—OH > CH_3—C(CH_3)(CH_3)—OH   in acidity
      1°              2°                  3°

See Section 4.3.1 for general comments on <u>physical properties</u> of organic compounds. The greater polarity (dipole moment) and, especially, hydrogen bonding account for the greater solubility of alcohols in water, and the higher boiling points than comparable alkanes, alkenes, aldehydes, ketones and alkyl halides. As the carbon chain gets longer this nonpolar hydrocarbon chain overshadows the -OH group and alcohols become less soluble in water.

The three major types of reactions of alcohols are dehydration, oxidation and substitution.

The <u>dehydration reaction</u> is,

alcohol $\xrightarrow[{-H_2O}]{+H^{\oplus}}$ $\xrightarrow{-H^{\oplus}}$ alkene

An intermediate carbonium ion is formed, and the faster reactions occur with the molecules that form the most stable carbonium ions (Section 4.4.1). The alkene formed is the most stable. Note that a phenyl group ( ⬡— ) takes preference over 1 or 2 alkyl groups. Otherwise, the most substituted (i.e., most alkyl groups) double bond is the most stable:

in rate of reaction

The <u>substitution reactions</u> are usually the replacement of the -OH by a halide (usually Cl or Br) using a variety of reagents (HCl, HBr, $PCl_3$). In the most common mechanism, an intermediate carbonium ion is formed; so, the fastest reacting molecules are those with the most stable carbonium ion (Section 4.4.1). The 1° alcohols, especially, require vigorous conditions and/or the addition of extra reagents such as $ZnCl_2$ or $H_2SO_4$ to make the reaction go. Examples:

$$H_2C = CH - CH_2 - OH \xrightarrow{\text{HCl}} H_2C = CH - CH_2 - Cl$$
$$(I)$$

$$CH_3 - CH_2 - \underset{\underset{CH_3}{|}}{\overset{\overset{CH_3}{|}}{C}} - OH \xrightarrow{\text{HBr}} CH_3 - CH_2 - \underset{\underset{CH_3}{|}}{\overset{\overset{CH_3}{|}}{C}} - Br$$
$$(II)$$

$$CH_3CH_2CH_2OH \xrightarrow[\Delta]{\text{HCl, ZnCl}_2} CH_3CH_2CH_2 - Cl$$
$$(III)$$

$$(I) > (II) > (III) \quad \text{in rate of reaction.}$$

Oxidation reactions can convert alcohols to aldehydes, ketones or carboxylic acids depending upon the structure of the alcohol ($1^O$ or $2^O$) and upon the reaction conditions. Primary ($1^O$) alcohols may be converted to carboxylic acids (Section 4.10.1) or aldehydes (Section 4.7.1):

$$R - CH_2 - OH \xrightarrow[H^{\oplus}]{\text{KMnO}_4 \text{ or K}_2\text{Cr}_2\text{O}_7} R - \overset{\overset{O}{\|}}{C} - OH$$
$$\text{carboxylic acid}$$

$$R - CH_2 - OH \xrightarrow[\Delta]{\text{CuO}} R - CHO \bullet$$
$$\text{aldehyde}$$

A secondary ($2^O$) alcohol is converted to a ketone (Section 4.7.1):

$$R - \underset{\underset{R'}{|}}{\overset{\overset{H}{|}}{C}} - OH \xrightarrow{\text{any of the above}} R - \underset{R'}{\overset{}{C}} = O \quad \text{Ketone}$$

Note that tertiary ($3^O$) alcohols are not oxidized under basic conditions but may be oxidized under acidic conditions by being dehydrated first and then by the double bond being oxidized.

Substitution reactions may be further separated into $S_N1$ and $S_N2$. The $S_N1$ (Substitution Nucleophilic Monomolecular) mechanism is:

$$R - L \xrightarrow{\text{slow}} R^{\oplus} + L^{\ominus}$$

$$Nu^{\ominus} + R^{\oplus} \xrightarrow{\text{fast}} Nu - R$$

for reactions above: R = carbon group, L = -OH, $Nu^- = Cl$, e.g.

The key features of the $S_N1$ are

(1)  the rate depends on $[R-L]$,
(2)  there is racemization of configuration (4.2.1),
(3)  a stable carbonium ion should be formed,
     benzyl $\approx$ allyl $>$ $3^O$ $>$ $2^O$ $>$ $1^O$ in terms of rate.

Note the benzyl, allyl, $3^O$ and $2^O$ alcohol substitutions are by this mechanism. The $S_N2$ (Substitution Nucleophilic Bimolecular) mechanism is:

$$Nu^{\ominus} + R - L \longrightarrow [Nu \ldots R \ldots L] \longrightarrow NuR + L^{\ominus}$$
$$\text{(symbolism as before).}$$

293

The key features of $S_N2$ are:

(1)    rate depends on $[R-L]$ and $[Nu^-]$.
(2)    there is inversion of configuration (the opposite enantiomer is formed) (Section 4.2.1) if the alcohol was optically active to begin with,
(3)    steric factors are important and not carbonium ions:

$$CH_3- \, > 1^O > 2^O \gg 3^O \quad \text{in terms of rate.}$$

So, the substitutions for $CH_3OH$ and $1^O$ alcohols are by the $S_N2$ mechanism.


### 4.6.2    QUESTIONS TO REVIEW ALCOHOLS

(1)    Alcohols have _HIGH_ boiling points and _HIGH_ solubility in water than corresponding alkanes and alkenes which is due to _H-BONDING_ .

   (a) lower, lesser, hydrogen bonding
   (b) higher, greater, hydrogen bonding
   (c) lower, lesser, polarity
   (d) none of these

(2)    In the dehydration reaction of alcohols, the _____ stable double bond is formed.

   (a) most                          (b) least

(3)    Which of the following alcohols undergoes a substitution reaction the fastest?

   (a) primary                       (b) secondary
   (c) allyl                         (d) tertiary

(4)    Which of the following types of alcohols is not normally oxidizable?

   (a) primary                       (b) secondary
   (c) tertiary                      (d) all of these are
                                         oxidizable

(5)    Which type of alcohol probably undergoes substitution by an $S_N2$ mechanism?

   (a) primary                       (b) tertiary
   (c) allyl                         (d) none of these

(6)    Name the following alcohol:

   (a) 2-Phenyl-4,4-dimethyl heptanol
   (b) 4,4 Dimethyl-6-phenyl-3-heptanol
   (c) Phenyl-2-heptanol
   (d) none of these

(7)    Select the strongest acid of the following:

(a)   $CH_3$—$\overset{\overset{\displaystyle CH_3}{|}}{CH}$—$OH$

(b)   $CH_3$—$CH_2$—$\overset{\overset{\displaystyle CH_3}{|}}{CH}$—$OH$

(c)   $CH_3$—$CH_2$—$\overset{\overset{\displaystyle CH_3}{|}}{\underset{\underset{\displaystyle CH_3}{|}}{C}}$—$OH$

(d)   $CH_3$—$CH_2$—$CH_2$—$OH$   ⟵ circled

(8)    Which alcohol is least soluble in water?

(a)   $CH_3$—$\overset{\overset{\displaystyle CH_3}{|}}{CH}$—$CH_2$—$OH$

(b)   $CH_3$—$CH_2$—$CH_2$—$CH_2$—$CH_2$—$CH_2$—$OH$   ⟵ circled

(c)   $CH_3$--$CH_2$--$OH$

(d)   $CH_3OH$

(9)    Which alcohol will be dehydrated the fastest?

(a)   [naphthalene ring]—$CH_2$—$CH_2$—$\overset{\overset{\displaystyle OH}{|}}{CH}$—$CH_3$

(b)   $CH_3$—$CH_2$—$CH_2$—$CH_2$—$\overset{\overset{\displaystyle CH_3}{|}}{\underset{\underset{\displaystyle CH_3}{|}}{C}}$—$CH_2OH$

(c)   $CH_3$—$\overset{\overset{\displaystyle CH_3}{|}}{CH}$—$CH_2$—$\overset{\overset{\displaystyle CH_3}{|}}{\underset{\underset{\displaystyle CH_3}{|}}{C}}$—$OH$   ⟵ circled

(d)   all at the same rate

(10)   What is the most likely (or greatest) product of the following reaction?

DEHYDRATION

$$CH_3-\overset{\overset{\displaystyle CH_3}{|}}{CH}-\overset{\overset{\displaystyle CH_2-CH_3}{|}}{\underset{\underset{\displaystyle OH}{|}}{C}}-CH_3 \xrightarrow{H^{\oplus}} ?$$

(a)   $\underset{H_3C}{\overset{H_3C}{>}}C=C\underset{CH_3}{\overset{CH_2-CH_3}{<}}$   ⟵ circled

(b)   $\underset{CH_3}{\overset{H_3C}{>}}CH-C\underset{CH_3}{\overset{CH-CH_3}{<}}$

(c)   $\underset{H_3C}{\overset{H_3C}{>}}CH-C\underset{CH_2}{\overset{CH_2-CH_3}{<}}$

(d)   all are equal

(11)   What is the most likely product of the following reaction:

$$CH_3-\overset{\overset{\displaystyle CH_3}{|}}{CH}-\overset{\overset{\displaystyle CH_2CH_3}{|}}{\underset{\underset{\displaystyle OH}{|}}{C}}-CH_2-[\text{ring}] \xrightarrow{H^{\oplus}} ?$$

(a)   $\underset{H_3C}{\overset{H_3C}{>}}C=C\underset{CH_2-[\text{ring}]}{\overset{CH_2CH_3}{<}}$

(b)   $\underset{CH_3}{\overset{CH_3}{>}}CH-C\underset{CH_2-[\text{ring}]}{\overset{CHCH_3}{<}}$

(c)   $\underset{CH_3}{\overset{CH_3}{>}}CH-C\underset{CH-[\text{ring}]}{\overset{CH_2CH_3}{<}}$   ⟵ circled

(d)   all are equal

**(12)  Which alcohol will undergo the fastest reaction with HBr?**

*1° slow*

(a)

HO

(b)  $CH_3CH_2OH$

(c)  $CH_3-CH$
         |        |
        $CH_3$  $OH$

(d)        $CH_2OH$

---

**4.6.3          ANSWERS TO QUESTIONS IN SECTION 4.6.2**

( 1)  b    (2)  a    (3)  c    (4)  c    (5)  a    (6)  b    (7)  d
( 8)  b    (9)  c    (10)  a   (11)  c   (12)  d


**4.6.4          DISCUSSION OF ANSWERS TO QUESTIONS IN SECTION 4.6.2**


**QUESTIONS #1 to #5:**  Adequately discussed in Section.


**QUESTION #6**  (Answer:  b)  The numbering is,

$$\text{C}-\underset{16}{\text{C}}-\underset{5}{\text{C}}-\underset{4}{\overset{\overset{\text{C}}{|}}{\text{C}}}-\underset{3}{\text{C}}-\underset{2}{\text{C}}-\underset{1}{\text{C}} \cdot$$

**QUESTION #7**  (Answer:  d)  Primary alcohols are stronger than similar $2°$ or $3°$ alcohols.

**QUESTION #8**  (Answer:  b)  The longer the carbon chain, the smaller the solubility in water.


**QUESTION #9**  (Answer:  c)  Tertiary alcohols undergo dehydration faster than the $1°$ or $2°$ alcohols shown.

**QUESTION #10**  (Answer:  a)  The most substituted double bond will be the one that is formed.


**QUESTION #11**  (Answer:  c)  The double bond will be most stable when conjugated with the benzene ring even though it is not the most substituted.

**QUESTION #12**  (Answer:  d)  Substitution reactions are faster for benzyl (shown) or allyl type alcohols.

296

_____ nomenclature of alcohols
_____ acidity of alcohols
_____ physical properties of alcohols

_____ dehydration reactions
_____ substitution reactions
_____ oxidation reactions


## 4.7    Aldehydes and Ketones


### 4.7.1    REVIEW OF ALDEHYDES AND KETONES

See Section 4.3.1 for the basics of nomenclature.  <u>Aldehydes</u> are generally symbolized as

$$R-\overset{\displaystyle O}{\overset{\|}{C}}-H,$$

and the suffix -al replaces the -e of alkanes:

$$H-\overset{\displaystyle \overset{H}{|}}{\underset{\underset{H}{|}}{C}}-\overset{\displaystyle O}{\overset{\|}{C}}-H$$

ethanal
(acetaldehyde)

$$CH_3-CH_2-\overset{\displaystyle \overset{CH_3}{|}}{CH}-CH_2-CH_2-\overset{\displaystyle O}{\overset{\|}{C}}-H$$

(6)    (5)    (4)    (3)    (2)    (1)

4-Methylhexanal
the aldehyde carbon is always #1

Ketones are generally symbolized as

$$R-\overset{\displaystyle O}{\overset{\|}{C}}-R'$$

and the suffix -one replaces the -e of alkanes:

$$CH_3-\overset{\displaystyle O}{\overset{\|}{C}}-CH_3$$

acetone <u>or</u>
2-Propanone
(the location of the $\left(\overset{\displaystyle O}{\overset{\|}{C}}\right)$
is always shown)

$$CH_3-CH_2-CH_2-\overset{\displaystyle O}{\overset{\|}{C}}-CH_2-CH_3$$

3-Hexanone <u>or</u>
Ethyl propyl ketone

The <u>carbonyl group</u>   ( $\overset{\displaystyle O}{\overset{\|}{C}}$ )   is the basis for the chemistry of aldehydes and ketones.  The key features are:

(1)    Polarity of C=O bond.  The oxygen is attacked by electrophiles (E$^{\oplus}$), and the carbon by nucleophiles (Nu:$^{\ominus}$).

Both of these disrupt the double bond:

large dipole moment

(2) The $\alpha$-hydrogen is acidic and can be abstracted by bases. It is even more acidic if between two carbonyls:

$H_2 > H_1$ in acidity

(3) The main reason for the acidity of the $\alpha$-H is that the resulting $\alpha$-carbanion is stabilized by resonance. This stabilization also allows for nucleophilic addition at the $\beta$-carbon in $\alpha$-$\beta$ unsaturated carbonyls:

resonance stabilization

carbanion

$\alpha,\beta$ unsaturated carbonyl

(4) The carbonyl exists in equilibrium with the enol form; this is tautomerization. Usually the carbonyl form predominates, but if the enol double bond can be conjugated with other double bonds, it can become very stable:

carbonyl

enol (undergoes reactions of the double bond)

(5) The O of the carbonyl forms hydrogen bonds with Hs attached to other O's or N's:

Most of the reactions and properties of carbonyls may be understood on the basis of the above features. In general, aldehydes oxidize easier and undergo nucleophilic addition easier than ketones.

The boiling point of carbonyls is higher than most other polar organic molecules but less than that of alcohols and acids (each can hydrogen bond to molecules of itself). The low molecular weight carbonyls are soluble in water because they can form hydrogen bonds with it--as the molecular weights increase, the hydrocarbon part dominates and solubility decreases.

Oxidation reactions of aldehydes are:

(1)

$$\underset{\text{(Ar)}}{\text{RCHO}} \xrightarrow[\text{(Tollen's Reagent)}]{\text{Ag(NH}_3)_2^{\oplus}} \underset{\text{(Ar)}}{\text{R-CO}_2\text{H}} + \text{Ag(mirror)}$$

Ar = Aromatic          Benedict's Reagent is also used

(2)

$$\underset{\text{(Ar)}}{\text{RCHO}} \xrightarrow[\text{(2)K}_2\text{Cr}_2\text{O}_7]{\overset{\text{(1)KMnO}_4}{\text{or}}} \underset{\text{(Ar)}}{\text{RCO}_2\text{H}}$$

(3) Ketones are rarely oxidized.

Reduction reactions of carbonyls

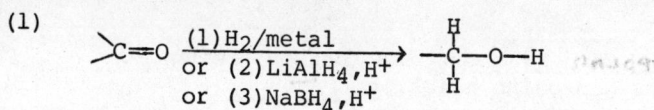

(1)

$$\text{>C=O} \xrightarrow[\text{or (3)NaBH}_4, \text{H}^+]{\overset{\text{(1)H}_2/\text{metal}}{\text{or (2)LiAlH}_4, \text{H}^+}} -\overset{\overset{\text{H}}{|}}{\underset{\underset{\text{H}}{|}}{\text{C}}}-\text{O}-\text{H}$$

Nucleophilic addition reactions (See #1 and #3 of second paragraph):

(1) Addition of nitrogen bases to carbonyls. The N needs two H's to add:

$$\text{>C=O} + \text{H}_2\text{N}-\text{R}' \longrightarrow \text{>C=N}-\text{R} \xrightarrow{\text{H}^{\oplus}} \text{>C=O}$$
Schiff base

e.g., of $\text{R}^{\angle}\text{NH}_2$

$\underset{\text{hydroxylamine}}{\text{H}_2\text{N}-\text{OH}}$     $\underset{\text{hydrazine}}{\text{H}_2\text{N}-\text{NH}_2}$     $\underset{\text{phenylhydrazine}}{\text{H}_2\text{N}-\text{N}-\bigcirc}$

$\underset{\text{semicarbazine}}{\text{H}_2\text{N}-\overset{\overset{\text{H}}{|}}{\text{N}}-\overset{\overset{\text{O}}{||}}{\text{C}}-\text{NH}_2}$     $\underset{\text{amino acids,}}{\text{R}-\overset{\overset{\text{NH}_2}{|}}{\text{C}}-\text{CO}_2\text{H}}$

(2) Acetal (Ketal) and hemiacetal (hemiketal) formation

$$\underset{\overset{\text{or}}{\text{Ketone}}}{\underset{\text{aldehyde}}{\text{>C=O}}} + \underset{\text{alcohol}}{\text{ROH}} \rightleftharpoons \underset{\overset{\text{or}}{\text{hemiketal}}}{\underset{\text{hemiacetal}}{-\overset{\overset{}{|}}{\underset{\underset{\text{OH}}{|}}{\text{C}}}-\text{O}-\text{R}}} \underset{}{\overset{\text{ROH}}{\rightleftharpoons}} \underset{\overset{\text{or}}{\text{ketal}}}{\underset{\text{acetal}}{\text{>C}\overset{\text{O-R}}{\underset{\text{O-R}}{}}}}$$

found in carbohydrate reactions,

(3) The Aldol condensation of carbonyls. The α-H is important:

$$\underset{\text{O}}{\overset{\text{C}'}{\underset{\text{(3)}}{||}}} + \underset{\text{H}}{\overset{|}{\underset{\text{(2)}}{\text{C}}}} \overset{|}{\underset{\text{(1)}}{\text{C}}} = \text{O} \xrightarrow[\text{acid}]{\text{base or}} -\overset{|}{\underset{\underset{\text{OH}}{|}}{\text{C}}}_{(3)} -\overset{|}{\underset{(2)}{\text{C}}}- \overset{\overset{\overset{\text{H}}{|}}{\text{C}}}{\underset{(1)}{}} = \text{O} \xrightarrow{\text{H}^{\oplus}} -\underset{(3)}{\overset{|}{\text{C}}} = \underset{(2)}{\overset{|}{\text{C}}} - \underset{(1)}{\overset{|}{\text{C}}} = \text{O}$$
usual product

(4) Nucleophilic addition to ∝,β-unsaturated carbonyls:

e.g., Nu:'s (do not have to be negative; need pair of electrons)

, amines, :CN.

active H's

## 4.7.2     QUESTIONS TO REVIEW ALDEHYDES AND KETONES

(1)    The carbonyl group is __POLAR__ with the carbon being
       slightly __+__ and the oxygen being slightly __−__.

       (a) polarized, negative, positive
       (b) polarized, positive, negative
       (c) neither (a) nor (b)

(2)    Which hydrogen is the most acidic?

       (a) $H_1$      (b)  $H_2$      (c)  $H_3$      (d)  $H_4$

(3)    Generally undergo   nucleophilic addition more easily:

       (a) aldehydes      (b)  ketones      (c)  both equally

(4)    Aldehydes and ketones have higher boiling points than
       corresponding compounds (similar carbon structures) of all the
       following except:

       (a) alkanes    (b)  alkenes    (c)  ethers    (d)  alcohols

(5)    Rarely oxidized:

       (a) aldehydes      (b)  ketones      (c)  neither

(6)    Name the following compound:

       (a) tert-chlorobutanal             (b)  tert-chlorobutyl
                                               ketone
       (c) hydrogen chloro-tert-butyl     (d)  3-chloro-3-methyl-
           ketone                              butanal

300

(7)  Name the following compound:

(a) 2-methyl-3-pentanone      (b) diethyl methyl ketone
(c) 2-methyl-3-butanal        (d) isobutyl ethyl ketone

(8)  Select the product of the following reaction:

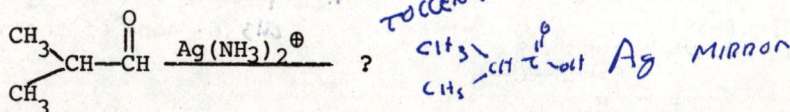

(a)

$$CH_3\text{-}CH(CH_3)\text{-}CH(OH)\text{-}CH(OH)\text{-}CH(CH_3)\text{-}CH_3$$

(b)

$$CH_3\text{-}CH(CH_3)\text{-}C(O\text{-}H)(H)$$

(c)

$$CH_3\text{-}C(CH_3)=CH_2$$

(d)

$$CH_3\text{-}CH(CH_3)\text{-}C(O)\text{-}OH$$

(9)  Select the product of the  following reaction:

$$\xrightarrow[\text{(2)} \ H^{\oplus}]{\text{(1)} \ LiAlH_4} \ ?$$

(a)

$$\text{Ph-}CH_2\text{-}CH_2\text{-}C(O)\text{-}OH \ + \ HO\text{-}C(O)\text{-}CH(CH_3)\text{-}CH_2CH_3$$

(b)

$$\text{Ph-}CH_2\text{-}CH_2\text{-}C(OH)(H)\text{-}CH(CH_3)\text{-}CH_2\text{-}CH_3$$

(c)

$$\text{Ph-}CH_2\text{-}CH_2\text{-}C(O)\text{-}H \ + \ H\text{-}C(O)\text{-}CH(CH_3)\text{-}CH_2\text{-}CH_3$$

(d) none of the above

(10)  Select the product of the following reaction:

$$CH_3\text{-}C(O)\text{-}CH_3 \ + \ \text{Ph-}NH\text{-}NH_2 \ \longrightarrow \ ?$$

(a)

$$CH_3\text{-}C(OH)(H)\text{-}CH_3$$

(b)

$$CH_3\text{-}C(CH_3)=N\text{-}NH\text{-}Ph$$

(c)

$$CH_3(H_3C)C=N\text{-}Ph(NH_2)$$

(d) none of the above

301

*(handwritten top:)* AcDol condensation

*(handwritten top right:)*
$CH_3-\overset{OH}{\underset{H}{C}}-H$

$\downarrow O4$

$CH_2=CH$

$HOH_3$  $H O4$

$CH_3-C=CH_2 \overset{H}{O}C-H$

$CH_2CH_3$

(11)    Select the product of the following reaction:

$$CH_3-\overset{O}{\overset{\|}{C}}-CH_2-CH_3 \;+\; CH_3-\overset{O}{\overset{\|}{C}}-H \;\xrightarrow{H^\oplus}\; ?$$

(a) no reaction

*(handwritten blue structure, labeled region near (b)):*
$CH_3-\overset{O}{\overset{\|}{C}}-\overset{\overset{H}{|}}{\underset{\underset{HO-\overset{|}{C}-H}{|}}{C}}\diagdown CH_3$

$CH_3$

(b)
$$CH_3-\overset{O}{\overset{\|}{C}}-\underset{\underset{CH_3}{|}}{HC}-CH_2-\overset{O}{\overset{\|}{C}}-H$$

(c) $CH_3 \diagup$
$\overset{}{\underset{H_3C-CH_2}{C}}=CH-\overset{O}{\overset{\|}{C}}-H$

(d) none of the above

---

**4.7.3        ANSWERS TO QUESTIONS IN SECTION 4.7.2**

( 1)  b   (2)  a   (3)  a   (4)  d   (5)  b   (6)  d   (7)  a
( 8)  d   (9)  b   (10)  b  (11)  c

---

**4.7.4        DISCUSSION OF ANSWERS TO QUESTIONS IN SECTION 4.7.2**

**QUESTIONS #1 to #5:**  Adequately discussed in Section.

**QUESTION #6**   (Answer:  d)  This is an aldehyde numbered as

$$C_4-\overset{\overset{\displaystyle C}{|}}{\underset{\underset{\displaystyle Cl}{|}}{C_3}}-C_2-\overset{O}{\overset{\|}{C_1}}-H.$$

**QUESTION #7**   (Answer:  a)  The numbering of this ketone is

$$\underset{C}{\overset{C_1}{}}\diagdown C_2-\overset{O}{\overset{\|}{C_3}}-C_4-C_5.$$

An alternate name is:  Ethyl isopropyl ketone

**QUESTION #8**   (Answer:  d)  This is an oxidation reaction as shown in the Section.

**QUESTION #9**   (Answer:  b)  This is a reduction reaction as shown in the Section.

**QUESTION #10**   (Answer:  b)  To add to the carbonyl, the N must have two H's (i.e., $-NH_2$).  The N attached to the benzene ring does not complete the reaction.

**QUESTION #11**   (Answer:  c)  There are many possible products of this reaction.  The key is that the $\alpha$-carbon of one carbonyl attacks the carbonyl of the other.  Other possible products are:

302

$$CH_3-CH_2-\overset{\overset{\text{O}}{\|}}{C}-CH_3 \qquad CH_3-\overset{\overset{\text{O}}{\|}}{C}-H$$
(1) (2) (3) (4)      (5) (6)

$$CH_3-CH=CH-\overset{\overset{\text{O}}{\|}}{C}-H$$
(4) (3) (5) (6)
$$(2)CH_2$$
$$(1)CH_3$$

$$\underset{(1)}{CH_3}\overset{(6)(5)}{-\underset{(2)}{C}=CH-CH_3}$$
$$(3)C=O$$
$$(4)CH_3$$

$$CH_3-CH_2-\overset{\overset{\text{O}}{\|}}{C}-CH=CH-CH_3$$
(1) (2) (3) (4) (6) (5)

(the answer given)

**4.7.5**      <u>VOCABULARY, CONCEPTS, ETC. CHECKLIST FOR ALDEHYDES AND</u>
<u>KETONES</u>

_____ nomenclature of aldehydes and ketones
_____ physical properties of aldehydes and ketones
_____ acidity of ∝-hydrogens
_____ carbanions
_____ nucleophilic addition reactions
_____ oxidation reactions
_____ carbonyl group

**4.8**      **Ethers**

**4.8.1**      <u>REVIEW OF ETHERS</u>

Ethers have the <u>general structure</u>:   R—O—R'

R, R' are aliphatic or aromatic but not H.   Ethers are named by
naming the R and R' and following these by 'ether':

$$CH_3-CH_2-O-CH_2-CH_3 \qquad CH_3-O-\underset{}{CH}\overset{CH_3}{\underset{CH_3}{<}}$$

     Diethyl ether        Methyl isopropyl ether
     (or 'ether')

The <u>physical properties</u> of ethers reflect the polar oxygen and the
nonpolar hydrocarbon component.   There is some solubility in water
due to the O hydrogen bonding with $H_2O$.   The boiling points are less
than alcohols and about the same as alkanes because there is no
hydrogen bonding between the molecules of ether.

**4.8.2**      Study the above brief section.   No questions, etc.

**4.9.1**     <u>REVIEW OF PHENOLS</u>

A phenol consists of a hydroxyl group attached to an aromatic ring. The <u>nomenclature</u> is as given in Section 4.5.1.  Some phenols which have counterparts in biochemistry and medicine are:

phenol     Cathechol     Resorcinol     Hydroquinone     Salicylic Acid

Important features of the chemistry of phenols are:

(1)     Phenols are acidic due to the dissociable hydrogen on the oxygen.  Phenols are more acidic than alcohols because of the electron withdrawing and resonance stabilization effects of the aromatic ring:

The resonance forms show that groups which stabilize electrons when placed at o-p positions should make the phenol more acidic.  Groups which can stabilize the negative charge are $-NO_2$, $-CN$, $-CO_2H$.  Groups which might tend to destabilize (and make less acidic) are alkyl groups or other o-p directors (see Section 4.5.1).

(2)     Phenols form intramolecular and intermolecular hydrogen bonds (see boiling point discussion below).

(3)     Phenols are powerful o-p directors.

<u>Physical properties</u> are understood by considering the hydrogen bond forming capacity and the hydrophobic nature of aromatic rings.  Even phenol itself is only slightly soluble in water (due to hydrogen bonding), but most other phenols are insoluble due to the aromatic ring.  Most phenols will have high boiling points, primarily due to hydrogen bonding between molecules.  Within the disubstituted phenols, the ortho compounds tend to have lower boiling points because they have the potential for intramolecular hydrogen bonding whereas meta and para have intermolecular hydrogen bonding (and higher boiling points):

ortho

intramolecular hydrogen bonding     meta (or para) intermolecular
                                    hydrogen bonding

**4.9.2**    <u>QUESTIONS TO REVIEW PHENOLS</u>

(1)    Name the following compound:

    (a) o,m-Hydroxynitrobenzene     (b)   2-Nitrophenol
    (c) o-Nitrophenol                 (d)   m-Nitrophenol

(2)    Which of the following is most acidic?

    (a) $CH_3CH_2$—OH            (b) $CH_3$—$\overset{\overset{\displaystyle CH_3}{|}}{\underset{\underset{\displaystyle CH_3}{|}}{C}}$—OH

    (c)      (d) all are probably equal

(3)    Which of the following is most acidic?

(4)    Which of the following compounds probably has the highest boiling point?

    (a) $CH_3(CH_2)_2$—$CH{=}CH_2$   (b) $CH_3$—O—$CH_3$   (c)    (d) $CH_3$—$CH_3$

(5)    Given the following two compounds

compound _____ probably has the lower boiling point because there is _____ hydrogen bonding possible.

    (a) I, intramolecular          (b)   II, intramolecular
    (c) II, intermolecular         (d)   none of these

**4.9.3**    <u>ANSWERS TO QUESTIONS IN SECTION 4.9.2</u>

(1)  d    (2)  c    (3)  d    (4)  c    (5)  a

QUESTION #1    (Answer:  d)  Name compound as a phenol with o-m-p as:

QUESTION #2    (Answer:  c)  Phenols are more acidic than alcohols.

QUESTION #3    (Answer:  d)  Electron withdrawing groups ($-NO_2$) at o-p positions increase the acidity of phenols.

QUESTION #4    (Answer:  c)  The phenol can hydrogen bond to itself which increases the boiling point; the others cannot.

QUESTION #5    (Answer:  a)  Intramolecular H-bonding is possible if the compound is ortho and this decreases the boiling point.

4.9.5         VOCABULARY, CONCEPTS, ETC. CHECKLIST FOR PHENOLS

        nomenclature of phenols
        physical properties of phenols
        acidity of phenols
        hydrogen bonding of phenols

4.10          Carboxylic Acids

4.10.1        REVIEW OF CARBOXYLIC ACIDS

See Section 4.3.1 on general nomenclature.   The -e of alkanes is replaced by -oic acid for carboxylic acids:

    $CH_3-CH_2-CH_2-CH_3$                    $CH_3-CH_2-CH_2-CO_2H$
                                              (4)  (3)  (2)  (1)
        Butane                                    Butanoic acid

The $-CO_2H$ carbon is always numbered #1 as above.  Other rules are as before.  For example:

5-Methyl-4-hexenoic acid

Some common carboxylic acids are (with trivial names)

Formic acid    Acetic acid    Benzoic acid

Oxalic acid    Succinic acid

The key functional group of these compounds is the carboxyl,

$$R-\underset{(1)\,(3)\,(2)}{\overset{\overset{O(4)}{\|}}{C}-O-H.}$$

Reactions of the carboxylic acids center around the four central features of the carboxyl group:

(1) The H(2) is acidic because it is weakly attached to the O(3) and because the resulting carboxylate anion is stabilized by resonance

Resonance forms

(2) The carboxyl carbon (1) is very susceptible to attack by nucleophilic agents (Nu; see Section 4.4.1) because of the attached electronegative oxygens and the carbonyl oxygen (4):

(3) The hydroxyl can become a good leaving group by appropriate solvent conditions (e.g., if basic) and/or by protonating, if acidic solution, and hence, this also promotes nucleophilic substitution,

(4) Hydrogen bonding is possible between molecules (intermolecular) and/or within the same molecule (intramolecular) because of the carbonyl and hydroxyl moieties,

Intermolecular (dimerization)        Intramolecular

Low molecular weight aliphatic carboxylic acids tend to be soluble in water due to hydrogen bonding with water; aromatic acids are not, in general, soluble. The acids are also soluble in dilute bases, NaOH or NaHCO₃, e.g., because of their acid properties. The boiling points are high because of the hydrogen bonding possible between molecules.

Carboxylic acids are the <u>acids</u> of organic chemistry. The only other compounds which approach their acid strength are substituted phenols (see Section 4.9.1). Organic classes of molecules by decreasing acid strength are:

$$RCO_2H > HOH > ROH > HC \equiv CH > NH_3 > RH$$

(substituted phenols may be stronger acids than $H_2O$).

The relative base strength is just the reverse. In order of decreasing base strength:

$$R^{\ominus} > NH_2^{\ominus} > HC \equiv C^{\ominus} > RO^{\ominus} > HO^{\ominus} > RCO_2^{\ominus}$$

The <u>relative acid strength</u> of carboxylic acids depends primarily on the groups attached and the distance of these groups from the carboxyl:

$$CH_3CH_2 - \overset{\overset{\text{Cl}}{|}}{\underset{\underset{\text{Cl}}{|}}{C}} - CO_2H > CH_3 - CH_2 - \overset{\overset{\text{H}}{|}}{\underset{\underset{\text{Cl}}{|}}{C}} - CO_2H \text{ in acid strength}$$

Cl is an electron withdrawer and stabilizes the carboxylate anion

$$CH_3 - \overset{\overset{\text{Cl}}{|}}{\underset{\underset{\text{Cl}}{|}}{C}} - CH_2 - CO_2H < CH_3 - CH_2 - \overset{\overset{\text{Cl}}{|}}{\underset{\underset{\text{Cl}}{|}}{C}} - CO_2H \text{ in acid strength}$$

The <u>nucleophilic substitution</u> reactions can involve a variety of nucleophiles (Nu) reacting under a variety of conditions,

$$R - \overset{\overset{\text{O}}{\|}}{C} - OH + Nu\!:^{\ominus} \longrightarrow R - \overset{\overset{\text{O}}{\|}}{C} - Nu + OH^{\ominus}$$

Nu: = $-OR'$  R' = $(1^{\circ} > 2^{\circ} > 3^{\circ})$, esters result
= $-NH_2$, amides result
= $-Cl$ from $SOCl_2$ or $PCl_3$ or $PCl_5$, acid chlorides result

In the ester reaction,

$$R - \overset{\overset{\text{O}}{\|}}{C} - O - H \quad + \quad R' - \overset{*}{O} - H \longrightarrow R - \overset{\overset{\text{O}}{\|}}{C} - \overset{*}{O} - R' + H_2O$$

acid                    alcohol                    ester
note the origin of the $O^{*}$

The major <u>reduction reaction</u> is with $LiAlH_4$:

$$R - \overset{\overset{\text{O}}{\|}}{C} - OH \xrightarrow{\text{LiAlH}_4} R - CH_2 - OH$$

alcohol

Acids can be converted to esters or amides and then reduced also.

The typical decarboxylation reaction involves β-diacids or β-Ketoacids:

$$\overset{\gamma}{C}-\overset{\beta}{C}-\overset{\alpha}{C}-C\overset{\displaystyle O}{\underset{\displaystyle OH}{}}$$

$$HO-\overset{\displaystyle O}{\underset{}{C}}-\overset{\displaystyle H}{\underset{\displaystyle R}{C}}-\overset{\displaystyle O}{\underset{}{C}}-OH \xrightarrow[\text{heat}]{\text{base}} H-\overset{\displaystyle H}{\underset{\displaystyle R}{C}}-\overset{\displaystyle O}{\underset{}{C}}-OH + CO_2$$

β- diacid

$$R-\overset{\displaystyle O}{\underset{}{C}}-CH_2-\overset{\displaystyle O}{\underset{}{C}}-OH \xrightarrow[\text{heat}]{\text{base}} R-\overset{\displaystyle O}{\underset{}{C}}-CH_3 + CO_2$$

β-Ketoacid

**4.10.2      QUESTIONS TO REVIEW CARBOXYLIC ACIDS**

(1)   Which atom below is susceptible to nucleophilic attack?

$$\underset{(I)}{CH_3}-\overset{\overset{\displaystyle O(III)}{\|}}{\underset{(II)}{C}}-\underset{}{O}-\underset{(IV)}{H}$$

(a) I      (b) II      (c) III      (d) IV

(2)   A high molecular weight carboxylic acid may be soluble in
_____ but probably not in _____.

(a) dilute acid, dilute base      (b)  water, dilute acid
(c) water, dilute base            (d)  dilute base, water

(3)   For comparable compounds, which of the following would be most
acidic?

(a) water    (b)  alcohol    (c)  alkene    (d)  carboxylic acid

(4)   Name the following compound:

$$CH_3-\overset{\overset{\displaystyle CH_3}{|}}{\underset{\underset{\displaystyle CH_3}{|}}{C}}-CH=\overset{\overset{\displaystyle Cl}{|}}{C}-CH_2-CO_2H$$

(a) 3-Chloro-5, 5-dimethylhexanoic acid
(b) 3-Chloro-5,5-dimethyl-3-hexenoic acid
(c) 2,2-Dimethyl-4-chloro-3-hexenoic acid
(d) none of the above

309

(5) Select the compound that is most acidic:

(a) 

$$Cl-\underset{\underset{Cl}{|}}{\overset{\overset{Cl}{|}}{C}}-CH_2-CO_2H$$

(b) $CH_3-CH_2-CO_2H$

(c) 

(d) all are equal

(6) Give the product of the following reaction:

$$\langle\text{ph}\rangle-CH_2-CH_2-\overset{\overset{O}{\|}}{C}-OH + CH_3-NH_2 \xrightarrow{\Delta} ?$$

(a) 
$$H_3C-\overset{\overset{H}{|}}{N}-\langle\text{ph}\rangle-CH_2-CH_2-\overset{\overset{O}{\|}}{C}-OH$$

(b) 
$$\langle\text{ph}\rangle-CH_2-CH_2-CH_2-OH$$

(c) 
$$\langle\text{ph}\rangle-CH_2-CH_2-CH_2-NH-CH_3$$

(d) none of the above

(7) Give the product of the following reaction:

$$CH_3-\underset{\underset{Cl}{|}}{\overset{\overset{Cl}{|}}{CH}}-CH_2-\overset{\overset{O}{\|}}{C}-OH + LiAlH_4 \longrightarrow ?$$

(a) 
$$CH_3-\underset{\underset{}{}}{\overset{\overset{Cl}{|}}{CH}}-CH_2-CH_2-OH$$

(b) 
$$CH_3-CH=CH-\overset{\overset{O}{\|}}{C}-OH$$

(c) 
$$CH_3-\overset{\overset{Cl}{|}}{CH}-CH_2-\overset{\overset{O}{\|}}{C}-O^{\ominus}Li^{\oplus}$$

(d) none of the above

(8) Which of the following compounds has the potential for decarboxylation?

(a) 
$$\langle\text{ph}\rangle-\overset{\overset{O}{\|}}{C}-\overset{\overset{O}{\|}}{C}-OH$$

(b) 
$$\langle\text{ph}\rangle-\overset{\overset{O}{\|}}{C}-CH_2-CO_2H$$

(c) 
$$CH_3-CH_2-CH\overset{CO_2H}{\underset{CH_2-CO_2H}{}}$$

(d) none of these

## 4.10.3  ANSWERS TO QUESTIONS IN SECTION 4.10.2

(1) b  (2) d  (3) d  (4) b  (5) c  (6) d  (7) a
(8) b

## 4.10.4  DISCUSSION OF ANSWERS TO QUESTIONS IN SECTION 4.10.2

QUESTIONS #1 to #3: Adequately discussed in Section.

QUESTION #4 (Answer: b) The numbering is:

$$
\begin{array}{ccccccc}
& C & & Cl & & & \\
| & | & & | & & & \\
C-C-C=C-C-CO_2H \\
(6)\ (5)\ (4)\ (3)\ (2)\ (1) \\
& | & & & & \\
& C & & & & \\
\end{array}
$$

Note how the double bond is handled.

QUESTION #5 (Answer: c) The benzene ring withdraws electrons, and, therefore, increases the acidity. The Cl's on option (a) are one carbon from the $-CO_2H$ and they are much less effective than a benzene ring attached to the carboxyl group.

QUESTION #6 (Answer: d) Correct product, ⬡$-CH_2-CH_2-\overset{\overset{O}{\|}}{C}-NHCH_3$

QUESTION #7 (Answer: a) Discussed in Section.

QUESTION #8 (Answer: b) Option (b) is the only $\beta$-Ketoacid (no $\beta$-diacids) given.


4.10.5    VOCABULARY, CONCEPTS, ETC. CHECKLIST FOR CARBOXYLIC ACIDS

___ nomenclature                    ___ key chemical features of carboxyl group
___ physical properties             ___ strengths of organic acids
___ reduction reactions             ___ nucleophilic substitution reactions


**4.11        Amines**


**4.11.1      REVIEW OF AMINES**


Amines are symbolized generally as:

$$R-\ddot{N}H_2 \qquad \underline{OR} \qquad Ar-\ddot{N}H_2 \qquad \underline{OR} \qquad R_1-\underset{\underset{R_3}{|}}{\overset{}{\ddot{N}}}-R_2.$$

R = aliphatic          Ar = aromatic

All the R's ($R_1$, $R_2$, $R_3$) or any combination can be carbon groups or hydrogens.  If R's are carbon groups,

$$R-\underset{\underset{H}{|}}{\overset{\overset{H}{|}}{N}} \qquad R-\underset{\underset{R'}{|}}{\overset{\overset{H}{|}}{N}} \qquad \underset{\underset{R''}{|}}{\overset{\overset{R\quad R'}{\diagdown\diagup}}{N}} \qquad R-\underset{\underset{R'}{|}}{\overset{\overset{R'''}{|}}{N^{\oplus}}}-R'', X^{\ominus}$$

$1^O$ amine      $2^O$ amine      $3^O$ amine      $4^O$ (quaternary) amine.

Amines may be named by locating the $-NR_2$ in a compound by numbers, e.g.,

$$\begin{array}{cc}
\overset{NH_2}{\underset{}{|}} & \overset{H-N-CH_3}{\underset{}{|}} \\
CH_3-CH_2-CH-CH_3 & CH_3-CH_2-CH-CH_3 \\
\text{2-Aminobutane} & \text{N-Methyl-2-amino butane}
\end{array}$$

Or by naming each group attached to the N,

⬡$-NH_2$        $CH_3-NH_2$        $CH_3-CH_2-\underset{\overset{|}{H}}{N}-CH_2-CH_3$        $\underset{H_3C}{\overset{H_3C}{\diagdown}}\underset{}{\overset{CH}{|}}\underset{\overset{|}{N}}{}\underset{H_3C\diagup\quad\diagdown CH_2CH_3}{}$

Aniline   Methylamine      Diethylamine        Methylethylisopropylamine

311

Nearly all the chemistry of amines depends upon the free pair of electrons upon nitrogen:

R = aliphatic, aromatic or H's.

Groups that withdraw electron density (aromatics, halides, e.g.) from nitrogen decrease the availability of this electron pair. Groups that donate electron density (especially alkyls) increase the availability.   The availability of the electrons is reflected in this sequence of decreasing base strengths:

The available electron pair classifies amines as Lewis bases. Amines are also nucleophiles.  Other important features of amines:

(1)    The N can form hydrogen  bonding via its electron pair with hydrogens attached to other N's or O's, and it can form hydrogen bonds from hydrogens attached to it with electron pairs of N, O, F or Cl:

Note that $1^O$ or $2^O$ amines can hydrogen bond with each other (intermolecularly) but $3^O$ amines cannot (no Hs attached to the N).  For this reason $1^O$ and $2^O$ amines have higher than expected boiling points for compounds of similar molecular weight (but lower than similar alcohols or carboxylic acids).   Low molecular weight amines are also soluble in $H_2O$ (due to H-bonding).

(2)    A dipole moment is possible:

(3)    Amines are ortho-para directors (Section 4.5.1).

Remember that the key reaction of amines is the nucleophilic attack (Section 4.4.1) by it upon an electron deficient carbon.

A very important reaction of 1° and 2° amines is with carboxylic acids (or usually their derivatives) to form <u>amides</u>:

$$R-\overset{\displaystyle O}{\overset{\|}{C}}-OH + R'-NH_2 \xrightarrow{\Delta} R-\overset{\displaystyle O}{\overset{\|}{C}}-\overset{\displaystyle H}{\overset{|}{N}}-R'$$

$$1°\ or\ 2°$$

Carboxylic acid                    Amide
(or Acyl chloride)

This is the reaction important in protein synthesis.

Another common reaction of amines is <u>alkylation</u> of amines by alkyl halides:

$$R-CH_2-Cl + R'-NH_2 \longrightarrow R-CH_2-\overset{\displaystyle H}{\overset{|}{N}}-R' + HCl$$

$$1°,2°\ or\ 3°$$

Both amide formation and alkylation make use of the nucleophilic character of the electrons on nitrogen.


## 4.11.2    QUESTIONS TO REVIEW AMINES

(1) Name the following compound:

$$CH_3-CH_2-CH=CH-CH-\overset{\displaystyle NH_2}{\overset{|}{CH}}-CH\overset{\nearrow CH_3}{\searrow_{CH_3}}$$

   (a) 6-Amino 7-methyl-3-octene       (b) Isononenyl amine

   (c) 2-Methyl-3-aminooctene        (d) none of the above

(2) Give the structure of Isopropyl diethyl amine:

   (a) H-N-CH$_2$CH$_3$            (b) CH$_3$CH$_2$-N-CH$_2$CH$_3$
            CH                          CH
     H$_3$C   CH$_3$                    H$_3$C   CH$_3$

   (c)     NH$_2$  CH$_2$CH$_3$     (d) none of the above
    CH$_3$-CH$_2$-CH$_2$

(3) Which compound has the greatest base strength?

   (a) CH$_3$-NH$_2$            (b) CH$_3$      CH$_3$
                              CH-C-NH$_2$
                          H$_3$C   CH$_3$

   (c) CH$_2$-CH$_2$-CH$_3$      (d) all are equal
    N-CH$_3$
    CH$_3$

**(4)** Which compound has the greatest base strength?

(a) $O_2N$—⬡—$NH_2$

(b) $NC$—⬡($\overset{CN}{\underset{NH_2}{}}$)

(c) $H_3C$—⬡—$NH_2$

(d) none of the above

**(5)** Which of the following compounds probably has the lowest boiling point?

(a) $CH_3$—$\overset{\displaystyle CH_2CH_2CH_3}{NH}$

(b) ⬡—$CH_2$—$NH_2$

(c) ⬡—$CH_2$—$\overset{}{\underset{CH_2CH_3}{N}}$—$CH_3$

(d) all are equal

**(6)** Give the product of the following reaction:

$CH_3$—$\overset{CH_3}{\underset{}{CH}}$—$\overset{O}{\underset{}{C}}$—$OH$ + $CH_3$—$CH_2$—$\overset{}{\underset{CH_3}{NH}}$ $\xrightarrow{\Delta}$ ?

(a) $CH_3$—$\overset{CH_3}{\underset{}{CH}}$—$\overset{H}{\underset{}{C}}$=$N$—$CH_2CH_3$

(b) $CH_3$—$\overset{CH_3}{\underset{}{CH}}$—$CH_2$—$OH$

(c) $CH_3$—$\overset{CH_3}{\underset{}{CH}}$—$\overset{\overset{N}{|}-CH_2CH_3}{\underset{CH_3}{CH}}$—$N$—$CH_2CH_3$

(d) $CH_3$—$\overset{CH_3}{\underset{}{CH}}$—$\overset{O}{\underset{}{C}}$—$\overset{}{\underset{CH_3}{N}}$—$CH_2CH_3$

**(7)** Give the product of the following reaction:

⬡—$CH_2$—$NH_2$ + $CH_3Cl$ $\longrightarrow$ ?

(a) ⬡—$CH_2$—$\overset{CH_3}{\underset{}{NH}}$

(b) ⬡($\underset{CH_3}{}$)—$CH_2$—$NH_2$

(c) ⬡($\underset{Cl}{}$)—$CH_2$—$NH_2$

(d) none of the above

**4.11.3** <u>ANSWERS TO QUESTIONS IN SECTION 4.11.2</u>

(1) a   (2) b   (3) c   (4) c   (5) c   (6) d   (7) a

DISCUSSION OF ANSWERS TO QUESTIONS IN SECTION 4.11.2

QUESTION #1   (Answer:  a)  The compound is named as an alkene and the amino group is considered to be a substituent (it could have been named as an amine also).  The numbering is,

$$C—C—C≡C—C—C—C \quad \begin{matrix} NH_2 \\ | \end{matrix} \quad \begin{matrix} C \\ 8 \end{matrix}$$

$$\underset{1}{C}—\underset{2}{C}—\underset{3}{C}=\underset{4}{C}—\underset{5}{C}—\underset{6}{C}—\underset{7}{C}$$

QUESTION #2   (Answer:  b)  The name is just taken literally.  Study it.

QUESTION #3   (Answer:  c)  Tertiary amines (option c) have greater base strength than primary (a or b) or secondary amines.

QUESTION #4   (Answer:  c)  Aromatic amines have low base strength in general, but electron withdrawing groups (-CN, -NO$_2$) placed ortho/para decreases it even more.  Electron donating groups (-CH$_3$) placed o/p can increase base strength.

QUESTION #5   (Answer:  c)  Tertiary amines have lower boiling points than 1$^o$ and 2$^o$ because there is no intermolecular hydrogen bonding.

QUESTION #6   (Answer:  d)  This is the amide forming reaction.

QUESTION #7   (Answer:  a)  This is the alkylation reaction.


4.11.5     VOCABULARY, CONCEPTS, ETC. CHECKLIST FOR AMINES

____ nomenclature of amines          ____ amide formation
____ physical properties of amines   ____ alkylation of amines
                                      ____ basicity of amines


4.12     Carboxylic Acid Derivatives


4.12.1     REVIEW OF CARBOXYLIC ACID DERIVATIVES


4.12.1.1     Review of Amides


See nomenclature of carboxylic acids (Section 4.10.1).  The -oic acid (or -ic acid) is changed to -amide, e.g.:

3-Methyl butanoic acid

$$\begin{matrix} H_3C \\ \phantom{x} \\ H_3C \end{matrix} CH—CH_2—\overset{\displaystyle O}{\overset{\|}{C}}—OH$$

$$\begin{matrix} CH_3 \\ \phantom{x} \\ CH_3 \end{matrix} CH—CH_2—\overset{\displaystyle O}{\overset{\|}{C}}—NH_2$$

3-Methyl butanamide

If the N is substituted, this feature is added as follows:

$$H_3C-\underset{\underset{H_3C}{|}}{CH}-CH_2-\underset{\underset{}{\overset{\overset{O}{\|}}{C}}}-N\underset{CH_3}{\overset{CH_3}{}}$$

N, N – Dimethyl –3– methyl butanamide

The boiling points of unsubstituted and monosubstituted amides are very high due to strong intermolecular hydrogen bonds. Disubstituted amides have boiling points like ketones or aldehydes (due to the carbonyl moiety). Amides have essentially no acidity (as compared to carboxylic acids) and no basicity (as compared to amines).

Amides are formed from carboxylic acids (or its derivatives) by,

$$R-\overset{\overset{O}{\|}}{C}-OH + NH_3 \text{ (or } R-NH_2, \text{ etc.)} \xrightarrow{\Delta} R-\overset{\overset{O}{\|}}{C}-NH_2$$

Amides are susceptible to nucleophilic substitution at the carbonyl carbon,

$$R-\overset{\overset{O}{\|}}{C}-NH_2 + NuH \longrightarrow R-\overset{\overset{O}{\|}}{C}-Nu + NH_3$$

Nu = nucleophile
(see Section 4.10.1).

Amides undergo hydrolysis back to the original acid and amine under basic or acidic conditions:

$$R-\underset{amide}{\overset{\overset{O}{\|}}{C}}-NHR \xrightarrow[H_2O]{H^\oplus} R-\underset{acid}{\overset{\overset{O}{\|}}{C}}-OH + \underset{amine}{RNH_2}$$

$$R-\overset{\overset{O}{\|}}{C}-NHR \xrightarrow{OH^\ominus} \underset{amine}{R-NH_2} + \underset{carboxylate}{R-\overset{\overset{O}{\|}}{C}-O^\ominus} \xrightarrow{H^\oplus} \underset{acid}{R-\overset{\overset{O}{\|}}{C}-OH.}$$

### 4.12.1.2    Review of Esters

See nomenclature of carboxylic acids (Section 4.10.1). The -oic acid of carboxylic acids is replaced by -oate and the carbon fragment of the ester precedes the base name:

$$\underset{H_3C}{\overset{H_3C}{}}CH-CH_2-\overset{\overset{O}{\|}}{C}-OH$$

3-Methyl butanoic
acid

$$\underset{CH_3}{\overset{CH_3}{}}CH-CH_2-\overset{\overset{O}{\|}}{C}-O-CH_2CH_3$$

Ethyl-3-methyl butanoate

Esters have no <u>acidity</u> (because no -OH) and have <u>boiling points</u> comparable to ketones and aldehydes because they have carbonyl groups but not hydrogen bonding.

Esters are formed from carboxylic acids (or derivatives) under acidic or basic conditions.

$$R-\overset{\overset{O}{\|}}{C}-OH \ + \ R'-\overset{*}{O}-H \ \longrightarrow \ R-\overset{\overset{O}{\|}}{C}-\overset{*}{O}-R.$$

acid      alcohol          ester

Esters undergo <u>nucleophilic</u> <u>substitution</u> at the carbonyl carbon,

$$R-\overset{\overset{O}{\|}}{C}-O-R' \ + \ NuH \ \longrightarrow \ R-\overset{\overset{O}{\|}}{C}-Nu \ + \ R'OH \quad Nu = nucleophile$$
(Section 4.10.1)

Esters are <u>hydrolized</u> by acid or base back to the original acid and alcohol:

$$R-\overset{\overset{O}{\|}}{C}-OR' \ \xrightarrow{H^{\oplus}} \ R-\overset{\overset{O}{\|}}{C}-OH \ + \ R'-OH$$
ester          acid     alcohol

$$R-\overset{\overset{O}{\|}}{C}-OR' \ \xrightarrow{NaOH} \ R-\overset{\overset{O}{\|}}{C}-O^{\ominus}Na^{\oplus} \ + \ R'OH \ \xrightarrow{H^{\oplus}} \ R-\overset{\overset{O}{\|}}{C}-OH$$
ester        carboxylate ion             acid.

<u>Fats</u> are a special class of esters of biologic importance. They are formed as follows:

$$CH_3(CH_2)_{14}CO_2H \ + \ \begin{matrix} CH_2OH \\ | \\ CH_2OH \\ | \\ CH_2OH \end{matrix} \ \longrightarrow \ \begin{matrix} CH_2-O-\overset{\overset{O}{\|}}{C}-(CH_2)_{14}-CH_3 \\ | \\ CH_2OH \\ | \\ CH_2OH \end{matrix} \ \longrightarrow \ II \ \longrightarrow \ III.$$

fatty acid    glycerol       monoglyceride
(long chain acids)        (a fat)

More fatty acids (FA) can be added to the glycerol to form di- (II) and tri-glycerides (III). Fats may be hydrolyzed back to FA's and glycerol by base (a process called <u>saponification</u>):

$$\begin{matrix} CH_2-O-\overset{\overset{O}{\|}}{C}-(CH_2)_{14}CH_3 \\ | \\ CH_2-O-\overset{\overset{O}{\|}}{C}-(CH_2)_{14}CH_3 \\ | \\ CH_2-O-\overset{\overset{O}{\|}}{C}-(CH_2)_{14}CH_3 \end{matrix} \ \xrightarrow{NaOH} \ \begin{matrix} CH_2OH \\ | \\ CH_2OH \\ | \\ CH_2OH \end{matrix} \ + \ 3 \ CH_3(CH_2)_{14}CO_2^{\ominus}Na^{\oplus}$$

a triglyceride               glycerol    salt of the FA
(a fat)

(1)    Amides have essentially no:

   (a) acidity                    (b)  basicity
   (c) hydrogen bonding           (d)  both (a) and (b)


(2)    Fats are _____ and are made of _____ and _____.

   (a) esters, glycerol, fatty acids
   (b) amide, an amine, fatty acids
   (c) ethers, glycerol, fatty acids
   (d) none of the above


(3)    Saponification is the _____ of _____.

   (a) alkaline hydrolysis, fats
   (b) acidic hydrolysis, fats
   (c) neutral hydrolysis, amides
   (d) none of the above


(4)    Name the following compound:

$$H_3C-C(CH_3)=C(H)-CH_2-C(=O)-N(H)-CH_3$$

   (a) N-Methyl-4-Methyl-3-pentenamide
   (b) 2-Methyl-2-pentenamide
   (c) Dimethyl pentenamide
   (d) none of the above


(5)    Which of the following compounds probably has a boiling point
       similar to comparable molecular weight   ketones or aldehydes?

   (a) $CH_3-C(=O)-N(CH_3)_2$          (b) $CH_3-C(=O)-NCH_3$ (with H)

   (c) $CH-C(=O)-NH_2$                 (d) none of the above


(6) Give the product of the following reaction:

$$CH_3-C(=O)-NH_2 + CH_3-CH_2-OH \xrightarrow[heat]{base} ?$$

   (a) $CH_3-CH_2-NH_2$              (b) $CH_3-C(=O)-OCH_2-CH_3$

   (c) $CH_3-C(=O)-N(H)-CH_2-CH_3$   (d) none of the above


318

(7) Give the product of the following reaction:

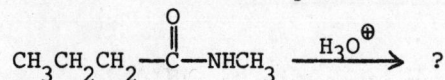

$$CH_3CH_2CH_2-\overset{\overset{\displaystyle O}{\|}}{C}-NHCH_3 \xrightarrow{\text{H}_3\text{O}^{\oplus}} ?$$

(a) $CH_3CH_2CH_2-\overset{\overset{\displaystyle O}{\|}}{C}-NH_2$

(b) $CH_3-CH_2CH_2-CH_2-NH_2$

(c) $CH_3-CH_2CH_2-CH_2-OH$

(d) none of the above

(8) Name the following compound:

$$\text{(benzene ring)}-CH_2-CH_2-\overset{\overset{\displaystyle O}{\|}}{C}-O-\overset{\overset{\textstyle CH_3}{|}}{\underset{\underset{\textstyle CH_3}{|}}{CH}}$$

(a) Isopropyl benzoate

(b) Isopropyl-3-phenyl propanoate

(c) Phenyl isopropyl ester

(d) none of the above

(9) Give the product of the following reaction:

$$CH_3-\overset{\overset{\displaystyle O}{\|}}{C}-O-CH_3 + CH_3-CH_2-CH_2-NH_2 \xrightarrow{\text{base}} ?$$

(a) $CH_3-\overset{\overset{\textstyle H}{|}}{C}=N-CH_2-CH_2-CH_3$

(b) $CH_3-\overset{\overset{\displaystyle O}{\|}}{C}-\overset{\overset{\textstyle H}{|}}{N}-CH_2CH_2CH_3$

(c) $CH_3-CH_2-CH_2-OH$

(d) none of the above

(10) Give the product of the following reaction:

$$\overset{\overset{\textstyle CH_3}{|}}{\underset{\underset{\textstyle CH_3}{|}}{CH}}-\overset{\overset{\displaystyle O}{\|}}{C}-O-CH_3 \xrightarrow{\text{NaOH}} ?$$

(a)
$$\overset{\textstyle CH_3}{\underset{\textstyle CH_3}{}}C=CH_2$$

(b)
$$\overset{\textstyle CH_3}{\underset{\textstyle CH_3}{}}CH-CH_2OH$$

(c)
$$\overset{\textstyle CH_3}{\underset{\textstyle H_3C}{}}CH-\overset{\overset{\displaystyle O}{\|}}{C}-O^{\ominus}Na^{\oplus}$$

(d) none of these

(11) The following compound is a:

$$\begin{array}{l} CH_2-O-\overset{\overset{\displaystyle O}{\|}}{C}-(CH_2)_8CH_3 \\ CH_2-O-\overset{\overset{\displaystyle O}{\|}}{C}-(CH_2)_{10}CH_3 \\ CH_2-O-\overset{\overset{\displaystyle O}{\|}}{C}-(CH_2)_{12}CH_3 \end{array}$$

(a) nucleotide

(b) monosaccharide

(c) amino acid

(d) triglyceride

**4.12.3** <u>ANSWERS TO QUESTIONS IN SECTION 4.12.2</u>

( 1)  d    (2)  a    (3)  a    (4)  a    (5)  a    (6)  b    (7)  d
( 8)  b    (9)  b   (10)  c   (11)  d


**4.12.4** <u>DISCUSSION OF ANSWERS TO QUESTIONS IN SECTION 4.12.2</u>

<u>QUESTIONS #1-#3</u>:  Adequately discussed in Section.

<u>QUESTION #4</u>   (Answer:  a)  The numbering is

<u>QUESTION #5</u>   (Answer:  a)  Disubstituted amides have boiling points similar to carbonyls because there is no intermolecular hydrogen bonding.

<u>QUESTION #6</u>   (Answer:  b)  Amides undergo nucleophilic substitution just like carboxylic acids.  An ester is formed in this case.

<u>QUESTION #7</u>   (Answer:  d)  This is an hydrolysis of an amide; the products are the original acid and amine:

<u>QUESTION #8</u>   (Answer:  b)  The numbering is:

<u>QUESTION #9</u>   (Answer:  b)  Esters undergo nucleophilic substitution just like carboxylic acids.  An amide is the product in this reaction.

<u>QUESTION #10</u>   (Answer:  c)  This is the alkaline hydrolysis of an ester, so a carboxylate anion results.

<u>QUESTION #11</u>   (Answer:  d)  Refer to Section.


**4.12.5** <u>VOCABULARY, CONCEPTS, ETC. CHECKLIST FOR CARBOXYLIC</u> <u>DERIVATIVES</u>

____  nomenclature of amides
____  nomenclature of esters
____  physical properties of amides
____  physical properties of esters

_____ nucleophilic substitution of amides
_____ nucleophilic substitution of esters
_____ hydrolysis of amides
_____ hydrolysis of esters
_____ fats
_____ saponification

## 4.13       Amino Acids and Proteins

### 4.13.1       REVIEW OF AMINO ACIDS AND PROTEINS

Amino acids (AA) are organic molecules with the common features of a carboxyl group and an $\alpha$(alpha) -amino group as shown and a side chain (R):

L-amino acid            D-amino acid

There are about 20 AA and all are in the L configuration. AA's serve primarily as the structural components of proteins. The types and sequence of AA in proteins determine their structural properties and acid-base behavior. The following AA's have R groups which are hydrocarbon in nature, are hydrophobic and are found in the interiors of proteins:

Valine        Leucine        Isoleucine

Phenylalanine        Methionine

Knowledge of these amino acids is not required for the MCAT.

Ionic and/or polar AA's are hydrophilic and tend to be found on the exterior of proteins:

Aspartic Acid        Glutamic Acid        Lysine
(and its amide)      (and its amide)

321

Arginine

Histidine

Certain amino acids can be found on the exterior or interior of proteins (these are polar also):

Serine

Threonine

Tyrosine

Tryptophan

Cysteine forms sulfur-sulfur covalent bonds with itself to stabilize the tertiary structure of proteins:

cysteine

cystine

Glycine, the smallest AA and the only one that is not optically active, is often found at the 'corners' of proteins:

$$H_2N—\overset{\overset{\displaystyle CO_2H}{|}}{\underset{\underset{\displaystyle H}{|}}{C}}—H$$

Glycine

Proline breaks the ∝-helix structure of proteins:

Proline

Alanine, being small, is usually found on the surface of proteins even though it is hydrophobic:

Alanine

The <u>basic amino acids</u> are lysine and arginine due to their extra amino ($-NH_2$) groups. The <u>acidic amino acids</u> are aspartic acid and glutamic acid due to their extra carboxyl ($-CO_2H$) groups. Histidine can act as a base or an acid depending upon the pH, and it is the best physiologic buffer of the AA's. All of the others are considered <u>neutral amino acids</u>.

Amino acids exist as <u>dipolar ions</u> due to the presence of both a basic part (the $-NH_2$) and an acidic part (the $-CO_2H$):

$$R-\overset{\overset{\oplus}{N}H_3}{\underset{H}{C}}-CO_2^{\ominus}$$

dipolar ion

The charge on the amino acid varies with the pH and the <u>isoelectric point</u>. The isoelectric point (pI) of an AA is the pH where the AA has no net charge:

$$R-\overset{\overset{NH_2}{|}}{\underset{\underset{H}{|}}{C}}-CO_2H$$

no net charge at isoelectric points

If the pH is above the isoelectric point or very basic, AA's have a net negative charge (anions):

$$R-\overset{\overset{\oplus}{N}H_3}{\underset{H}{C}}-CO_2^{\ominus} \quad \xrightarrow[\text{(basic)}]{OH^{\ominus}} \quad R-\overset{\overset{NH_2}{|}}{\underset{H}{C}}-CO_2^{\ominus}$$

anionic form

If the pH is below the isoelectric point or very acidic, AA's have a net positive charge (cations):

$$R-\overset{\overset{\oplus}{N}H_3}{\underset{H}{C}}-CO_2^{\ominus} \quad \xrightarrow[\text{(acidic)}]{\overset{\oplus}{H}} \quad R-\overset{\overset{\oplus}{N}H_3}{\underset{H}{C}}-CO_2H$$

cationic form

Proteins also have isoelectric points. Whether proteins are basic or acidic depends on the relative numbers of basic and acidic AA's present. If there is an excess of acidic AA's, the proteins are acidic and have an isoelectric point at a pH less than 7 (neutrality for water). So, at pH =7, they have a net negative charge. If there is an excess of basic AA's, proteins are basic and have an isoelectric point at a pH greater than 7. At pH = 7, they have a net positive charge. Proteins undergo electrophoresis just like amino acids. In other words, if the pH of the medium is less than the pI of the protein, the protein must have a net positive charge. Or, if the pH of the medium is greater than the pI, the protein must have a net negative charge. Proteins are composed of AA's linearly linked by peptide bonds. A <u>peptide bond</u> is an amide bond (See Section 4.12.1.1.) formed by the ∝-amino group of an AA and the 1-carboxyl group of a second AA. Water is released when a peptide bond is formed and is added when it is hydrolyzed:

$$R_1 \underset{\underset{AA_1}{\overset{|}{H}}}{\overset{\overset{NH_2}{|}}{C}} - CO_2H \ + \ R_2 \underset{\underset{AA_2}{\overset{|}{H}}}{\overset{\overset{NH_2}{|}}{C}} - CO_2H \ \longrightarrow \ H - \underset{\underset{}{\overset{|}{R_1}}}{\overset{\overset{NH_2}{|}}{C}} - \overset{\overset{O}{\parallel}}{C} - NH - \underset{\underset{}{\overset{|}{R_2}}}{\overset{\overset{H}{|}}{C}} - \overset{\overset{O}{\parallel}}{C} - OH \ + \ H_2O$$

formation of peptide bond          peptide bond

$$H_2N - \underset{\underset{}{\overset{|}{R_1}}}{\overset{\overset{H}{|}}{C}} - \overset{\overset{O}{\parallel}}{C} - NH - \underset{\underset{}{\overset{|}{R_2}}}{\overset{\overset{H}{|}}{C}} - CO_2H \ + \ H_2O \ \xrightarrow{H^\oplus} \ H_2N - \underset{\underset{}{\overset{|}{R_1}}}{\overset{\overset{H}{|}}{C}} - \overset{\overset{O}{\parallel}}{C} - OH \ + \ NH_2 - \underset{\underset{}{\overset{|}{R_2}}}{\overset{\overset{H}{|}}{C}} - CO_2H$$

hydrolysis of peptide bond

The structure of proteins is divided into primary ($1^O$), secondary ($2^O$), tertiary ($3^O$) and quaternary ($4^O$). The $\underline{1^O \text{ structure}}$ of a protein is the sequence of AA as determined by DNA (Section 2.4.1) and it determines the higher structures. $\underline{\text{Secondary structure}}$ is the orderly intermolecular or intramolecular hydrogen bonding of the protein chain assuming an $\alpha$-helix (e.g. in keratin) or $\beta$-pleated sheet (e.g. in silk), respectively. The $\underline{3^O \text{ structure}}$ is the further folding of the protein (many parts of it still remain $\alpha$-helical) onto itself. The molecule is stabilized by hydrogen bonding, van der Waals bonding, hydrophobic bonding, electrostatic bonding (see Section 3.4.1) and, especially, covalent bonding in the form of disulfide bonds (by cysteine). Globular proteins result and usually have an interior that is hydrophobic and an exterior that is hydrophilic; enzymes are examples. $\underline{\text{Quaternary structures}}$ is when two or more separate protein chains bind together by noncovalent bonds (e.g., hemoglobin).

4.13.2          QUESTIONS TO REVIEW AMINO ACIDS AND PROTEINS

(1)   What characteristics of amino acids determine the primary structure of proteins?

   (a) acid-base properties          (b)  side chain composition
   (c) hydrogen bonding properties   (d)  sequence in proteins

(2)   Which is an $\alpha$-amino acid?

 (a), (b), (c), (d) structures for question 2

324

(3)    The peptide bond would be described chemically as which type
       of bond?

       (a) ester    (b) amide    (c) ether    (d) anhydride

(4)    When a peptide bond is hydrolyzed (split):

       (a) water is released from the amino acid(s)
       (b) water is added to the amino acid(s)
       (c) oxidation of the amino acid occurs
       (d) reduction of amino acid occurs

(5)    Primary structure of amino acids is:

       (a) exemplified by $\alpha$-helical structure
       (b) not found in quaternary proteins
       (c) coded for by DNA
       (d) all of the above

(6)    Secondary structure of proteins is associated with:

       (a) sequence of amino acids
       (b) not in globular proteins
       (c) coded for by DNA
       (d) $\alpha$-helix

(7)    Select the type(s) of bonding important in maintenance of
       tertiary structure of proteins:

       (a) hydrophobic               (b)  van der Waals
       (c) covalent                  (d)  all are important

(8)    The highest level of protein structure found in monomeric
       globular proteins is:

       (a) primary   (b) secondary   (c) tertiary   (d) quaternary

(9)    Which of the following would be considered a hydrophilic amino
       acid?

       (a)     (b)

       (c)     (d)  none of the above

(10)   Select the basic amino acid:

       (a)     (b)

       (c)     (d)  none of the above

(11)  **Select the acidic amino acid:**

(a) $HO_2C-CH_2-CH_2-\overset{\overset{\displaystyle NH_2}{|}}{CH}-CO_2H$

(b) $H_2N-(CH_2)_4-\overset{\overset{\displaystyle NH_2}{|}}{CH}-CO_2H$

(c) $\langle \bigcirc \rangle-CH_2-\overset{\overset{\displaystyle NH_2}{|}}{CH}-CO_2H$

(d)  none of the above

(12)  **Which amino acid in question #12 will most likely be found on the interior of globular proteins?**

(a)        (b)        (c)        (d)

(13)  **Which of the following peptides probably has the highest pI?**

(a) $H_2N-\overset{\overset{\displaystyle H}{|}}{\underset{\underset{\displaystyle CH_2OH}{|}}{C}}-\overset{\overset{\displaystyle O}{||}}{C}-NH-\overset{\overset{\displaystyle H}{|}}{C}-NH-\overset{\overset{\displaystyle H}{|}}{\underset{\underset{\displaystyle CH_3}{|}}{C}}-\overset{\overset{\displaystyle O}{||}}{C}-OH$

(b) $H_2N-\overset{\overset{\displaystyle H}{|}}{\underset{\underset{\displaystyle CH_2CO_2H}{|}}{C}}-\overset{\overset{\displaystyle O}{||}}{C}-NH-\overset{\overset{\displaystyle H}{|}}{\underset{\underset{\displaystyle CH_2-CH_2-CO_2H}{|}}{C}}-\overset{\overset{\displaystyle O}{||}}{C}-NH-\overset{\overset{\displaystyle H}{|}}{C}-\overset{\overset{\displaystyle O}{||}}{C}-OH$

(c) $H_2N-\overset{\overset{\displaystyle H}{|}}{\underset{\underset{\displaystyle CH}{|}}{C}}-\overset{\overset{\displaystyle O}{||}}{C}-NH-\overset{\overset{\displaystyle H}{|}}{\underset{\underset{\displaystyle HO-CH}{|}}{C}}-\overset{\overset{\displaystyle O}{||}}{C}-NH-\overset{\overset{\displaystyle H}{|}}{\underset{\underset{\displaystyle CH_2OH}{|}}{C}}-\overset{\overset{\displaystyle O}{||}}{C}-OH$

(d) $H_2N-\overset{\overset{\displaystyle H}{|}}{\underset{\underset{\displaystyle (CH_2)_4-NH_2}{|}}{C}}-\overset{\overset{\displaystyle O}{||}}{C}-NH-\overset{\overset{\displaystyle H}{|}}{\underset{\underset{\displaystyle CH_3}{|}}{C}}-\overset{\overset{\displaystyle O}{||}}{C}-NH-\overset{\overset{\displaystyle H}{|}}{\underset{\underset{\displaystyle (CH_2)_3-NH-C-NH_2}{|}}{C}}-\overset{\overset{\displaystyle O}{||}}{C}-OH$

(14)  **Which of the peptides in #14 will probably migrate to the cathode at pH = 7.0?**

(a)        (b)        (c)        (d)

(15)  **Which of the peptides in #14 will probably migrate to the anode at pH = 7.0?**

(a)        (b)        (c)        (d)

4.13.3        ANSWERS TO QUESTIONS IN SECTION 4.13.2

( 1)  d    (2)  d    (3)  b    (4)  b    (5)  c    (6)  d    (7)  d
( 8)  c    (9)  b    (10) a    (11) a    (12) c    (13) d    (14) d
(15)  b

326

QUESTIONS #1-#8:  Adequately discussed in text.

QUESTIONS #9-#11:  Look at the R groups to determine the neutrality, basicity, acidity or hydrophilicity.  Refer to Section if necessary.

QUESTION #12  (Answer:  c) Hydrophobic AA's are found on the interior.  The AA in option (c) with the phenyl group is hydrophobic.

QUESTION #13  (Answer:  d) (a) and (c) have only polar or hydrophobic AA's, so its pI is around 7.  (b) has two acidic AA's and one AA that may be basic or acidic; therefore, its pI is less than 7.  (d) has two basic amino acids and, therefore, has a pI greater than 7.  See Section for discussion.

QUESTION #14  (Answer:  d)  The cathode attracts the positive ion.  Therefore, the peptide must be positively charged at pH = 7.0.  This means pH = 7 must be acidic relative to the pI and that the pI must be greater than 7, which means it must contain basic AA's.

QUESTION #15  (Answer:  b)  The anode attracts the basic ion.  Therefore, the peptide must be negatively charged at pH = 7.0.  This means that pH = 7 must be alkaline relative to the pI, or that the pI must be less than 7.  Therefore, there must be an excess of acidic AA's.  See discussion in Section.


4.13.5    VOCABULARY, CONCEPTS, ETC. CHECKLIST FOR AMINO ACIDS
          AND PROTEINS


_____   classes of amino acids
_____   protein structure
_____   peptide linkage and hydrolysis
_____   dipolar ions
_____   isoelectric point, pI
_____   basic amino acids
_____   acidic amino acids
_____   primary structure
_____   secondary structure
_____   tertiary structure
_____   quaternary structure
_____   classes of amino acids

## 4.14.1     REVIEW OF CARBOHYDRATES

Carbohydrates have the general formula $C_n(H_2O)_m$ where n and m are whole numbers. <u>Monosaccharides</u> are the basic units of carbohydrates. They are classified by the number of carbons they contain, i.e., <u>hexoses</u> ($C_6$), <u>pentoses</u> ($C_5$), etc. Hexoses and pentoses exist in predominantly ring forms called <u>pyranoses</u> (six membered rings) or <u>furanoses</u> (five membered rings) in equilibrium with the open-chain forms. Ring forms are hemiacetals (see Section 4.7.1); open-chain forms are polyhydroxy aldehydes. In the ring forms, ∝ or β-anomers are possible. The pyranoses exist in the stable chair conformation with most, if not all, of the hydroxyls in equatorial positions. When two monosaccharides differ by the configuration of one hydroxyl group, they are called <u>epimers</u>. If n is the number of asymmetric carbons, then $2^n$ is the number of optical <u>isomers</u> (based on open chain). Hexoses usually have n = 4 and pentoses usually have n = 3. Sugars are given a relative <u>configuration</u> on the basis of the orientation of the next to last carbon's hydroxyl group as compared to D-glyceraldehyde. Most naturally occuring sugars have the <u>D</u> configuration. A <u>ketose</u> is a carbohydrate with a ketone group; an <u>aldose</u> has an aldehyde group. Illustrations of the above points with the common monosaccharides are in Fig. 4.7.

**Fig. 4.7 - Monosaccharides**

Monosaccharides bond together to form __disaccharides__. The new bond formed is called a __glycosidic bond__ and is between the hemi-acetal carbon and an hydroxyl group of the other sugar; water is released when the bond is formed. Hydrolysis (breaking) of the bond requires water. The glycosidic bond is an acetal grouping (see Section 4.7.1) (Fig. 4.8). __Sucrose__ (common sugar) is made of glucose and fructose. __Lactose__ (milk sugar) is made of galactose and glucose. __Maltose__ ($\alpha$-1,4 bond) is made of two glucose units and is an hydrolysis product of starch or glycogen. __Cellobiose__ ($\beta$-1,4 bond) is also made of two glucoses, and it is the breakdown product of cellulose.

Fig. 4.8 - Glycosidic Bond

__Polysaccharides__ are many monosaccharides joined by glycosidic bonds; they may be branched also. __Starch__ (plant energy storage), __glycogen__ (animal short-term energy storage), and __cellulose__ (plant structural component) are all made from glucose. Cellulose has $\beta$-1,4 bonds not found in the other two. Starch and glycogen both have $\alpha$-1,4 bonds but differ in the frequency and position of branch points ($\alpha$-1,6 bonds).

Inulin is a polymer of fructose.

### 4.14.1 QUESTIONS TO REVIEW CARBOHYDRATES

(1) Which disaccharide has the __incorrect__ monosaccharide components listed by it?

(a) maltose--mannose and glucose
(b) lactose--galactose and glucose
(c) sucrose--fructose and glucose
(d) cellobiose--two glucoses

(2) Which of these is not a monosaccharide?

(a) ribose     (b) galactose     (c) maltose     (d) mannose

(3) Which compound is the reference for the relative configuration of sugars and amino acids?

(a) d-glucose                    (b) d-glyceraldehyde
(c) l-glycine                    (d) d-alanine

(4) Both glycogen and cellulose are polymers of glucose. The main factor that makes them different is

(a) cellulose has more glucose units;
(b) glycogen has more branch points;
(c) glycogen has ∝-1,4 bonds and cellulose has β-1,4 bonds between glucose units;
(d) cellulose has more glucose units and more branch points.

(5) For monosaccharides, the ring forms (pyranose or furanose) are:

(a) acetals  (b) hemiacetals  (c) carbonyls  (d) esters

Use the following structures for questions (6) - (12).

(6) Which structure is a furanose?

(a) III    (b) VI    (c) VIII    (d) IX

(7) Which structure is a ketose?

(a) I    (b) II    (c) III    (d) VI

(8) Which structure is the anomer of III?

(a) I    (b) IV    (c) V    (d) none of these

(9) Which structure is an epimer of IV?

(a) III    (b) V    (c) VI    (d) none of these

(10) Which conformation is more stable?

(a) VI    (b) VII    (c) both equal

(11) Which compound is a pentose?

(a) I    (b) II    (c) III    (d) VIII

(12) Which compound has an ∝-1,4 glycosidic bond?

(a) IX    (b) X    (c) both    (d) neither

330

**4.14.3** <u>ANSWERS TO QUESTIONS IN SECTION 4.14.2</u>

( 1) a (2) c (3) b (4) c (5) b (6) c (7) b
( 8) c (9) a (10) a (11) a (12) a


**4.14.4** <u>DISCUSSION OF ANSWERS TO QUESTIONS IN SECTION 4.14.2</u>

<u>QUESTIONS #1 to #5</u>: Adequately discussed in Section.

<u>QUESTION #6</u> (Answer: c) A furanose is a ring form which contains five atoms.

<u>QUESTION #7</u> (Answer: b) A ketose is a sugar which has a ketone functional grouping. (Section 4.7.1).

<u>QUESTION #8</u> (Answer: c) Anomers are compounds in the ring that differ in configuration only at the former carbonyl carbon:

<u>QUESTION #9</u> (Answer: a) Epimers are optical isomers that are different in configuration at a carbon other than the anomeric. III differs from IV at Carbon #4.

<u>QUESTION #10</u> (Answer: a) The more stable conformation is where the maximum number of substituents, especially the larger substituents, are in equatorial positions.

<u>QUESTION #11</u> (Answer: a) A pentose has a total of five carbons. See Section for symbolism.

<u>QUESTION #12</u> (Answer: a) To have an $\alpha$ bond the compound must be an $\alpha$-anomer:

**4.14.5** <u>VOCABULARY CONCEPTS, ETC. CHECKLIST FOR CARBOHYDRATES</u>

____ cyclic structures                    ____ ketose
____ conformations of hexoses             ____ aldose

_____ epimers
_____ anomers
_____ glycosidic bonds, hydrolysis
_____ monosaccharides
_____ hexoses
_____ pentoses
_____ pyranoses
_____ furanoses
_____ starch
_____ nomenclature and classification
of carbohydrates

_____ glucose
_____ fructose
_____ galactose
_____ mannose
_____ maltose
_____ sucrose
_____ lactose
_____ glycogen
_____ cellulose

## 4.15    References for Review of Organic Chemistry

Hendrickson, J. B., Cram, D. J., and Hammond, G. S. Organic Chemistry. McGraw-Hill, Inc.

Morrison, R. T., and Boyd, R. N. Organic Chemistry. Allyn and Bacon, Inc.

Both of the above texts are excellent introductory texts with the latter being easier to follow upon first reading. Both, however, are too detailed for the requirements of the MCAT. A selective review might be valuable.

# C H A P T E R   5:

# R E V I E W

# O F

# P H Y S I C S

### 5.1.1        REVIEW OF TRANSLATIONAL MOTION

Distance depends upon the path taken, has an inconstant direction, and has magnitude only. Speed is the distance traveled divided by the change in time. Both speed and distance are scalar quantities-- have magnitude but not direction. They have positive values only. Displacement is independent of the path taken (i.e., depends only on initial and final positions of the object) and has a constant direction and magnitude. Velocity is the displacement divided by the change in time. Both velocity and displacement are vector quantities (i.e., have direction and magnitude). Acceleration is the change in velocity divided by the change in time, and it is a vector also. (Fig. 5.1.)

note that displacement has a constant direction
and magnitude and is independent of the path
taken (there are many paths from A to B but
the displacement is the same regardless of
the path taken)

$$\text{speed} = \frac{\Delta \text{distance}}{\Delta \text{time}} = \frac{d_f - d_i}{t_f - t_i} \qquad \begin{array}{l} f = \text{final} \\ i = \text{initial} \end{array}$$

$$\text{velocity} = \frac{\text{displacement}}{\Delta \text{ time}}$$

$$\text{acceleration} = \frac{\Delta \text{ velocity}}{\Delta \text{ time}} = \frac{v_f - v_i}{t_f - t_i}$$

$$\Delta \text{ (delta)} \equiv \text{change}$$

**Fig. 5.1 — Translational Motion Parameters**

The units of distance and displacement are length such as feet (ft), meters (m), miles and kilometers (km). The units of speed and velocity then become length divided by time such as feet/sec., miles/hour or meters/sec. Acceleration has the units of length/time/time (length/time$^2$) and examples are feet/sec$^2$, meters/sec$^2$ and miles/hour$^2$. Note the sign (+ or –) of displacement, velocity or acceleration depends on the system under study and the specific values of the final (f) and initial (i) values. A displacement is negative if it is opposite to the direction designated as positive. The velocity is negative if the displacement is negative. The acceleration is negative if the velocity is decreasing. Instantaneous velocity or acceleration is for a given point in time. For velocity, it is the slope of the graph of distance vs. time at the given time. The average velocity or acceleration is for a period of time, and is conveniently taken as:

$$\bar{v} = \frac{v_f + v_i}{2} \quad \text{if acceleration is constant,}$$

$$\bar{a} = \frac{a_f + a_i}{2} \quad \text{if the force is constant.}$$

Note that these are different from the equations presented earlier.

Forces (Section 5.3.1) act upon objects to cause an acceleration. If a constant force is acting there is a constant (unchanging) acceleration. The motion produced in this case is called <u>uniform motion</u>. The acceleration (a) is causing a change in velocity (v) over time (t): if $a = 10$ m/sec$^2$ and 5 secs elapse

$$\text{then } v = at = \left(10\frac{m}{\text{sec}^2}\right) (5 \text{ secs}) = 50 \text{ m/sec after 5 seconds.}$$

The changing acceleration and velocity are both causing a change in displacement (d)--the directions of acceleration, velocity and displacement are all in the same direction:

$d_{vo} = v_o t$ displacement due to the initial velocity ($v_o$) at time $= t$;

$d_a = \frac{1}{2} at^2$ displacement due to the acceleration at time $= t$

$d_o =$ initial displacement (if any) from a reference.

The total displacement (d) in a time (t) for uniform motion (equation for uniform linear motion) is:

$\mathbf{d = d_o + v_o t + \frac{1}{2}at^2}$ (memorize)
or, final displacement (d) = initial displacement from a reference point ($d_o$) + change in displacement due to initial velocity ($v_o t$) + change in displacement due to acceleration ($\frac{1}{2}at^2$).

<u>Translational motion</u> is the motion of an object through space. The above equations illustrate uniform translational motion along a straight line.

Displacements, velocity and accelerations are added (or subtracted) by methods of <u>vectors</u>.

5.1.2       QUESTIONS TO REVIEW TRANSLATIONAL MOTION

(1)   Which of the following depends upon the path taken?

(a) distance   (b) displacement   (c) both   (d) neither

(2)   Which of the following is a vector?

(a) distance   (b) speed   (c) velocity   (d) all of these

(3)   The quantity below with the dimension of length/time$^2$ is:

(a) displacement              (b) velocity
(c) acceleration              (d) force

335

(4)  A constant acceleration is caused by a:

(a) constant force                    (b) changing force
(c) constant displacement             (d) either (a) or (b)

(5)  An object was moving at 10m/sec; then a force was applied for
10 sec and the final velocity was 60m/sec.  The acceleration
was:

$\frac{50}{10}$

(a) 3 m/sec$^2$                       (b) 5 m/sec$^2$
(c) 7 m/sec$^2$                       (d) none of the above

$V = V_0 + at$
$60 = 10 + a(10)$
$50/10 = 5$

(6)  An object initially moving at 15m/sec is accelerated at the
rate of 5m/sec$^2$ for 5 sec, the final velocity of the object is:

$15 + 5*5 = 40$

(a) 15 m/sec                          (b) 25 m/sec
(c) 40 m/sec             25           (d) 100 m/sec

$V = V_0 + at$
$V = 15 + 5(5) = 40$

(7)  An object starts 5m from a reference point with an initial
velocity of 10 m/sec and an acceleration of 5 m/sec$^2$.  After 5
secs, the object is how far from the reference point?

$S = S + vt + \frac{1}{2}at^2$
$= 50 + \ldots = 5$

(a) 75m    (b) 80m    (c) 117.5m    (d) 180.5m

$\Delta x = V_0 t + \frac{1}{2}at^2$
$x = 10(5) + \frac{1}{2} 5(25)$
$x = 50 + \frac{125}{2}$
$x = 110$

Use the following graph for Questions #8 through #12.  The motion is
initially to the right and is in a straight line.

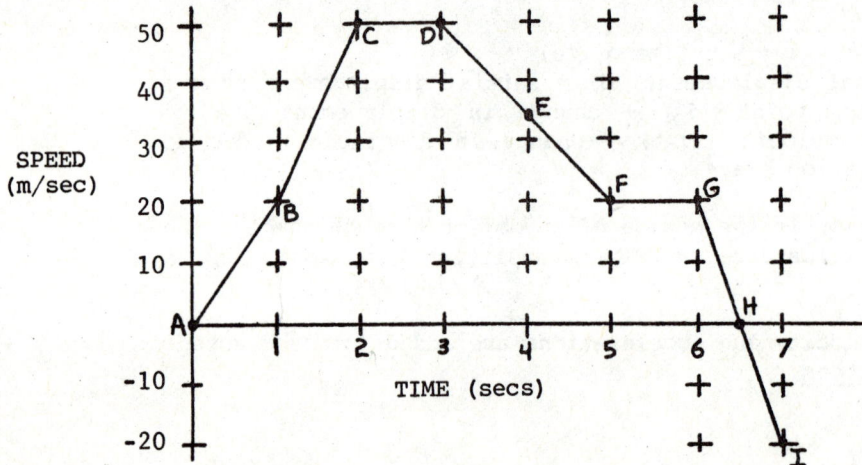

(8)  The slope of the graph at any point represents:

(a) acceleration                      (b) displacement
(c) force                             (d) kinetic energy

(9)  The instantaneous speed at point B is:

(a) 20 m/sec                          (b) 25 m/sec
(c) 10 m/sec                          (d) 35 m/sec

(10)  The instantaneous acceleration at point E is:

(a) 15 m/sec$^2$                      (b) -15 m/sec$^2$
(c) 30 m/sec$^2$                      (d) -30 m/sec$^2$

336

(11)  At point I, the object is:

   (a) to the left of the origin
   (b) moving to the right
   (c) moving to the left
   (d) not moving

(12)  The average speed from 0 to 2 secs is:

   (a) 12.5 m/sec                    (b) 20 m/sec
   (c) 22.5 m/sec                    (d) 25 m/sec


5.1.3          ANSWERS TO QUESTIONS IN SECTION 5.1.2

( 1)  a   (2)  c   (3)  c   (4)  a   (5)  b   (6)  c   (7)  c
( 8)  a   (9)  a   (10)  b   (11)  c   (12)  c


5.1.4          DISCUSSION OF ANSWERS TO QUESTIONS IN SECTION 5.1.2

QUESTIONS #1 to #4:  Adequately discussed in the Section.

QUESTION #5  (Answer:  b)  Use the formula for acceleration (a),

$$a = \Delta V/\Delta t = V_f - V_i/t_f - t_i = 60-10/10-0 = 50/10 = 5 \text{ m/sec}^2$$

QUESTION #6  (Answer:  c)  The final velocity ($v_f$) is:

$v_f$ = initial velocity + velocity change due to acceleration
   = 15 m/sec + at = 15 + (5 m/sec$^2$)(5 sec) = 15 + 25 = 40 m/sec

QUESTION #7  (Answer:  c)  Use the formula for distance:

$$d = d_o + v_o t + \tfrac{1}{2} at^2 = 5 + (10)(5) + \tfrac{1}{2}(5)(5)^2$$
$$= 5 + 50 + (\tfrac{1}{2})(5)(25) = 55 + \tfrac{1}{2}(125)$$
$$= 55 + 62.5 = 117.5$$

QUESTION #8  (Answer:  a)  The slope of the curve of any graph is the ratio of the change in the y-axis ($\Delta y$) to the corresponding change in the x-axis ($\Delta x$).  In this case,

$\Delta y$ = change in speed = $\Delta v$

$\Delta x$ = change in time  = $\Delta t$

then:
     slope = $\Delta y/\Delta x = \Delta v/\Delta t$ = acceleration.

QUESTION #9  (Answer:  a)  The answer is 20 m/sec as read from the graph.  Instantaneous speed is the speed at a given point in time.

QUESTION #10  (Answer:  b)  Since E is on the line $\overline{DF}$, the instantaneous acceleration (i.e., the slope at a given point) at E is the same as the slope of line $\overline{DF}$:

337

acceleration at E = 20 - 50/5 - 3 = -30/2 = -15 m/sec$^2$

QUESTION #11 (Answer: c) Initially, a positive speed meant the object was moving to the right. A negative speed now means the object is moving to the left. The area between the curve and the time axis is the distance traveled. Since the area from A to H is much greater than the area from H to I, the object could not have moved back to the origin as (a) states. Also, only at points A and H is the object motionless.

QUESTION #12 (Answer: c) The average speed is,

average speed = total distance/total time.

The total distance is the area under the graph from A to C.

Total area = distance = Area #1 + Area #2 + Area #3
    = (½)(20)(1) + (20)(1)+(½)(30)(1)
    = 10 + 20 + 15 = 45m

Then: avg speed = 45m/2 sec. = 22.5 m/sec. The formula $\bar{v} = \dfrac{V_f + V_i}{2}$

cannot be used because the acceleration is not constant over this interval.

5.1.5    VOCABULARY, CONCEPTS, ETC. CHECKLIST FOR TRANSLATIONAL MOTION

____ units and dimensions of distance, speed (velocity), acceleration
____ equation for uniform linear motion
____ speed
____ distance
____ displacement
____ velocity
____ acceleration
____ translational motion

5.2    Equilibrium

5.2.1    REVIEW OF EQUILIBRIUM

When a force (Section 5.3.1) acts upon an object, the object will undergo translational motion or rotational motion. Translational motion is the motion of the object through space when the force is acting along an axis and/or the center of mass (that point whose motion can be described like a particle, Section 5.3.1). Rotational motion is the rotation of an object about an axis caused by a force not directed along that axis. The effective force causing rotation about an axis is the torque (L) (Fig. 5.2).

L = (force)(moment arm)
    moment arm is the perpendicular distance
    from the force to the axis
F = force
r = moment arm
c = center of mass or an axis
$L_1 = (F_1)(r_1)$ = counterclockwise (1) = positive
$L_2 = (F_2)(r_2)$ = clockwise (2) = negative

Fig. 5.2 - Torque


To determine the direction of rotation caused by the torque, imagine the direction the object would rotate if the force is pushing against its moment arm (at right angles). The net forces acting on an object is best determined by analysis of them into the x and y components.* The net torques acting on an object is obtained by summing the counterclockwise (+) and clockwise (-) torques. An object is at equilibrium when the net forces and torques acting on it is zero. Note that this means there is no acceleration but does not mean there is no velocity; it means either the object is motionless or moving with a constant velocity. The conditions of equilibrium are:

for translational equilibrium
$\Sigma F_x = 0$      ( $\Sigma$ = sum over all)
$\Sigma F_y = 0$
for rotational equilibrium
$\Sigma L = 0$      (in a given geometric plane, must hold for three
                    mutually perpendicular planes).

If the torques sum to zero about one point in an object, they will sum to zero about any point in the object. If the point chosen as reference includes the line of action of one of the forces, that force need not be included in calculating the torques.

Newton's First Law states that objects at rest or in motion tend to remain as such unless acted upon by an outside force. That is, objects have inertia (resistance to motion). For translational motion, the mass (m) is a measure of inertia. For rotational motion, a quantity derived from mass called the moment of inertia (I) is the measure of inertia. The $I = \Sigma mr^2$ in general, but its exact formulation depends on the structure of the object. See Section 5.6.1 for compressive and tensile forces.

Momentum (M) is a vector quantity. Its formulation for magnitude is:

$$M = mv$$
m = mass
v = velocity


(For a discussion of vectors, refer to Volume II of A COMPLETE PREPARATION FOR THE MCAT.)

Linear momentum is a measure of the tendency of an object to maintain motion in a straight line. Notice that $\underline{M}$ is directly proportional to the mass of the object and its velocity (not acceleration). The larger the $\underline{M}$, the greater the tendency of the object to remain moving along a straight line (in the same direction). The $\underline{M}$ is also a measure of the force needed to stop or change direction of the object. The impulse (I) is given by:

$$I = F \, \Delta t = \underline{M} = mv$$
$$F = \text{force acting}$$
$$\Delta t = \text{elapsed time which force is acting over}$$

The I is a measure of the force required to impart or change momentum of an object. The I is also a vector.

Just like energy, momentum is also conserved. The total linear momentum of a system is constant when the resultant external force acting on the system is zero.

Collisions are a form of interaction of matter during which momentum (remember, it is a vector) is conserved. During an elastic collision (objects do not stick), there is conservation of momentum and conservation of the kinetic energy. During an inelastic collision (objects stick together), there is conservation of momentum but not of kinetic energy (the remainder of the energy is lost as heat or sound, so total energy is conserved).

Two special collisions will be mentioned. In the explosion of an object at rest, the total momentum of all the fragments must sum to zero (original momentum was zero). If one object collides elastically with a second identical object that is at rest, the first object comes to rest and the second moves off with the momentum of the first.

5.2.2      QUESTIONS TO REVIEW EQUILIBRIUM

(1)   Rotational motion:

(a) movement of an object along a curved line
(b) movement of an object through space
(c) motion of an object about a fixed point
✓(d) motion of an object about an axis

(2)   "An object at rest tends to remain at rest while objects in motion tend to remain in motion...;" this is Newton's First Law and it reflects the property of:

(a) velocity                          (b) weight
(c) potential energy          ✓(d) inertia

(3)   If a force is acting on an object, but off an axis, what type of motion results?

✓(a) rotational                          (b) translational

340

(4)    The product of force times the moment arm is the:

(a) energy                          (b) work
(c) torque ✓                        (d) force


(5)    The net force (in newtons) on the following object  (answers in nts) is:

$F_2 = 100$ nts  $y(+)$

$F_1 = 20$ nts

(-) _ _ _ _ _ 60° __ 30° _ _ _ (+) / X    m = 10 kg

weight
(-)

(a) zero                            (b) $F_x = -32.7$; $F_y = -1.5$
(c) $F_x = -15.4$; $F_y = +98.3$    (d) $F_x = -80$; $F_y = -98.3$

$F_y = \dfrac{100}{\sqrt{3}} + \dfrac{20}{2} - 98$

$= 50 + 10$

① $F_x = 20\cos 30° = 10\sqrt{3}$
$F_y = 20\sin 30° = 10$

② $F_x = 100\cos 120 = -50$
$F_y = 100\sin 120 = 50\sqrt{3}$

③ $F_y = 10 \times (-9.8) = -98$

TOT:  $F_y = 10 + 50\sqrt{3} - 98$
$= -1.397$

$F_x = 10\sqrt{3} - 50 = -32.6$


(6)    What is the net force on the following object?

$F_1$ 10 nts          5 nts  $F_2$

(a) 15 nts                          (b) 5 nts to the right
(c) 5 nts compressive force         (d) none of these

$F_x = +10$
$F_x = -5$  = 5


(7)    What is the net torque acting about the axis through the center A (perpendicular to the paper) of the square with sides equal to 4m?

$F_1 = 10$ nts
45°      90°
$F_4 = 10$ nts
A
$F_3 = 20$ nts  ←90°→  $F_2 = 5$ nts

$2\sqrt{2}$

$\dfrac{4}{\sqrt{2}}$    $2\sqrt{2} = 2.8$      0

$2.8\sqrt{\phantom{x}}$

$28 + 2\sqrt{2} \cdot \dfrac{20}{\sqrt{2}} - \dfrac{N}{\sqrt{2}} 2\sqrt{\phantom{x}} \dfrac{5}{\sqrt{2}} 2\sqrt{2}$

$28 + 40 - 20$
$.68 - 30 =$

(a) 38.2 nt-m counterclockwise     (b) 76.4 nt-m clockwise
(c) 38.2 nt-m clockwise            (d) none of the above


(8)    The object below is in static and rotational equilibrium. What are the components of the force, $F_1$?

(+)
y
(-) ___ (+)
x
(-)

$F_3 = 10$ nts
$F_2 = 50$ nts
mass = 10 Kgs
$F_1 = ?$

$F_1$

$F_3$   $F_x = 0$          $0 + 50 + F_x = 0$
$F_y = 10$          $F_x = 50$
$F_2$   $F_x = 50$
$F_y = 0$    $-98 \cdot 10 + 0 + F_y = 0$

$F_y = -8$

(a) $F_x = -50$ nts; $F_y = -10$ nts     (b) $F_x = -50$ nts; Fy = +88 nts
(c) $F_x = +50$ nts; $F_y = -108$ nts    (d) none of the above

$w = 98$ y

341

(9)   The object below is in rotational equilibrium.  What force,
$F_1$, is required for this equilibrium (neglect the weight)?

A = axis of potential rotation

(a) counterclockwise, 17.5 nts     (b) clockwise, 5 nts
(c) clockwise, 35 nts              (d) none of the above

**5.2.3**          ANSWERS TO QUESTIONS IN SECTION 5.2.2

(1)  d   (2)  d   (3)  a   (4)  c   (5)  b   (6)  b   (7)  c
(8)  b   (9)  d

**5.2.4**          DISCUSSION OF ANSWERS TO QUESTIONS IN SECTION 5.2.2

QUESTION #1 to #4:  Adequately discussed in the text.

QUESTION #5   (Answer:  b)  The forces may be rediagrammed as:

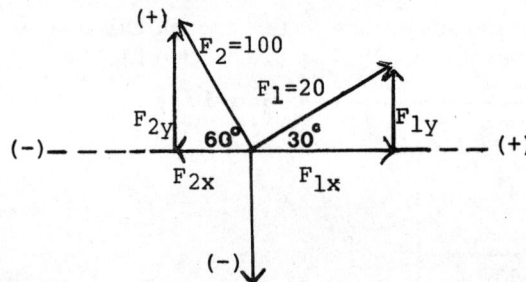

$W_y = mg = (10)(9.8) = 98$ nts
(Weight has no x-component in this case.)

For a 30°-60° right triangle (see also A COMPLETE PREPARATION FOR
THE   MCAT,   Volume   II:   Skills   Development   in   Reading   and
Quantitative) use:

Then: for $F_1$:  $F_{1y} = +(1/2)(20) = +10$       $F_{1x} = +(\sqrt{3}/2)20 = +10\sqrt{3}$
      for $F_2$:  $F_{2y} = +(\sqrt{3}/2)(100) = +50\sqrt{3}$     $F_{2x} = -(1/2)(100) = -50$

Then: $\Sigma F_x = F_{1x} + F_{2x} + W_x = 10\sqrt{3} - 50 + 0 = 17.3 - 50 = -32.7$ nts
                   $(\sqrt{3} \sim 1.73)$
      $\Sigma F_y = F_{1y} + F_{2y} + W_y = +10 + 50\sqrt{3} - 98 = +50(1.73) - 88$
             $= 86.5 - 88 = -1.5$ nts.

The net force (F) would be:

$$F^2 = F_x^2 + F_y^2$$
$$F = \sqrt{F_x^2 + F_y^2} = \sqrt{(-32.7)^2 + (-1.5)^2} = 32.7 \text{ nts}$$
(calculation on calculator)

QUESTION #6 (Answer: b)  These are opposing forces acting along the same line of action.  The net force is the algebraic sum (assume positive is to the right):

net force = +10 nts − 5 nts = +5 nts.

QUESTION #7 (Answer: c)  The forces, their moment arms (r) and directions of rotation (R) are:

(Refer to **Volume II: Skills Development in Reading and Quantitative** mentioned above.)

The torques are:

Counterclockwise (+)
$L_1 = F_1 \times r_1 = (10)(2) = +20 \text{ nt-m}$
$L_2 = F_2 \times r_2 = (5)(2) = +10 \text{ nt-m}$

Clockwise (−)

$L_3 = F_3 \times r_3 = -(20)(2) = -40 \text{ nt-m}$

$L_4 = F_4 \times r_4 = -(10)(2\sqrt{2}) = -20\sqrt{2} = -28.2 \text{ nt-m}$

The net torque (L) is:

$L = L_1 + L_2 + L_3 + L_4 = +20+10-40-28.2 = +30 - 68.2$
$L = -38.2 \text{ nt-m}$ (which is clockwise).

QUESTION #8   (Answer:  b)   The force diagram is:

$$W\text{(weight)} = mg = (10)(9.8) = 98 \text{ nts}$$

$$W\text{ (weight)} = mg = (10)(9.8) = 98 \text{ nts}$$

Components of forces:

$F_1 : F_{1x} = ?$          $F_{1y} = ?$
$F_2 : F_{2x} = +50$      $F_{2y} = 0$
$F_3 : F_{3x} = 0$       $F_{3y} = +10$
$W : W_x = 0$       $W_y = -98$

Net force (F):

$$\Sigma F_x = 0 = F_{1x} + F_{2x} + F_{3x} + W_x = F_{1x} + 50 + 0 + 0 = F_{1x} + 50$$
$$\text{then,}\quad F_{1x} + 50 = 0$$
$$F_{1x} = -50 \text{ nts}$$

$$\Sigma F_y = 0 = F_{1y} + F_{2y} + F_{3y} + W_y = F_{1y} + 0 + 10 - 98 = F_{1y} - 88$$
$$\text{then,}\quad F_{1y} - 88 = 0$$
$$F_{1y} = 88 \text{ nts.}$$

QUESTION #9   (Answer:  d)   The directions of rotations are:
    $F_2$ causes counterclockwise (+) motion
    $F_3$ causes counterclockwise (+) motion

The individual torques are:
    $L_1 = F_1 \times r_1 = (F_1)(2) = 2F_1$     (sign unknown)
    $L_2 = +F_2 \times r_2 = +(5)(3) = +15$ nt-m
    $L_3 = +F_3 \times r_3 = +(20)(1) = +20$ nt-m.

Since rotational equilibrium exists the torques sum to zero:
    $\Sigma L = L_1 + L_2 + L_3 = 0$
      $2F_1 + 15 + 20 = 0$
      $2F_1 + 35 = 0$
      $2F_1 = -35$
      $F_1 = -17.5$ nts and motion is clockwise.

5.2.5       VOCABULARY, CONCEPTS, ETC. CHECKLIST FOR EQUILIBRIUM

\_\_\_\_  conditions for translational equilibrium
       conditions for rotational equilibrium
\_\_\_\_  separation of forces into their components
\_\_\_\_  Newton's First Law
\_\_\_\_  torque

5.3.1     REVIEW OF FORCE, MOTION AND GRAVITATION

The center of mass (COM) of an extended body is that point whose
motion can be described like a particle (e.g., as linear, circular,
parabolic) even if the motion of the extended object cannot be so
described.  In collisions, the COM velocity (of the system) is not
changed.   The center of gravity (COG) is the COM but is
conceptualized as that point where the sum of gravitational forces
acting on an extended object can be represented by a summation force
(acting at the COM).   An object suspended from the COG is in
rotational equilibrium (Section 5.2.1).  The COG can be determined
experimentally by suspending an object by a string at different
points and noting that the direction of the string passes through the
COG.   The intersections of the projected lines in the different
suspensions is the COG.  The COG of a regular geometric object is the
geometric center.  The COG of an irregular object may be inside or
outside the object. An object is in stable equilibrium if the COG is
as low as possible, and any change in orientation will lead to an
elevation of the COG.  Unstable equilibrium is when the COG is high
(relative to a surface supporting it, e.g.), and any change in
orientation would lead to a lowering of the COG.  Neutral equilibrium
is an intermediate location of the COG and a change in orientation
would not change the level of the COG.  A force acting through the
COG causes translational motion.  A force acting off the COG causes
rotational motion.  Mass is a dimension that cannot be broken down
into simpler units.  This is to be contrasted with weight which is a
force.  Units of mass are slugs (weight in pounds divided by g = 32
ft/sec$^2$), kilograms, grams, etc.   Units of weight are pounds
(defined differently from the pounds of mass), dynes (gms·cm/sec$^2$)
and newtons (kg·m/sec$^2$).

Newton's Second Law involves an unbalanced force acting upon an
object and producing an acceleration in the direction of the force
that is directly proportional to the force and inversely
proportional to the mass of the body:

$$a = F/m$$
$$\text{or, } F = ma.$$

For every action, there is an equal and opposite reaction.  This is
Newton's Third Law.  If one object exerts a force, F, on a second
object, the second object exerts a force, -F, on the first.  These
forces cannot neutralize each other because they act on different
objects.  Every force arises from three basic forces.  These are
gravitational (below), electromagnetic (Section 5.7), and nuclear
(Section 5.13).

Newton also formulated the Law of Gravitation as:

$$F = K_G (m_1 m_2 / r^2)$$

This states that there is a gravitational force existing between any
two bodies of masses $m_1$ and $m_2$.  The force is proportional to the
product of the masses:

$$F \propto m_1 m_2$$

and inversely proportional to the square of the distance between them:

$$F \propto 1/r^2$$

The $K_G$ is the universal constant of gravitation, and its value depends upon the units being used.

Free fall motion. This is vertical motion (in reference to the earth), that is, upward or downward in a straight line. It is always uniformly accelerated motion with the acceleration equal to g. Values of g are:

$$32 \text{ ft/sec}^2 \text{ or } 980 \text{ cms/sec}^2 \text{ or } 9.8 \text{ m/sec}^2.$$

The equations for uniform linear motion (Section 5.1.1) are applicable when the g is substituted for a:

$$d = d_0 + v_0 t + \tfrac{1}{2} gt^2$$
$$V = gt.$$

The reference point (origin) and positive and negative directions must be defined. As an example, in $g = 32 \text{ ft/sec}^2$, what the g means is that for every second an object is falling under the influence of gravity (neglecting air resistance), the velocity is increasing by 32 ft/sec. For an object thrown straight up, its speed is decreasing by 32 ft/sec for every second.

In the free fall of actual objects, the value of g is modified by buoyancy of air and resistance of air. What results is drag force and depends on the location on earth, weight, shape and size of the object, and the velocity of the object (as free fall velocity increases, the drag force increases). When the drag force reaches the force of gravity, the object reaches a final velocity called the terminal velocity and continues to fall at that velocity.

Projectile motion is conveniently thought of as having vertical (affected by g) and horizontal (independent of g) components. The vertical component is described by free fall motion (as above) and the horizontal component is described by uniform linear motion (Section 5.1.1) with a = 0. The projectile is generally fired at some angle ($\theta$) to the horizontal, and the motion is parabolic (see Fig. 5.3).

Fig. 5.3 – Projectile Motion

<u>Vertical component (free fall)</u>

initial speed $\quad\quad\quad V_{oy} \quad = V_o \sin\Theta$

distance at time $= t \quad y \quad = V_{oy}t + \frac{1}{2}gt^2$

speed at any time $= t \quad V_y = V_{oy} + gt$

(note that g is negative if it is opposite to the original displacement)

<u>Horizontal component (linear with constant speed)</u>

initial speed $\quad\quad\quad V_{ox} = v_o\cos$

distance at any time $= t \quad x = V_{ox}t$

speed at any time $= t \quad\quad V_x = V_{ox}$ (speed is constant)

<u>Initial velocity vector ($\vec{V}$) at any time $= t$</u>

magnitude $\quad V^2 = (V_{ox})^2 + (V_{oy})^2$ (Pythagorean Theorem)

direction ($\Theta$) $\tan\Theta = V_{oy}/V_{ox}$

Points to note about the above are:

(1) $V_{ox}$ is constant

(2) $V_y$ is zero at $Y_{max}$, then $V_y = 0 = V_{oy} + gt$
$-V_{oy} = gt$ (and can solve for t)

(3) at O and F, the V's are equal but opposite in sign

(4) the maximum range is attained when $\Theta = 45^o$

<u>Frictional forces</u> are illustrated in Fig. 5.4.

W = weight = mg = N (neglecting signs)

**Fig. 5.4 - Frictional Forces**

$F = \mu N$, this is the maximal frictional force

$\mu$ = coefficient of friction

N = normal (perpendicular) force to the surface the object rests on.

Frictional forces are nonconservative (mechanical energy is not conserved) and are caused by molecular adhesions between tangential surfaces but are independent of the area of contact of the surfaces. Frictional forces always oppose the motion. Static friction is when the object is not moving, and it must be overcome for motion to begin. The coefficient of static friction, $\mu_s$, is given as:

$$\mu_s = \tan\Theta ,$$

where $\Theta$ is the angle at which the object first begins to move on an inclined plane as the angle is increased from $0^o \longrightarrow \Theta^o$:

there is also a coefficient of kinetic friction, $\mu_k$, which exists when surfaces are in motion. The $\mu_s > \mu_k$ always.

The analysis of <u>motion on an incline</u> is shown in Fig. 5.5.

W = weight = mg

components of forces
N = normal to surface
$W_y = W_{\cos\theta}$    $W_x = W_{\sin\theta}$

**Fig. 5.5 – Motion on an Incline I**

The weight (W) due to gravity (g) may be sufficient to cause motion if friction is overcome.  The reference axes are usually chosen as shown such that one (the x) is along the surface of the incline. Additional forces on the object added to the basic set above is shown in Fig. 5.6.

$$\left.\begin{array}{l} \text{net } F_x = m_1g - W_{2x} \\ \text{net } F_y = -W_{2y} \end{array}\right\} \text{net } F = \sqrt{F_x{}^2 + F_y{}^2}$$

**Fig. 5.6 – Motion on an Incline II**

Note that N is the reactive force to $W_{2y}$, the axes are assigned  + and - as one desires.

5.3.2            QUESTIONS TO REVIEW FORCE, MOTION AND GRAVITATION

(1)    One of Newton's Laws of Motion:

(a) An unbalanced force acting upon an object produces an acceleration of that object.

(b) Objects moving in circles at constant tangential velocity have no force acting upon them.

(c) The square of the period of revolution is proportional to the cube of the radius of revolution.

(d) Objects falling to earth describe a hyperbolic projectory

(2)    The analysis of projectile motion is greatly simplified by:

(a) using the formula for describing the motion as a parabola;

(b) realizing that the time of ascent is one-half the time of descent;

(c) neglecting the effect of gravity if the object is considered a point mass;

(d) separating the motion into vertical (free fall) and horizontal (uniform linear motion) components.

(3) The maximum horizontal distance an object can attain is when the object is thrown at what angle to the horizontal?

(a) 15⁰     (b) 30⁰     (c) 45⁰     (d) 60⁰

(4) An unbalanced force acting upon an object causes

(a) a change in the mass of the object;
(b) an acceleration of the object;
(c) the object to maintain a constant velocity;
(d) none of the above.

(5) In order for any object to undergo an acceleration, it must

(a) lose energy;
(b) gain energy;
(c) be acted upon by balanced (net zero) forces;
(d) be acted upon by unbalanced forces.

(6) Newton's Second Law:

(a) $E = \frac{1}{2} mv^2$        (b) $F = -kx$
(c) $U = mgh$           (d) $F = ma$

(7) Frictional forces exist between an object and the surface it is on, and they

(a) are proportional to the normal force to the surface that the object rests on;
(b) are dependent on the area of contact between the surfaces;
(c) always augment the motion of the object;
(d) are conservative forces.

(8) For $\mu_s$ (coefficient of static friction) and $\mu_k$ (coefficient of kinetic friction)

(a) $\mu_s > \mu_k$        (b) $\mu_s = \mu_k$
(c) $\mu_s < \mu_k$        (d) any of the above

(9) The motion of the center of mass is like a(n):

(a) particle          (b) extended object
(c) both               (d) neither

(10) The force of gravity between two objects is

(a) inversely proportional to the products of the masses;
(b) inversely proportional to the distance between them;
(c) directly proportional to the square of the radius;
(d) inversely proportional to the square of the distance between them.

(11) A force of 15 newtons acting upon a 5 kg object will produce an acceleration equal to:

(a) $1/3$ m/sec$^2$        (b) $1/75$ m/sec$^2$
(c) 3 m/sec$^2$          (d) 75 m/sec$^2$

(12) An object has an acceleration of 2 m/sec$^2$ and a mass of 5 kg. The force necessary to impart this acceleration is:

(a) 0.4 newtons        (b) 2.5 newtons
(c) 5 newtons           (d) 10 newtons

(13) If F = force, $\Delta U$ = potential energy change, $\Delta x$ = displacment over which $\Delta U$ occurs, then:

(a) $F = \Delta U \Delta x$  (b) $F = 1/ \Delta U \Delta x$
(c) $F = - \Delta x/ \Delta U$  (d) $F = - \Delta U/ \Delta x$

(14) An object is thrown vertically upward at an initial velocity of 49 m/sec. It will rise to what height?

(a) 122.5 m  (b) 245 m
(c) 490 m  (d) the time must be given

(15) An object dropped from the edge of a cliff will fall how far in 10 seconds?

(a) cannot be determined; need the mass of the object
(b) 98 m
(c) 980 m
(d) 490 m

(16) An object first begins to slide down an inclined plane when the angle with the horizontal is 45°. The coefficient of static friction ($\mu$s) of the object-surface is:

(a) 0.5  (b) 1.0

(c) $\sqrt{2}/2$  (d) need more information

Use the following graph for Questions #19 through #23.

The above is a graph for a 2 kg object moving along a straight line to the right initially.

(17) The area under the graph represents:

(a) distance  (b) acceleration
(c) force  (d) velocity

(18) The greatest force is acting at:

(a) $\overline{AB}$  (b) $\overline{BC}$  (c) $\overline{CD}$  (d) $\overline{EF}$

(19) No force is acting along:

(a) $\overline{AB}$  (b) $\overline{BC}$  (c) $\overline{CD}$  (d) $\overline{EF}$

350

(20)  The distance traveled from A to B is:

   (a) 5 m     (b) 10 m     (c) 15 m     (d) 20 m

(21)  At point F, the object is:

   (a) motionless              (b) moving backward
   (c) moving forward          (d) at the origin

**Use the following information for Questions #22 and #23.**

An object is thrown with an initial speed of 19.6 m/sec at an angle of 30° with the horizontal.

(22)  The maximum height the object reaches is:

   (a) 2.45 m                  (b) 4.9 m
   (c) 9.8 m                   (d) 98 m

(23)  The range (horizontal distance) of the object is:

   (a) 19.6 m                  (b) $19.6\sqrt{3}$ m

   (c) 9.8 m                   (d) $9.8\sqrt{3}$ m

(24)  What value of Weight ($W_1$) is required such that the object (A) does not move down the incline (assume no friction)

mass of A is 10 kg

   (a) 5 newtons               (b) 10 newtons
   (c) 49 newtons              (d) none of the above

5.3.3    ANSWERS TO QUESTIONS IN SECTION 5.3.2

( 1)  a   ( 2)  d   ( 3)  c   ( 4)  b   ( 5)  d   ( 6)  d   ( 7)  a
( 8)  a   ( 9)  a   (10)  d   (11)  c   (12)  d   (13)  d   (14)  a
(15)  d   (16)  b   (17)  a   (18)  d   (19)  b   (20)  c   (21)  a
(22)  b   (23)  b   (24)  c

5.3.4    DISCUSSION OF ANSWERS TO QUESTIONS IN SECTION 5.3.2

QUESTIONS #1 to #10:  Adequately discussed in the Section.

QUESTION #11  (Answer:  c)  F = ma
       a = F/M = 15 newtons/5 Kgs = 3(nts/Kg)
              = 3 $\left[(Kg\text{-}m/sec^2)/Kg\right]$  = 3 m/sec$^2$

351

QUESTION #12   (Answer:  d)

$$F = ma = (5 \text{ kg}) (2 \text{ m/sec}^2) = 10 \text{ kg-m/secs}^2 = 10 \text{ newtons.}$$

QUESTION #13   (Answer:  d)   If the relationship is not already known to you, it may be determined (in this case) by knowing unit interrelations (i.e., by doing dimensional analysis):

$$\text{energy} = \text{work} = \text{Fd} \quad \text{(Section 5.4.1)}$$

then to get force equal to some combination of energy and displacement:

Force $\propto$ energy/displacement, which is the <u>form</u> of
answer (d).

Or, since Force = newtons and energy = joules = <u>newtons-meters</u> and d = meters, the only way to combine the units of energy and displacement to yield the units of force is:

$$\text{newtons (force)} \propto \frac{\text{newtons-meters (energy)}}{\text{meters(displacement)}} = \text{newtons}$$

$$\text{or} \qquad \text{Force} \propto \frac{\text{energy}}{\text{displacement}}.$$

Note that the best that can be said from this analysis is that force is proportional to energy over displacement.   The exact form of answer (d) could not be arrived at in this manner.

QUESTION #14   (Answer:  a)   The object will rise for as long as it takes the downward acceleration (due to gravity-g) to overcome the initial upward velocity, i.e.:

$$V_O = gt$$

$$t = \frac{V_O}{g} = \frac{49 \text{ m/sec}}{9.8 \text{ m/sec}^2} = 5 \text{ secs.}$$

Then using the formula for uniform linear motion (Section 5.1.1):

$$d = d_o + v_o t + \tfrac{1}{2} gt^2 = 0 + 49 (5) + \tfrac{1}{2} (-9.8)(5)^2 = 245 - 122.5$$
$$d = 122.5 \text{ m.}$$

Note that the g is negative because it opposes the original motion.

QUESTION #15   (Answer:  d)   Using the equations for linear motion (Section 5.1.1) and the fact that gravity is the accelerative force:

$$d = d_o + v_o t + \tfrac{1}{2} gt^2$$
$$= 0 + (0)(10) + (\tfrac{1}{2})(9.8)(10)^2 = (4.9)(100) = 490 \text{ m.}$$

This is an example of free fall motion.

QUESTION #16   (Answer:  b)   The $\mu_s$ is found by:

$$\mu_s = \tan \theta$$
$$\mu_s = \tan 45^\circ$$
$$\mu_s = 1/1 = 1$$

$$\tan \theta = \text{opposite/adjacent.}$$

**Refer to Volume II:  Skills Development in Reading and Quantitative.**

QUESTION #17 (Answer: a) The area under any curve is proportional to the product of the axes:

         y-axis is speed (v)
         x-axis is time (t)
    product = (v)(t) = distance.

QUESTION #18 (Answer: d) The greatest force is acting where the greatest acceleration (whether positive or negative) is also. This is because:

         F = ma and F $\propto$ a.

The greatest acceleration is where the slope $\Delta v/\Delta t$ is the greatest in absolute value (neglecting signs). For each of the above line segments, the slope, and acceleration, is:

$$a = \Delta v/\Delta T = (V_f - V_i)/(t_f - t_i)$$

$\overline{AB}$:  $a = (20-10)/(1-0) = 10/1 = 10$
$\overline{BC}$:  $a = (20-20)/(2-1) = 0/1 = 0$
$\overline{CD}$:  $a = (50-20)/(3-2) = 30/1 = 30$
$\overline{EF}$:  $a = (0-50)/(6-5) = -50/1 = -50.$

Hence, $\overline{EF}$ has the largest acceleration and the largest force.

QUESTION #19 (Answer: b) Again, since F = ma and F$\propto$a, a zero acceleration gives a zero force. A zero acceleration occurs where the slope is zero. See the discussion in Question #18 for the slopes of the segments. $\overline{BC}$ is the only one with a zero slope and, therefore, a zero acceleration and a zero force.

QUESTION #20 (Answer: c)

(I) By geometry:

Area (1) = ($\frac{1}{2}$)(10)(1) = 5m
Area (2) = (10)(1) = 10 m
total = 5 + 10 = 15 m

(II) By formulas:

$$d = d_0 = v_0 t + \tfrac{1}{2} a t^2 \quad \text{(Section 5.1.1)}$$
$$d_0 = 0 \quad v_0 = 10 \text{ m/sec}$$
$$a = \Delta v/\Delta t = (20-10)/(1-0) = 10/1 = 10 \text{ m/sec}^2$$
$$t = 1 \text{ sec}$$
$$d = 0 + (10)(1) + (\tfrac{1}{2})(10)(1)^2 = 10 + 5 = 15 \text{ m.}$$

QUESTION #21 (Answer: a) The speed is zero at point F, so the object must not be moving. Also, note that at no point is the speed negative, so the object could not have returned to the origin.

QUESTION #22 (Answer: b) The maximum height would correspond to the height reached if the object was thrown vertically upward with the vertical component of the initial velocity ($v_0$)

$$v_y = v_0 \sin 30^\circ = (19.6)(\tfrac{1}{2}) = 9.8 \text{ m/sec}$$

$$v_x = v_0 \cos 30^\circ = (19.6)(\sqrt{3}/2) = 9.8\sqrt{3} \text{ m/sec}$$

Remember:     $\sin \theta$ = opposite/hypotenuse

$\cos \theta$ = adjacent/hypotenuse

The distance can be calculated using the formula for linear motion (Section 5.1.1):

$$d = d_0 + v_0 t + \tfrac{1}{2}gt^2.$$

But the time is needed. This is found by reasoning that the object continues to rise until its upward motion is offset by the downward acceleration of gravity (g): $v_y = gt$

$$t = \frac{v_y}{g} = \frac{9.8 \text{ m/sec}}{9.8 \text{ m/sec}^2} = 1 \text{ sec.}$$

Note that 1 sec is the time required for half the trajectory. Using the above:    $d = d_0 + v_0 t + \tfrac{1}{2}gt^2$
$$d = 0 + (9.8)(1) + (\tfrac{1}{2})(-9.8)(1)^2 = 9.8 - 4.9 = 4.9 \text{m}.$$

QUESTION #23   (Answer:  b)  From question #22, the time for half the trajectory was 1 sec, so the total time is two secs. To find the range, use the horizontal component of the initial velocity ($v_x$) as calculated in question #22. There is no force in the horizontal direction so the acceleration is zero in this direction. Then using the equation for linear motion applied in the horizontal direction (Section 5.1.1):

$$d = d_0 + v_0 t + \tfrac{1}{2} at^2$$

$$d = 0 + (9.8 \sqrt{3})(2) + (\tfrac{1}{2})(0)(2)^2$$

$$d = 19.6 \sqrt{3} \text{ m.}$$

QUESTION #24   (Answer:  c)  The schematic showing the forces is:

$W_A = mg = (10)(9.8) = 98 \text{nts}$
$W_{Ax} = W_A \sin 30^\circ = (98)(\tfrac{1}{2}) = 49 \text{nts}$
Remember:

$\sin 30^\circ = 1/2$

In order for the object not to move, the $W_1$ should balance $W_{Ax}$. The $W_{Ay}$ has no effect on motion along x (the incline). Therefore, a $W_1$ of 49 nts is required. The mass would be:

$$m = W_1/g = 49/9.8 = 5 \text{ kgs.}$$

5.3.5        VOCABULARY, CONCEPTS, ETC. CHECKLIST FOR FORCE, MOTION, GRAVITATION

| | |
|---|---|
| ____ center of mass | ____ projectile motion |
| ____ center of gravity | ____ Newton's Third Law |
| ____ Newton's Second Law | ____ Law of Gravitation |
| ____ motion on an incline | |

____ friction
____ mass
____ weight
____ free fall motion

**5.4**      **Work and Energy**

**5.4.1**      REVIEW OF WORK AND ENERGY

Energy is a scalar (see **Volume II: Skills Development in Reading and Quantitative**) and is generally conceptualized as the ability to do work. Note that objects exert forces upon other objects, and if a displacement results, work (see below) is performed which is not contained within the object. Energy, by contrast, is contained by the object (or system), and if work is performed, this energy either increases or decreases (for negative or positive work respectively).

Mechanical energy is divided into kinetic energy (K) and potential energy (U). Kinetic energy is the energy associated with the motion of objects. It is formulated as $K = \frac{1}{2} mv^2$, where m = mass and v = speed. Potential energy is the energy which results by position or configuration (of a system); there is no motion. When motion begins, potential energy is converted into kinetic energy. The formulation of potential energy depends upon the system. For gravity (g) one gets,

    U = mgh
    m = mass
    h = height above earth's surface.

Additional features of potential energy are: (1) potential energy cannot be defined for frictional forces, and (2) the potential energy of a system is independent (in contrast to work) of the path to reach that system.

The Law of Conservation of Energy is:
       Total Energy (TE) = kinetic energy ( K ) + potential energy ( U )
              + energy due to dissipative forces (e.g., friction).

In the absence of dissipative forces, this can be taken as:

                         TE = K + U

Work (W) is a scalar also. Work results when a force (F) causes displacement (d):

    $W = Fd \cos\theta$

Note that $F \cos\theta$ is the component of F along the displacement (d). When $\theta = 0°$, then $\cos 0° = 1$, and W = Fd which is the result for forces in the same direction as the displacement. When $\theta = 90°$, then $\cos 90° = 0$ and W = 0. That is, forces perpendicular to the displacement do no work.

Another way of looking at work is as the change in mechanical energy of an object. Remember that the potential energy between two points (or positions) is the amount of work that would be required to move an object between those two points. The change in kinetic energy of an object is the work performed by the object assuming all the energy goes into work. To summarize:

$$W = E_f - E_i = \Delta E$$
$$E = K + U = \text{mechanical energy}$$
$$f = \text{final} \quad i = \text{initial} \quad \Delta = \text{change.}$$

This means work and energy have the same units:

$$W = (\text{force})(\text{distance}) = \text{newtons-meters} \equiv \text{Joules}$$
$$= \text{dynes-cms} \equiv \text{ergs.}$$

Joules and ergs are units of work or energy.
Pressure (P) times volume (V) also yields work (W): $W = (P)(V)$.

<u>Power</u> (P) is a scalar and is the rate at which work is done:

$$P = \text{work}(w)/\text{time}(t) = w/t$$

The units of power are:

$$P = \text{work/time} = \text{Joules/secs} \equiv \text{watts.}$$

5.4.2        <u>QUESTIONS TO REVIEW WORK AND ENERGY</u>

(1)    When a system does work or work is done on a system

   (a) the force of the system changes;
   (b) the momentum of the system changes;
   (c) the torque of the system changes;
   (d) the energy of the system changes.

(2)    All of the following statements are correct concerning potential energy (PE) except:

   (a) PE depends on the configuration rather than the motion of a system;
   (b) PE may be converted to kinetic energy;
   (c) PE cannot be defined for frictional forces;
   (d) PE depends upon the path taken to reach a certain state.

(3)    The Law of Conservation of Energy takes into account all of the following except:

   (a) conversion of mass into energy
   (b) potential energy
   (c) kinetic energy
   (d) energy loss due to dissipative forces

(4)    If W = work and t = time, then power (P) is:

   (a) $P = W/t$          (b) $P = t/W$
   (c) $P = Wt$           (d) $P = 1/Wt$

(5)    At what angle to the direction of the displacement would a force perform no work?

   (a) $0°$     (b) $45°$     (c) $90°$     (d) $180°$

(6)   All are expressions of work except:

(a) changes in mechanical energy
(b) momentum times mass
(c) force times distance ✓
(d) pressure times volume ✓

(7)   A 5kg object is moving in a straight line at a velocity of 4 meters/sec.  The kinetic energy (K) is:

(a) 40 Joules                    (b) 20 Joules
(c) 10 Joules                    (d) 80 Joules

$K = \frac{1}{2}mv^2$
$\frac{1}{2}(5)(16) = 40$

$\frac{1}{2}mv^2 = \frac{1}{2} \cdot 5 \cdot 16$
$= (40)$

(8)   An object weighing 10 kg is at a distance of 10 m above the earth's surface.  The potential energy (U) of this object is:

(a) 980 Joules                   (b) 100 Joules
(c) 9.8 Joules                   (d) 1000 Joules

$U = mgH$
$10(9.8)10$

$mgh = 10 \cdot 9.8 \cdot 10$
$= 100 = 980$

(9)   If a 5 kg object is 20 meters above the earth's surface and it falls to 10 meters above the surface, what is the change in potential energy (U)?

(a) gains 490 Joules
(b) loses 490 Joules
(c) loses 50 Joules
(d) only the kinetic energy changes, the potential energy does not change

$10 \times 5 \times 9.8$

$mgh =$
$5(9.8)(20)$  980
$5(9.8)(10)$
$98$   490
$\frac{5}{490}$

(10)  The shaded area under the graph might represent:

Force
Displacement

(a) momentum                     (b) force field
(c) work                         (d) pressure

(11)  A person does 20 Joules of work in 10 seconds; the power (P) generated is:

(a) 2000 watts                   (b) 200 watts
(c) 2 watts                      (d) 0.5 watts

$W = Fd = 20(20)$
$400$

(12)  A force of 20 newtons is used to move a 10 kg object 20 meters in 10 seconds; the power (P) generated is:

(a) 40,000 watts                 (b) 4,000 watts
(c) 400 watts                    (d) 40 watts

$W = Fd$
$P = \frac{Fd}{t} = \frac{20 \cdot 20}{10}$
$= 40$

(13)  A force of 10 newtons pushes a 5 kg object 20 meters.  The work performed is:

(a) 200 Joules                   (b) 40 Joules
(c) 10 Joules                    (d) 2.5 Joules

$10$
$\frac{10}{20}$
$\overline{200}$

357

(14)  How much work is performed in the diagram below?

F = 10 nts

60°

displacement = 5m

W = 10(5)cos 60°

25

(a) 50 Joules            (b) 50 cos 30° Joules
(c) 25 Joules            (d) 50  sin 60° Joules

(15)  A 5 kg object moving at 4 m/sec strikes a second object. After
the collision, the first object is moving at 2 m/sec.  Assuming
all the energy (E) was used to perform work (W) on the second
object, the work performed is:

(a) 30 Joules            (b) 60 Joules
(c) 90 Joules            (d) 120 Joules

$\frac{1}{2}mv^2 = mgh$

$\frac{1}{2}mv^2 - \frac{1}{2}mv^2$

$= \frac{1}{2}5 \cdot 8 - \frac{1}{2}5 \cdot 4 \cdot 2 = 40 - 10 = 30$

## 5.4.3 ANSWERS TO QUESTIONS IN SECTION 5.4.2

( 1) d    (2) d    (3) a    (4) a    (5) c    (6) b    (7) a
( 8) a    (9) b    (10) c   (11) c   (12) d   (13) a   (14) c
(15) a

## 5.4.4 DISCUSSION OF ANSWERS TO QUESTIONS IN SECTION 5.4.2

QUESTIONS #1 to #6:  Adequately discussed in the Section.

QUESTION #7  (Answer:  a)

$K = \frac{1}{2}mv^2 = (\frac{1}{2})(5)(4)^2 = (5/2)(16) = 40$ Joules.

QUESTION #8  (Answer:  a)

$U = mgh = (10$ kg$)(9.8$ m/sec$^2)(10m) = 980$ Joules.

QUESTION #9  (Answer:  b)

$\Delta U = U_2 - U_1 = mgh_2 - mgh_1 = mg(h_2 - h_1)$
$= (5)(9.8)(10-20) = (5)(9.8)(-10) = -490$ Joules.

The minus sign means U is lost.

QUESTION #10  (Answer:  c)  The area under the graph is given by the
product of the axes.  This is (force)(displacement), which is work
(or energy).

QUESTION #11  (Answer:  c)

$P = $ work/time $= 20$ Joules/10 secs $= 2$ Joules/sec $= 2$ watts.

358

QUESTION #12   (Answer:  d)

P = work/time = **400** Joules/10 secs = 40 Joules/sec = 40 watts.

work = (force)(distance) = (20)(20) = 400 Joules.

QUESTION #13   (Answer:  a)

W = Fd cos $\theta$
    $\theta$ must be $0^o$ so cos $\theta$ = 1
W = Fd = (10)(20) = 200 Joules.

QUESTION #14   (Answer:  c)   Remember that:

cos $60^o$ = ½

Then:  W = Fd cos $\theta$ = (10)(5) cos $60^o$ = 50(½) = 25 Joules.

QUESTION #15   (Answer:  a)

$\Delta E = W = E_f - E_i$
$E = \frac{1}{2} mv^2$
$W = \frac{1}{2}mv_f^2 - \frac{1}{2}mv_i^2 = \frac{1}{2}m(v_f^2 - v_i^2)$
$W = \frac{1}{2}(5)(4^2 - 2^2) = (5/2)(16-4) = (5/2)(12) = 30$ Joules.


5.4.5        VOCABULARY,  CONCEPTS,  ETC.  CHECKLIST  FOR  WORK  AND
             ENERGY


\_\_\_\_   work
\_\_\_\_   kinetic energy
\_\_\_\_   gravitational potential energy
\_\_\_\_   Law of Conservation of Energy
\_\_\_\_   power
\_\_\_\_   Joules
\_\_\_\_   watts


5.5        **Thermodynamics**


5.5.1        REVIEW OF THERMODYNAMICS


Heat is a form of energy.  Bodies do not contain heat; they either
emit or absorb energy as heat.  When a body absorbs or emits energy,
all of the energy need not be in the form of heat.  For example, a
body emitting energy may emit some as heat and some as light energy.
A body does contain thermal energy (or internal energy) which is the
sum of the potential and kinetic energies associated with the
position or motion, respectively, of the molecules.

Thermal equilibrium results when the average kinetic energies per molecule of two bodies are equal.  This is also when the heat flow between the bodies is zero, and when the temperatures of the two bodies are equal.  Temperature is taken to be a measure of the average thermal energy of a body; it is also a measure of the amount of energy absorbed or emitted as heat by a body.  Thus when temperature rises, the average kinetic energy per molecule rises, and the object absorbs more energy as heat, and vice versa.

Measurement of temperature is by thermometers.  A thermometer has (1) a thermometric property (e.g. pressure, density, resistance) which varies directly as temperature; (2) a lower fixed point (e.g., freezing point (FP) of water); (3) a higher fixed point (e.g., boiling point (BP) of water); and (4) a scale calibrated between these two points and extrapolated beyond them.  Relative temperature scales are the Celsius or Centigrade (FP of water = 0°C, BP of water = 100°C) and the Fahrenheit (FP of water = 32°F, BP of water = 212°F).  Absolute scales (the zero point of the scale is the true absolute zero) are the Rankine (°R) calibrated in °F units and the Kelvin (°K) calibrated in °C units.  Interconversions of the scales are:

$$°C = 5/9 \ (°F-32) \quad \text{or} \quad °F = (9/5) \ °C + 32 \text{ and 5 units Celcius} =$$
$$°K = °C + 273 \quad\quad\quad °R = °F + 460 \quad\quad\quad 9 \text{ units Fahrenheit}$$

The Celsius and Fahrenheit scales are equal at -40°.

Heat capacity is a measure of the amount of heat a body can gain (or lose) per change in temperature ($\Delta t$),

$$\text{heat capacity} = \text{heat gained/temperature change} = Q/\Delta t.$$

Specific heat capacity (C) is the heat capacity per unit mass of substance:

$$C = (Q/\Delta t)/m = Q/m\Delta t.$$

This can be rearranged to give the amount of heat exchanged (gained or lost) by a substance:

$$Q = (C)(m)(\Delta t).$$

The units of heat most commonly used are calories.  A calorie is the amount of heat required to raise 1 gram of water one degree Celsius.  A kilocalorie is 1000 calories.  Since heat is a form of energy, its units must be equivalent to the unit of other energies (kinetic or potential) or work which is the Joule (or other similar units).  The interconversion of calories and Joules is:

    4.184 Joules = 1 kilocalorie
    4.2 Joules $\approx$ 1 kilocalorie.

The specific heat of water is then:

    1 (calorie/gm - °C).

360

It is in the understanding of <u>phase transitions</u> that specific heat, heat of fusion and heat of vaporization have particular value. Below are the important features of phase transitions (See Sections 3.41 and 3.51):

<u>Phase Transition</u>　　　　　<u>Conditions</u>　　　　　　　<u>Heat Associated</u>

(1) solid $\underset{\text{freeze}}{\overset{\text{melt}}{\rightleftarrows}}$ liquid

Solid and liquid vapor pressure in equilibrium. Temperature called melting (or freezing) point (MP or FP).

heat of fusion ($H_f$)
$H_f = Q/m$ at MP
or $Q = m\ H_f$
$Q$ = heat transferred
$m$ = mass

(2) liquid $\underset{\text{condense}}{\overset{\text{evaporate (boil)}}{\longrightarrow}}$ gas

Gas and liquid vapor pressure in equilibrium. Temperature called the boiling point (BP)

Heat of evaporation ($H_v$)
$H_v = Q/m$ at BP
or $Q = H_v\ m$

Note that $H_v > H_f$ because usually more kinetic energy per molecule is required to separate liquid molecules to become gaseous than to separate solid molecules to become liquid. As a substance gains or loses energy as heat, it passes through the various phases. A scheme for substances gaining heat is:

| Phases & Temps | Solid Below MP | (1) | Solid at MP | (2) | Liquid at MP | (3) | Liquid at BP | (4) | Gas at BP | (5) | Gas above BP |
|---|---|---|---|---|---|---|---|---|---|---|---|
| | (1) | | (2) | | (3) | | (4) | | (5) | | |
| Heat changes | Heat is absorbed to raise the temperature as the specific heat of the solid:<br><br>$Q=C\ m\ \Delta\ t$<br>C=of solid | | Heat is absorbed as heat of fusion to cause solid to melt to the liquid. Note that the temperature does not change:<br>$Q=H_f\ m$ | | Heat is absorbed as the specific heat of the liquid to raise its temperature:<br><br>$Q=C\ m\ \Delta\ t$<br>C=of liquid | | Heat is absorbed as heat of vaporization to cause the liquid to be converted to gas. The temperature does not change.<br>$Q=H_v\ m$ | | Heat is absorbed as the specific heat of the gas to raise its temperature<br><br><br><br><br>$Q=C\ m\ \Delta\ t$<br>C=of gas | | |

The reverse steps would hold if the substance was losing energy as heat. To summarize, heat is used to change the phase or the temperature of a substance. When two objects are in contact and at different temperatures, heat flows from the one with the higher temperature to the one with the lower temperature until the temperatures are equal. The above equations can be used to calculate heat flows and temperatures by using:

heat loss = heat gain.

When substances gain (or lose) heat they usually undergo <u>expansion (or contraction)</u>. Expansion (contraction) can be by linear dimensions, by area, or by volume. These are:

| Type | Final | Original | Change caused by heat |
|------|-------|----------|----------------------|

(1) Linear L     $L_O$                     $\alpha \Delta t L_O$

$L = L_O + \alpha \Delta t L_O = L_O(1 + \alpha \Delta t)$

$\alpha$ = coefficient of linear thermal expansion, $\Delta t$ = change in temp

(2) Area     A     $A_O$                     $\gamma \Delta t A_O$

$A = A_O + \gamma \Delta t A_O = A_O(1 + \gamma \Delta t)$

= coefficient of area thermal expansion = $2\alpha$

(3) Volume V     $V_O$                     $\beta \Delta t V_O$

$V = V_O + \beta \Delta t V_O = V_O(1 + \beta \Delta t)$

$\beta$ = coefficient of volume thermal expansion = $3\alpha$

Heat flows between substances by three mechanisms: conduction, convection and radiation. Conduction is a process in which heat energy is transferred by adjacent molecular collisions throughout a material medium--the medium does not move. The heat energy is carried off by the motion of the electrons. Good electrical conductors, therefore, are usually good heat conductors. The rate of heat transfer (H) by conduction is:

$$H = Q/T = kA(\Delta t/L)$$

Q = heat exchanged
T = time elapsed
A = cross-sectional area
L = length over which transfer occurs
$\Delta t$ = temperature difference
k = thermal conductivity of the material.

Note that the rate (H) is directly proportional to A and $\Delta t$ and inversely proportional to L. The k is a property of the substance.

Convection is a process in which heat energy is transferred by the actual mass motion of a fluid (gas or liquid). Convection currents are set up which may be natural (caused by density differences, e.g. wind) or forced (as in a house ventilation system). The rate of energy transfer (H) is:

$$H = Q/T = hA\Delta t \quad \text{(note the relations shown)}.$$

The h is the convection coefficient but is not a property of the substance.

Radiation is a process in which heat energy is transferred by electromagnetic waves absorbed or emitted at the atomic level. All substances radiate heat regardless of the temperature. In general, as the absolute temperature (T) increases, the wavelength of the emitted heat decreases. The rate of emission (R) is:

$$R = e \delta T^4 \quad \text{(Stephan-Boltzmann Law)}$$

T = absolute temperature
e = emissivity = the ability to absorb or emit thermal radiation
$\delta$ = Stephan's Constant.

The key relation is that the R is proportional to the fourth power of the absolute temperature. A body at the same temperature as its surroundings will radiate and absorb heat at the same rate. If not at the same temperature, the net rate of radiation is:

net rate of radiation = rate of energy emission - rate of energy absorption

$$R = e\delta T_1^4 - e\delta T_2^4 = e\delta (T_1^4 - T_2^4)$$

$T_1$ = temperature of body

$T_2$ = temperature of surroundings.

Thermodynamics is concerned with the energy states of molecules and chemical reactions. A system is the object under study. It is the reference point. When the system gains (e.g. energy), the (energy) change is positive. The environment is everything outside the system. Systems exchange energy by the processes of work or heat exchange. The systems do not contain work or heat. Work or heat exchange depends upon the path from the initial to the final state. This is in contrast to state functions which are independent of the path taken but depend upon the initial and final states only. The state functions to be discussed are pressure (P), volume (V), temperature (T), internal energy (E) and entropy (S). See section 3.8.1 for the discussion of other state functions, enthalpy (H) and free energy (G).

Energy is a property of a system and not a process (like heat or work). Specifically, the internal energy change ($\Delta E$), of a system depends on the work done and heat exchanged as follows:

$\Delta E$ = q-w       First Law of Thermodynamics

q = + if heat is added to the system

q = - if heat is lost from the system

w = +p$\Delta V$ if work is done by the system

   p = external pressure

   $\Delta V = V_f - V_i$  change in volume of the system

        Note: this gives the sign to the work.

The internal energy depends on the kinetic energies of the molecules, on the potential energies of forces between molecules, and the kinetic and potential energies of the electrons and nuclei. The First Law of Thermodynamics is a restatement of the Law of Conservation of Energy. The $\Delta E$ of a reaction is determined by running the reaction at constant volume and measuring the amount of heat exchanged:

$$\Delta E = q - w = q - p\Delta V = q_V$$

$$\Delta V = 0$$

$q_V$ = heat at constant volume.

A reversible process is one that occurs in such small increments that it can be reversed at any point. An irreversible process is one that cannot be easily reversed. As a concrete example, if you walked down a flight of stairs one step at a time, it would be fairly easy to reverse your direction at any step--this would be a reversible process. But if you jumped out of a window, equivalent to that flight of stairs, you could not reverse yourself--this would be an irreversible process. For reversible (rev) and irreversible (irrev) processes, the following are true:

$W_{rev} > W_{irrev}$

$q_{rev} > q_{irrev}.$

These concepts lead into entropy (S) and the Second Law of Thermodynamics which is

$\Delta S$ =(q rev/T) for a reversible path

363

Note:   (1)   $\Delta S$ is still independent of a particular
              reversible path,
       (2)   $\Delta S = \Delta S \text{ system} + \Delta S \text{ environment} = 0$,
       (3)   $\Delta S$ exists for an irreversible path but it is
              not equal to $(q \text{ rev}/T)$
       (4)   $\Delta S$ is increasing for an irreversible path.

Entropy is further discussed in Section 3.8.1.


## 5.5.2   QUESTIONS TO REVIEW THERMODYNAMICS


(1)   Heat:

      (a) is contained by an object
      (b) is absorbed or emitted by an object
      (c) both (a) and (b)
      (d) neither (a) nor (b)

(2)   Temperature:

      (a) is a measure of the average thermal energy of a body
      (b) is a measure of the amount of heat a body absorbs or emits
      (c) increases when the average kinetic energy per molecule
          increases
      (d) all of the above

(3)   Thermal equilibrium occurs when:

      (a) the average kinetic energy per molecule of two bodies is
          equal
      (b) the heat flow between two bodies is zero
      (c) the temperature between two bodies is equal
      (d) all are correct


(4)   Heat capacity is:

      (a) the amount of heat a body contains per degree of
          temperature
      (b) the amount of heat a body can gain or lose per degree
          change in temperature
      (c) represented as:  temperature/heat
      (d) both (a) and (c)

(5)   Specific heat capacity:

      (a) the amount of heat contained by a substance
      (b) the amount of heat contained per unit change of
          temperature by a substance
      (c) the heat capacity per unit change in temperature
      (d) the heat capacity per unit mass

(6)   If C = specific heat capacity, $\Delta t$ = change in temperature and
      m = mass, then the amount of heat (Q) exchanged is:

      (a) $Q = C/m \Delta t$          (b) $Q = C m \Delta t$
      (c) $Q = Cm/ \Delta t$          (d) $Q = C \Delta t /m$

$J \, K^{-1} \, Kg^{-1}$

(7)    Heat of fusion refers to the phase change between:

(a) gas and solid            (b)  liquid and gas
(c) liquid and solid         (d)  all phases

(8)    When a solid is converted to a liquid:

(a) heat is released         (b)  heat is required
(c) temperature increases    (d)  both (a) and (c)

(9)    A net release of heat to the environment occurs during:

(a) condensation             (b)  sublimation
(c) evaporation              (d)  melting

(10)   Heat flows between substances by all the following processes except:

(a) conjugation              (b)  conduction
(c) convection               (d)  radiation

(11)   The process whereby heat is transferred by adjacent molecular collisions throughout a medium is:

(a) convection               (b)  conduction
(c) radiation                (d)  momentum

(12)   In heat transfer in a substance (e.g., a rod) by conduction, the rate of heat transfer is:

(a) directly proportional to the length of heat transfer (end to end of the rod, e.g.)
(b) indirectly proportional to the temperature difference
(c) directly proportional to the cross-sectional area (e.g., of the rod)
(d) independent of the nature of the substance

(13)   The process of transferring heat energy by the mass motion of a fluid is called:

(a) bulk flow                (b)  radiation
(c) conduction               (d)  convection

(14)   Heat loss or gain by the process of radiation:

(a) occurs in all substances regardless of temperature
(b) occurs only if the temperature is above the critical temperature of a substance
(c) is independent of the nature of a substance
(d) only (b) and (c)

(15)   As the absolute temperature increases, the wavelength of radiation emitted by a substance tends to:

(a) increase                 (b)  decrease
(c) remain the same          (d)  totally unpredictable

(16)   The reference point in thermodynamics is called the:

    (a) surroundings           (b) environment
    (c) state                (d) system

(17)   Which of the following is independent of the path taken for its value?

    (a) internal energy       (b) work
    (c) heat                (d) none of these

(18)   A statement of the First Law of Thermodynamics is:

    (a) $\Delta S = q\ rev/T$        (b) $\Delta G = \Delta H - T\Delta S$

    (c) $\Delta E = q-w$         (d) none of these

(19)   The internal energy ($\Delta E$) depends upon:

    (a) kinetic energy of molecules
    (b) potential energy of forces between molecules
    (c) kinetic and potential energies of electrons and nuclei
    (d) all of these

(20)   The Second Law of Thermodynamics involves a definition of:

    (a) internal energy       (b) enthalpy
    (c) entropy            (d) free energy

(21)   During the step of conversion of a liquid to a gas, the heat is

    (a) used to overcome intermolecular forces between liquid
        molecules and convert them to gaseous molecules;
    (b) used to raise the temperature of the gas;
    (c) used to raise the temperature of the liquid;
    (d) all of the above.

(22)   The conversion of 10 grams of a solid to 10 grams of its liquid at the freezing point (25°C) requires 100 cals of heat. The heat of fusion of this substance is:

$Q = \frac{cal}{mas}$

    (a) 0.40 cals/gm-°C      (b) 40 cals-gm/°C
    (c) 10 cals/gm          (d) 250 cals-°C/gm

$Q = mC\Delta T$

(23)   An object weighing 10 gms has a specific heat of 2 cals/gm/°C. To raise its temperature from 10°C to 60°C would require how many calories?

$\Delta H = 2 \cdot 10 \cdot 50$
$= 500 \cdot 2$
$= 1000$

    (a) 10 cals           (b) 100 cals
    (c) 1000 cals        (d) 5000 cals

$Q = 10(2)(50) = 1000$

(24)   A substance weighing 5 gms has its temperature raised from 25° to 75°C without a phase change while absorbing 45 calories of heat. Its specific heat capacity is:

$\frac{45-9}{50 \cdot 8} = \frac{90}{50}$

    (a) 11,250 cals/gm-°C    (b) 450 cals/gm-°C
    (c) 0.18 cals/gm-°C     (d) 4.50 cals/gm-°C

$45 = 5(c)(50)$

$c = \frac{45}{5(50)} = \frac{9}{50} =$

(25) The amount of heat required to convert 10 gms of water (solid) at 0°C to water (liquid) at 50°C (specific heat of solid water is 0.5 cals/gm-°C; specific heat of liquid water is 1.0 cals/gm-°C; heat of fusion of water is 80 cals/gm) is:

(a) 1300 kilocalories      (b) 350 cals
(c) 1300 cals            (d) 1500 cals

(26) If a heating coil is supplying 50 cals/min to a tank containing water (ice) at 0°C, the amount of water (as a liquid) that can be formed in 10 min. (use specific heat and heat of fusion from question #25) is:

(a) 3.5 gms         (b) 6.25 gms
(c) 420 gms        (d) 500 gms

(27) A temperature of 50°C (Celsius) corresponds to what temperature Fahrenheit (F)?

(a) 122°F          (b) 90°F
(c) 82°F           (d) 27.8°F

(28) At what temperature are the Celsius (°C) and Fahrenheit (°F) scales equal?

(a) 100            (b) 37
(c) -40            (d) 0

(29) The coefficient of linear expansion ($\alpha$) of a substance is $2 \times 10^{-5}$°C$^{-1}$  The coefficient of volume expansion ($\beta$) would be:

(a) $6 \times 10^{-5}$°C$^{-1}$      (b) $8 \times 10^{-5}$°C$^{-1}$
(c) $2 \times 10^{-15}$°C$^{-3}$     (d) need more information

(30) An object with a linear expansion coefficient ($\alpha$) of $2 \times 10^{-4}$°C$^{-1}$  has the volume of 10.000 liters. If the temperature increases 100°C, the new volume will be:

(a) 10.020 liters      (b) 10.008 liters
(c) 10.600 liters      (d) no change to three decimal places

(31) Heat is being conducted through a square-faced metal block 4 meters long with sides 2 meters in length. If another block of the same metal is constructed but with a square face of 4 meters on a side and 8 meters long, what is the rate of heat conduction through it, compared with the first block, for a given temperature difference?  Note: the heat is passing through the square faces along the complete length.

(a) The second is four times the first.
(b) The second is twice the first.
(c) The second is one-half the first.
(d) The second is one-fourth the first.

(32)    If the temperature of an object is changed from 20°C to 10°C, the rate of radiational heat loss is how much of the original?

(a) slightly more than 1.0        (b) slightly less than 1.0
(c) 1/2 as much                   (d) 1/16 as much

## 5.5.3    ANSWERS TO QUESTIONS IN SECTION 5.5.2

( 1)  b   (2)  d   (3)  d   (4)  b   (5)  d   (6)  b   (7)  c
( 8)  b   (9)  a   (10) a   (11) b   (12) c   (13) d   (14) a
(15) b   (16) d   (17) a   (18) c   (19) d   (20) c   (21) a
(22) c   (23) c   (24) c   (25) c   (26) b   (27) a   (28) c
(29) a   (30) c   (31) b   (32) b

## 5.5.4    DISCUSSION OF ANSWERS TO QUESTIONS IN SECTION 5.5.2

QUESTIONS #1 to #20:  Adequately discussed in Section.

QUESTION #21  (Answer:  a)  During a phase conversion step, energy is used to break intermolecular bonds and is not used to increase the average kinetic energy of the molecules (raise the temperature).

QUESTION #22  (Answer:  c)

heat of fusion = calories required for phase change/mass undergoing phase change
$$= 100 \text{ cals}/10 \text{ gms} = 10 \text{ cals/gm}$$

QUESTION #23  (Answer:  c)

$Q = C \, m \, \Delta t = (2 \text{ cals/gm-°C})(10 \text{ gms})(60-10°C) = (2)(10)(50) \text{ cals}$
$Q = 1000 \text{ cals}$

QUESTION #24  (Answer:  c)

$C = Q/m\Delta t = 45 \text{ cals}/(5 \text{ gms})(75-25°C) = 9/50 = 0.18 \text{ (cals/gm-°C)}$

QUESTION #25  (Answer:  c)  The scheme is:

water (solid) at 0°C $\xrightarrow{(1)}$ water (liquid) at 0°C $\xrightarrow{(2)}$ water (liquid) at 50°C
(1)  heat of fusion ($H_f$) of water for phase change
     cals = ($H_f$)(mass) = (80 cals/gm)(10 gms) = 800 cals
(2)  SH of water (liq) to raise temperature
     cals = (SH)(mass)(temp change) = $C \, m \, \Delta t$
          = (1.0)(10)(50 − 0) = (10)(50) = 500 cals

Total:      (1) + (2) = 800 + 500 = 1300 cals.

QUESTION #26  (Answer:  b)  The total heat delivered in 10 mins is:

cals = 50 cals/min)(10 mins) = 500 cals.

The scheme for water changes is:

water (solid) at 0°C $\xrightarrow{(1)}$ water (liquid) at 0°C
(1)  heat of fusion ($H_f$) of water for phase change
     $H_f$ = heat change/mass = $Q/m$
     $m = Q/H_f = 500 \text{ cals}/(80 \text{ cals/gm}) = 6.25 \text{ gms}.$

368

QUESTION #27 (Answer: a) Use ratio and proportion and known facts about temperature scales:

°C        °F
100 — BP — 212
$(50-0)/(100-0) = (F-32)/(212-32) = (F-32)/180$
$(50)(180)/100 = F-32$
$90 = F-32$
$122 = F$

50 — ?°F

0 — FP — 32

BP = boiling point
FP = freezing point

(The key to understanding this is noting that the distances on the scales are equal even though the calibrations differ.

QUESTION #28 (Answer: c) This is similar to Question#27:

°C    BP    °F
100 ——— 212
$C-0/100-0 = F-32/212-32$
$C/100 = F-32/180$
now $C = F$ for problem
$F/100 = F-32/180$
$180F/100 = F-32$
$9F/5 = F-32$
$9F = 5F-160$
$4F = -160$
$F = -40° = C$

?°C — ?°F

0 ——— 32
FP

QUESTION #29 (Answer: a) The following relationship holds:

$$\beta = 3\alpha = 3(2 \times 10^{-5}°C^{-1}) = 6 \times 10^{-5}°C^{-1}.$$

QUESTION #30 (Answer: c) The coefficient of volume expansion ($\beta$) is: $\beta = 3\alpha = (3)(2 \times 10^{-4}°C^{-1}) = 6 \times 10^{-4}°C^{-1}.$

The formula for volume expansion is:

$$V = V_o (1+\beta \Delta t)$$

$$= (10.000) \left[ 1 + (6 \times 10^{-4})(100) \right] = 10.00 \left[ 1 + (6 \times 10^{-4})(10^2) \right]$$

$$= (10.000)(1 + 6 \times 10^{-2}) = (10.000)(1 + 0.06)$$
$$= (10.000)(1.06) = 10.600 \text{ liters.}$$

QUESTION #31 (Answer: b) The formula for heat rate in conduction is:

$$H = k\left(A/L\right) \Delta t \quad \text{(see in section),}$$
or could remember that,
$H \propto A$ and $H \propto 1/L$ or,
$H \propto A/L$.
Then k and $\Delta t$ are constants. And,
$A_1 = (2)(2) = 4 \text{ m}^2$ (area of a square)
$L_1 = 4 \text{ m}$
$A_2 = (4)(4) = 16 \text{ m}^2$
$L_2 = 8 \text{ m}$
Putting these in either of the formulas above

$$\frac{H_2}{H_1} = \frac{k\frac{A_2}{L_2}\Delta t}{k\frac{A_1}{L_1}\Delta t} = \frac{\frac{A_2}{L_2}}{\frac{A_1}{L_1}} = \frac{A_2}{L_2} \cdot \frac{L_1}{A_1} = \frac{(16)}{(8)} \cdot \frac{(4)}{(4)} = 2$$

$$H_2 = 2H_1$$

QUESTION #32   (Answer:  b)  Using the Stephan-Boltzman Law:

$$R = e \delta T^4$$

1 = original    2 = final

$$T_1 = 20^{\circ}+273^{\circ} = 293^{\circ} \quad T_2 = 10^{\circ}+273^{\circ} = 283^{\circ}$$

$$\frac{R_2}{R_1} = \frac{e\delta t_2^4}{e\delta t_1^4} = \frac{T_2^4}{T_1^4} = (283)^4/(293)^4 = (283/293)^4 = 0.89$$

$$R_2 = 0.89R_1$$

5.5.5        <u>VOCABULARY, CONCEPTS, ETC. CHECKLIST FOR THERMODYNAMICS</u>

| | |
|---|---|
| ____ First Law of Thermodynamics | ____ conduction |
| ____ Second Law of Thermodynamics | ____ convection |
| ____ equivalence of Joules and calories | ____ radiation (of heat) |
| ____ Celsius (Centigrade) | ____ specific heat |
| ____ Fahrenheit | ____ heat capacity |
| ____ Rankine | ____ heat of fusion |
| ____ Kelvin | ____ heat of vaporization |
| ____ interconversions of temperature scales | ____ internal energy |
| | ____ entropy |
| ____ coefficients of thermal expansion | |

## 5.6        Solids and Fluids

### 5.6.1        <u>REVIEW OF SOLIDS AND FLUIDS</u>

#### 5.6.1.1        <u>Review of Solids</u>

When a force acts on a solid, the solid is deformed. If the solid returns to its original shape, it is called <u>elastic</u>. The effect of a force depends on the area over which it acts. Stress is defined as the ratio of the force to the area over which it acts. Strain is defined as the relative change in dimensions or shape of the object caused by the stress. This is embodied in the definition of the modulus of elasticity (ME) as:

$$ME = stress/strain,$$

Some different types of stresses are <u>tensile stress</u> (equal and opposite forces directed away from each other), <u>compressive stress</u> (equal and opposite forces directed toward each other), and <u>shearing stress</u> (equal and opposite forces which do not have the same line of action).  There are two commonly useful moduli of elasticity:

(1) Young's Modulus (Y) for compressive or tensile stress:

$$Y = \text{longitudinal stress/longitudinal strain} = (F/A)/(\Delta l/l)$$
$$= Fl/A\Delta l$$

The A is the area normal (perpendicular) to the force

**Fig. 5.7(a) – Tensile Stress**

**Fig. 5.7(b) – Compressive Stress**

(2) Shear modulus (S) or the modulus of rigidity is:

S = shearing stress/shearing strain = $(F/A)/\phi$ = $(F/A)/\tan \phi$ = $(F/A)/(d/l)$ = $Fl/dA$ (see Fig. 5.8)

The A is the area tangential to the force.

**Fig. 5.8 – Shear Stress**

5.6.1.2    Review of Fluids

Density is defined as:  density = mass/volume.

This holds for solids or fluids.  Solids, in general, are more dense than liquids which are more dense than gases.  The specific gravity (SG) is defined as:

$$SG = \left(\frac{\text{density of a substance}}{\text{density of water}}\right) \text{ at a given temperature}$$

The density of water is about 1 gm/ml over most common temperatures. So in most instances the specific gravity of a substance is the same as its density.  Note that the units of density are mass/volume, whereas SG has no units.

Density is one of the key properties of fluids (liquids or gases) and the other is pressure.  Pressure (P) is defined as force (F) per unit area (A):

$$P = F/A.$$

The F is the normal (perpendicular) force.  Fluids can only exert P at an enclosed surface or body.  Otherwise, fluids will flow under a shearing stress instead of being deformed elastically as solids would (see above).  Pressure is also formulated as potential energy

371

per unit volume as follows:

$$P = F/A = mg/A = (mg/A)(h/h) = mgh/V = \rho gh$$

$\rho$ = density    h = depth below surface.

Characteristics of force and pressure of fluids are:

(1)    Forces exerted by fluids are always perpendicular to the container.

(2)    The fluid pressure (hydrostatic) is directly proportional to the depth of the fluid and to its density:
$$P \propto \rho h.$$

(3)    At any particular depth, the fluid pressure is the same in all directions.

(4)    Fluid pressure is independent of the shape or area of its container.

(5)    An external pressure applied to an enclosed fluid is transmitted uniformly throughout the volume of the liquid (Pascal's Law).

(6)    An object which is completely or partially submerged in a fluid experiences an upward force equal to the weight of the fluid displaced (Archimede's Principle). This buoyant force ($F_B$) is:
$$F = V\rho g = mg$$
buoyant force = weight of displaced fluid.
An object that floats must displace its own weight (not volume) in fluid.

Fluids in motion are described by two equations, the continuity equation and Bernoulli's Equation. Fluids are assumed to have streamline flow which means that the motion of every particle in the fluid follows the same path as the particle that preceded it. Turbulent flow occurs when one path is not followed, molecules collide, energy is dissipated and frictional drag is increased. Rate of flow (R) is:

$$R = \text{volume past a point/time} = Avt/t = Av$$
$$\text{volume} = (\text{cross-sectional area})(\text{length}) = (A)(vt) = Avt$$
$$\text{length} = \text{distance} = (\text{velocity})(\text{time}) = vt$$

The equation can also be written as (the continuity equation):

$$A_1v_1 = A_2v_2 = \text{constant}$$

where subscripts 1 and 2 refer to different points in the line of flow. Note that the velocity of the fluid is faster where the cross-sectional area is smaller and vice versa. Also, where the velocity is faster, the pressure (P) exerted is smaller and vice versa.

Bernoulli's Equation is an application of the Law of Conservation of energy and is:
$$P + \rho gh + \tfrac{1}{2}\rho v^2 = \text{constant}$$
pressure energy + potential energy + kinetic energy = constant

This can be equivalently written as:
$$P_1 + \rho gh_1 + \tfrac{1}{2}\rho v_1^2 = P_2 + \rho gh_2 + \tfrac{1}{2}\rho v_2^2.$$
where the subscripts 1 and 2 refer to different points in the flow. All symbols are as defined previously.

Another important property of fluids is viscosity. Viscosity is analogous to friction between moving solids. It may, therefore, be viewed as the resistance to flow of layers of fluid (as in streamline or laminar flow) past each other. This also means that viscosity, as friction, results in dissipation of mechanical energy. As one layer flows over another, its motion is transmitted to the second layer and causes this layer to be set in motion. Since a mass (m) of the second layer is set in motion (v) and some of the energy of the first layer is lost, there is a transfer to momentum (mv) between the layers. The greater the transfer of this momentum from one layer to another, the more energy ($\propto v^2$) that is lost and the slower the layers move. The viscosity coefficient ($\eta$) is a measure of the efficiency of transfer of this momentum. Therefore, the higher the viscosity coefficient, the greater the transfer of momentum and loss of mechanical energy and, thus loss of velocity. The reverse situation holds of low viscosity coefficients. Then a high viscosity (coefficient) substance flows slowly (e.g., molasses), and a low viscosity (coefficient) substance flows relatively fast (e.g., water or, especially, helium). Note that the transfer of momentum to adjacent layers is, in essence, the exertion of a force upon these layers to set them in motion (Newton's 1st Law--5.2.1). Whether flow is streamline (laminar) or turbulent (loss of layers flowing past each other and their replacement with eddies and whirlpool, etc., with the resultant dissipation of much mechanical energy) depends on a combination of factors already discussed. A convenient measure is Reynolds Number (R):

$$R = vd\rho /\eta$$

v = velocity of flow; d = diameter of tube; $\rho$ = density of fluid; $\eta$ = viscosity coefficient. In general, if R<2000 the flow is streamline; if R>2000 the flow is turbulent. Note that as v↑ , d↑ , $\rho$↑ or $\eta$↓, the flow becomes more turbulent.


## Surface Tension

Molecules of a liquid exert attractive forces toward each other (cohesive forces), and exert attractive forces toward surfaces they touch (adhesive forces). If a liquid is in a gravity-free space without a surface, it will form a sphere (smallest area relative to volume). If the liquid is lining an object, the liquid surface will contract (due to cohesive forces) to the lowest possible surface area. The forces between the molecules on this surface will create a membrane-like effect. Due to the contraction, a potential energy (PE) will be present in the surface. This PE is directly proportional to the surface area (A). An exact relation is formed as follows:

$$PE = \gamma A$$
$$\gamma = \text{surface tension} = PE/A = Joules/m^2$$

An alternative formulation for surface tension ($\gamma$) is:

$$\gamma = F/\ell$$
F = force of contraction (of surface)
$\ell$ = length along surface.

Because of the contraction, small objects which would ordinarily sink in the liquid may "float" on the surface membrane.

The liquid will rise or fall on a wall or in a capillary tube if the adhesive forces are greater than cohesive or cohesive are greater than adhesive forces, respectively:

cohesive > adhesive          adhesive > cohesive

The distance the liquid rises or falls in the tube is directly proportional to the δ and inversely proportional to the liquid density and radius of the tube.

5.6.2          QUESTIONS TO REVIEW SOLIDS AND FLUIDS

(1)   Stress, as used in physics, is defined as:

(a) the maximum weight an object can support
(b) the force per unit length
(c) the ratio of the force to the area over which it acts
(d) the relative change in dimensions of an object caused by a force

(2)   When an object is deformed by forces acting on an object along the same line of action but in the opposite directions, the stress resulting is called:

(a) tensile stress                    (b) traction stress
(c) compressive stress                (d) shearing stress

(3)   If D = density, m = mass and V = volume occupied by that mass, then density is:

(a) D = (m)(V)          $D = m/V$          (b) D = 1/(m)(V)
(c) D = m/V                                (d) D = V/m

(4)   Pressure is defined as:

(a) force per unit volume
(b) force per unit area
(c) mass per unit volume
(d) work times volume

(5)   Pressure may be formulated as:

(a) force per unit volume
(b) work times volume
(c) potential energy per unit volume
(d) weight per unit volume

374

(6) All are characteristics of forces and pressures exerted by fluids except:

(a) forces are always perpendicular to the container walls
(b) pressure is directly proportional to the product of depth and fluid density
(c) pressure depends on the shape and size of the container
(d) buoyant force of submerged object equals the weight of the displaced fluid

(7) Pascal's Law (of fluids):

(a) an external pressure applied to an enclosed fluid is transmitted uniformly through the volume of the fluid
(b) at any depth, the fluid pressure is the same in all directions
(c) fluid pressure is dependent of the shape or area of its container
(d) an object completely or partly submerged in a fluid experiences an upward force equal to the weight of the fluid displaced

(8) Bernoulli's Equation is an application of:

(a) the 2nd Law of Thermodynamics
(b) the Law of Conservation of Momentum
(c) the Law of Conservation of Mass
(d) the Law of Conservation of Energy

(9) All are true of viscosity except:

(a) it is analogous to friction
(b) there is no dissipation of mechanical energy
(c) there is transfer of momentum between adjacent layers
(d) as viscosity increases, rate of flow decreases

(10) A certain metal has a mass (m) = 36 gm and occupies a volume (V) = 4 mls. The density (d) of it is:

(a) 144 gm-mls
(b) 9 gms/ml
(c) 1/9 mls/gm
(d) 1/444 $gms^{-1} mls^{-1}$

(11) A substance has a density (d) of 7 gms/ml. If 42 gms are required, what volume (V) of the substance is this?

(a) 1/6 mls
(b) 6 mls
(c) 294 mls
(d) need more information

(12) A fluid has a density (d) of 5 gms/ml and fills a container up to a height (h) of 10 cm's. The pressure (P) on the floor of the container is:

(a) 49,000 dynes/$cm^2$
(b) 50 nts/$m^2$
(c) 50 V dynes/$cm^2$ where V = volume in ml/s
(d) need more information

(13) If an object is moved from 4 meters to 8 meters beneath the surface of a large tank of water, the pressure on it will:

(a) remain the same
(b) quadruple
(c) halve
(d) double

375

(14) At a depth of 10 meters in a large container of water, 3 sheets of glass are placed parallel to the surface. Sheet A is 3mx5m, sheet B is 4x4 and sheet C is 2x9. Which sheet has the greatest fluid pressure on its surface?

(a) A    (b) B    (c) C    (d) all are equal

(15) The buoyant force ($F_B$) on an object that has a mass of 10 gms, a volume of 10 mls and displaces 2 mls of a liquid with a density of 5 gms/ml is:

(a) 10 dynes              (b) 9800 dynes
(c) 1000 dynes           (d) 40 dynes

(16) In order for an object to float in a fluid, it must

(a) be made of a substance more dense than the fluid;
(b) be made of a substance less dense than the fluid;
(c) displace its own weight in the fluid;
(d) displace its own volume in the fluid.

(17) The key feature of an object that sinks when placed in a fluid is that

(a) it displaced its weight in the fluid;
(b) it displaced less than its weight in the volume it displaced;
(c) it displaced its weight before it displaced its volume;
(d) both (a) and (b).

(18) A pipe has a section A of diameter = 10 meters and a section B of 5 meters. A given quantity of fluid flowing through it would

(a) move at the same speed at A and B;
(b) move faster at A;
(c) move faster at B;
(d) would need volume of fluid to evaluate.

(19) Fluid is flowing as shown in the pipe below. At what point is the pressure exerted by the fluid the highest (pipe is filled with fluid at all points)?

(a) A        (b) B        (c) C        (d) D

(20) At which point is the pressure exerted by the fluid the least in the constant diameter pipe below?

(a) A        (b) B        (c) C        (d) D

(21) The relative diameters of the blood vessels of the body and the relative flows are:

$$arteries > arterioles > capillaries.$$

In which of the above is turbulent flow most likely?

(a) artery    (b) arteriole    (c) capillary    (d) all equal

## 5.6.3    ANSWERS TO QUESTIONS IN SECTION 5.6.2

( 1)  c  ( 2)  a  ( 3)  c  ( 4)  b  ( 5)  c  ( 6)  c  ( 7)  a
( 8)  d  ( 9)  b  (10)  b  (11)  b  (12)  a  (13)  d  (14)  d
(15)  b  (16)  c  (17)  b  (18)  c  (19)  c  (20)  d  (21)  a

## 5.6.4    DISCUSSION OF ANSWERS TO QUESTIONS IN SECTION 5.6.2

QUESTIONS #1 to #9:   Adequately discussed in the text.

QUESTION #10: (Answer: b)

$$d = m/v = 36 \text{ gms}/4 \text{ mls} = 9 \text{ gms/ml}$$

QUESTION #11: (Answer: b)

$$d = m/v$$
$$V = m/d = 42 \text{ gms}/7 \text{gms per ml} = 6 \text{ mls}$$

QUESTION #12: (Answer: a)

$$F = F/A = \rho gh$$
$$P = (5 \text{ gms/cm}^3)\left[(980)(\text{cms/sec}^2)\right](10 \text{ cms}) = 49,000 \quad (\text{gm-cm/sec}^2)/\text{cm}^2$$
$$P = 49,000 \text{ dynes/cm}^2$$
$$\text{dyne} = (\text{gm} - \text{cm})/\text{sec}^2.$$

QUESTION #13: (Answer: d)  The pressure (P) exerted by the fluid is:

$$P = \rho gh \text{ or } P \propto h$$
$$h = \text{depth under surface.}$$
So, P is directly proportional to h and if h doubles (8/4 = 2)
Then P doubles.  OR
$$P_1 = \rho gh_1 = \text{original depth}$$
$$P_2 = \rho gh_2 = \text{final depth}$$
$$P_2/P_1 = \rho gh_2/\rho gh_1 = h_2/h_1 = 8m/4m = 2$$
$$P_2 = 2P_1.$$

QUESTION #14: (Answer: d)  Fluid pressure (P) is independent of the area or shape of its container or objects.  The $P \propto \rho h$ where $\rho$ = density and h = depth.  So at any particular depth the presure is equal in all directions.

QUESTION #15   (Answer:  b)   From Archimedes Principle:

$$F = V\rho g$$

   $V$ = volume displaced = 2 mls
   $\rho$ = density of fluid = 5 gms/ml
   $g$ = 980 cms/sec$^2$
$F = (2)(5)(980) = 9800$ dynes.

QUESTION #16   (Answer:  c)   If (b) were true, large ships would never float by virtue of their shape which makes the density of the whole object (not the steel material) less than that of water.

QUESTION #17   (Answer:  b)   According to Archimedes Principle an object must displace its weight to float.  The maximum volume of fluid that an object can displace is its (the object's) own volume. If a weight of fluid displaced in that maximum volume is not greater than the weight of the object, then it will sink.

QUESTION #18   (Answer:  c)   The continuity equation is:
$$A_1 v_1 = A_2 v_2.$$
Note that the larger the cross section, the smaller the fluid velocity and vice versa.

QUESTION #19   (Answer:  c)   The velocity (v) is slowest where the cross-sectional area (A) is greatest from the continuity equation ($A_1 v_1 = A_2 v_2$).  At faster velocities, the pressure is lower, and at slower velocities the pressure (P) is higher from Bernoulli's Equation:
$$P + \rho g h + \tfrac{1}{2}\rho v^2 = \text{constant}$$
   $\rho g h$ does not change if h = constant
      then $\tfrac{1}{2}\rho v^2$ increases as v increases, and P must decrease
         because the whole expression is constant.
As the fluid moves faster, pressure energy (P) is converted to kinetic energy ($\tfrac{1}{2}\rho v^2$) and the pressure drops.

QUESTION #20   (Answer:  d)   Since the diameter is constant, the velocity of fluid flow is constant by the continuity equation ($A_1 v_1 = A_2 v_2$).  From Bernoulli's equation:
$$P + \rho g h + \tfrac{1}{2}\rho v^2 = \text{constant}$$
   $\tfrac{1}{2}\rho v^2$ does not change
      $\rho$ = density   v = velocity
   $\rho g h$ changes because h (height above some arbitrary reference point) is changing, the larger h means the larger this term; the larger $\rho g h$ means the smaller the P term becomes; then, the higher the pipe (due to h), the smaller the pressure (P).

QUESTION #21   (Answer:  a)   Turbulence is best estimated using Reynolds number (R) or by remembering the relations from R.  The viscosity and density of the fluid (i.e., the blood) is constant. Since diameter (d) and velocity (v) are greatest in the arteries and
      — turbulence $\propto$ (v)(d) —
they have the highest turbulence.  The velocity is greater in the arteries because the total cross-sectional area of the arteries is less than the total cross-sectional area of the capillaries.

_____ density                        _____ Pascal's Law
_____ elastic properties             _____ viscosity
_____ specific gravity               _____ Bernoulli's Equation
_____ buoyancy                       _____ tensile forces
_____ hydrostatic pressure           _____ compressive forces


## 5.7      Electrostatics


### 5.7.1      REVIEW OF ELECTROSTATICS


The elementary charges are called positive (+) or negative (−). Each has a charge of $1.6 \times 10^{-19}$ coulombs but differ in sign. The electron is the negative charge carrier, and the proton is the positive charge carrier. Substances with an excess of electrons have a net negative charge. Substances with a deficiency of electrons have a net positive charge. One way of charging substances is by rubbing them (i.e., by contact). For example, glass rubbed on fur becomes positive and rubber rubbed on fur becomes negative. Objects can also be charged by induction which occurs when one charged object brought near another causes a charge redistribution in the latter to give net charge regions. Conductors transmit charge readily. Insulators resist the flow of charge.

Charges exert forces upon each other. Like charges repel each other and unlike charges attract. For two charges the force is given by Coulomb's Law:

$$F = k(q_1 q_2/r^2) = (1/4\pi E_o)(q_1 q_2/r^2)$$

q = charges      k = constant = $9.0 \times 10^9$ nt-m$^2$/coul$^2$
$E_o$ = permittivity of air to the forces = $8.85 \times 10^{-12}$ coul$^2$/nt-m$^2$
r = distance between the charges.

A charge generates an electric field (E) in the space around it. Fields (force fields) are vectors (have direction and magnitude). A field is generated by an object and is that region of space around an object that will exert a force on a second object when it is brought into the field. The field exists independently of the second object and is not altered by its presence. The force exerted on the second object depends upon that object and the field. The electric field (E) is:

$$E = F/q = kQ/r^2 \qquad (i.e., F = kQq/r^2)$$

E and F are vectors
Q = charge generating the field
q = charge placed in it.

Charges exert forces upon each other through fields. The direction of a field is the direction a positive charge would move if placed in it. Electric field lines are imaginary lines which are in the same direction as E at that point. The direction is away from positive charges and toward negative charges (Fig. 5.9).

**Fig. 5.9 – Electric Field Lines**

The <u>potential energy (PE)</u> of a charged object in a field would equal the work done on that object to bring it from infinity to a distance (r) from the charge setting up the electric field or,

$$PE = work = Fr = (qE)r = kQq/r$$

Q = charge setting up field
q = charge brought in to a distance r.

When a +q moves against E, its PE increases. When a –q moves against E, its PE decreases. Realize that if you brought two positive charges together, work would have to be done to the system (and PE would increase), and vice versa for a +q and a –q.

The <u>electric potential (V)</u> is a scalar, and it is defined at each distance (r) from a charge (Q) generating an electric field. It represents the negative of the work per unit charge in bringing a +q from infinity to r:

$$V = PE/q = kQ/r = volts = Joules/coulomb$$

$$V = Ed \text{ for a parallel plate capacitor (Section 5.8.1)}.$$

Lines (and surfaces) of equal V are perpendicular to electric field lines. Work can only be done when moving between surfaces of Vs and is, therefore, independent of the path taken. No work is done when a charge (q) is moved along an equal potential (equipotential) surface (or line), because the component of force is zero along it. Potential (V) is defined in terms of positive charges such that V is positive when due to a +Q and negative when due to a –Q. Potential (V) is added algebraically at a point (because it is a scalar). (Fig. 5.10).

(1) $V_1$, $V_2$ are two potential surfaces perpendicular to E and F;
(2) $V_2-V_1$ (or $V_1-V_2$) is the potential difference (PD, see below);
(3) charge (q) moved from A to B has work (W) done on it
 $$W = q (V_1-V_2) = q (PD) \text{ see below};$$
(4) charge (q) moved from A to C has no work done because this is along an equipotential surface and the component of force (F) is perpendicular to it;
(5) the lines of F are along the lines of E.

**Fig. 5.10 – Electrical Potential**

The potential difference (PD) is the difference in V between two points, or it is the work per unit positive charge done by electric forces moving a small test charge from the point of higher potential to the point of lower potential (Fig. 5.10):

$$PD = V_A - V_B = \text{volts} = \text{work/charge}$$
$$\text{Work} = q (V_A - V_B) = q (PD).$$

An electric dipole consists of two charges separated by some finite distance (d). Usually the charges are equal and opposite. The laws of forces, fields etc., above, apply to dipoles. A dipole is characterized by its dipole moment (D.M.) which is the product of the charge (q) and d. Dipoles tend to line up with the electric field. Motion of dipoles against an electric field requires energy as discussed above (Fig. 5.11).

Dipole with equal and opposite charges     Alignment of dipole with E

E = electric field
F = forces exerted by E on the dipole

dipole moment = (distance)(charge) = qd.

**Fig. 5.11 - Dipoles**

5.7.2     QUESTIONS TO REVIEW ELECTROSTATICS

(1)   Concerning fields, which is incorrect?

(a) They exist in space and are generated by objects (e.g. mass).
(b) Gravitational and electrical fields are examples.
(c) They are scalars.
(d) They exist independently of other objects.

(2)   Coulomb's Law of electrical forces     (q = charge, r = distance between charges, k = constant, F = force) is:

(a) $F = k(q_1q_2/r^2)$          (b)  $F = k(q/r^2)$
(c) $F = k(q_1q_2/r)$            (d)  $F = k(q^2/r)$

(3)   If $F = \text{force} = kq_1q_0/r^2$ and $q_0$ = an electric charge, then $F/q_0$ is:

(a) the electric field generated by $q_1$
(b) the force acting on $q_0$
(c) the electric potential set up by $q_0$
(d) the work done by the force on $q_1$

(4)   Electric field lines are

(a) directed away from negative charges;
(b) directed away from positive charges;
(c) directed toward positive charges;
(d) any of the above may be correct.

381

(5) The electric potential:

(a) represents the negative of the work per unit charge in bringing a positive charge from infinity to a distance (r) from an object generating an electric field;
(b) is a vector;
(c) has the units of henries;
(d) all of the above.

(6) Formulations for electric potential (V) include all except: (q = charge, r = distance, E = electric field, F = force)

(a) $V = (1/4\pi E_o)(q/r)$      (b) V = potential energy/ charge

(c) V = Er      (d) V = Fq

(7) A volt is a:

$\frac{E}{r}$

(a) newton/coulomb      (b) Joule/coulomb
(c) coulomb/newton      (d) coulomb/Joule

(8) Electrical work is:

(a) dependent on the path taken by a charge between equipotential surfaces;
(b) zero when a charge is moved along an equipotential (electric potential) line;
(c) zero when a charge moves between surfaces of different electric potential;
(d) both (a) and (c).

(9) The potential difference as used in electricity is

(a) the difference in potential energy between two points;
(b) the difference in electric potential between two points;
(c) the difference in work between two points;
(d) both (a) and (c).

(10) Which of the following is a correct formulation of electrical work (W) done on moving a charge (q) in an electric field (E)? (V = electric potential, PD = potential difference, F = electrical force, r = distance between charges)

(a) W = q(PD)      (b) W = Fq
(c) W = Vr      (d) W = Eq

(11) All are true about electric dipoles except:

(a) they consist of two charges separated by finite distance
(b) the dipole moment is a product of the charge and the distance between them
(c) the motion of dipoles against an electric field requires no energy
(d) the positive end of the dipole points in the direction of the electric field

(12) If the distance between two electrical charges is doubled, the force between them is:

(a) decreased by 1/4      (b) decreased by 1/2
(c) doubled      (d) quadrupled

(13) The charge (q) on each of two objects is doubled and they are moved twice as far apart (r); the force between them is:

(a) increased by a factor of 8
(b) increased by a factor of 4
(c) increased by a factor of 2
(d) unchanged

(14) As two electrical charges move further apart, the force between them:

(a) increases proportionally to the inverse square of their separation
(b) increases proportionally to their separation
(c) decreases proportionally to the inverse square of their separation
(d) decreases proportionally to their separation

(15) If charge #1 ($q_1$) is doubled in size and charge #2 ($Q_2$) is tripled in size and the distance (r) between them is not changed, the force (F) between them is:

(a) decreased by a factor of 36
(b) increased by a factor of 36
(c) increased by a factor of 6
(d) unchanged

(16) What is the force between charge #1 ($q_1$) and charge #2 ($q_2$) in the diagram below?

$q_1$ = 2 couls                    $q_2$ = 4 couls

(a) repulsive, 2 nts              (b) attractive, 2 nts
(c) repulsive, 2k nts            (d) attractive, 2k nts

(17) The net force on charge C ($q_C$) is:

(a) zero
(b) horizontally and to the right, ½k nts
(c) horizontally and to the left, ½k nts
(d) vertical and down, ½k nts

(18) The electric field (E) generated by a charge

(a) is constant at all distances from the charge;
(b) decreases directly as distance from the charge increases;
(c) decreases proportional to the inverse square of the distance from the charge;
(d) decreases proportional to the inverse distance from the charge.

(19) All of the following are correct formulations for the potential energy (PE) of a charged object (q) in an electric field except:

(F = force on charge, V = electric potential, E = electric field, r = distance of charge from object setting up the electric field)

(a) $PE = V_q$                    (b) $PE = Fr$
(c) $PE = E_q$                    (d) $PE = qEr$

(20) A positive charge is moved against (in the opposite direction of) an electric field. The potential energy of this object:

(a) remains the same          (b) decreases
(c) increases                 (d) cannot be evaluated

(21) A negative charge is moved against (in the opposite direction of) an electric field. The potential energy of this negative charge:

(a) stays the same            (b) increases
(c) decreases                 (d) cannot be evaluated
                                  from the information
                                  given

(22) What is the electrical potential (V) at point A?

$\longleftarrow$ 1 meter $\longrightarrow$
$\oplus$                              A

q = 4 couls

(a) +4 volts                  (b) -4 volts
(c) +4k volts                 (d) -4k volts

(23) Determine the electric potential at point A.

$\oplus$ —— 1m —— A —— 2m —— $\ominus$

$V = \frac{1}{4\pi\varepsilon_0}\frac{q}{r}$

$q_1 = +4$ couls        $+4k - \frac{16k}{2}$        $q_2 = -16$ couls

(a) -28 volts                 (b) +28 volts
(c) +4k volts                 (d) -4k volts

(24) What is the work done in moving a charge $q_1$ from A to B?

$\oplus$ - - - 2m - - - $\ominus$ - - 1m - - $\bullet$
q=8 couls        $q_1=2$ couls

$-\frac{16}{3}k + 8k$

(A) $\longrightarrow$ (B)

$\frac{8}{3}k$

(a) -10 $\pi$ Joules           (b) +10 $\pi$ Joules

(c) +(8/3)k Joules             (d) -(8k/3) Joules

5.7.3        ANSWERS TO QUESTIONS IN SECTION 5.7.2

( 1)  c   (2)  a   (3)  a   (4)  b   (5)  a   (6)  d   (7)  b
( 8)  b   (9)  b   (10) a   (11) c   (12) a   (13) d   (14) c
(15)  c   (16) d   (17) d   (18) c   (19) c   (20) c   (21) c
(22)  c   (23) d   (24) c

384

QUESTIONS #1 to #11:  Adequately discussed in Section.

QUESTION #12   (Answer:  a)  From Coulomb's Law:

$$\frac{F_f}{F_o} = \frac{k\frac{q_1 q_2}{r_f^2}}{k\frac{q_1 q_2}{r_o^2}} = \frac{\frac{1}{r_f^2}}{\frac{1}{r_o^2}} = \frac{\frac{1}{r_f^2}}{\frac{r_o^2}{1}} = \frac{r_o^2}{r_f^2} = \frac{r_o^2}{(2r_o)^2} = \frac{r_o^2}{4r_o^2} = \frac{1}{4}$$

$$(r_f = 2r_o)$$

$$\frac{F_f}{F_o} = \frac{1}{4}$$

$$F_f = \frac{1}{4}F_o. \qquad f = final \qquad o = original$$

Or reason from Coulomb's Law that force is proportional to the inverse square of distance ($1/r^2$); this is $(\frac{1}{2})^2 = \frac{1}{4}$ for this case.

QUESTION #13   (Answer:  d)  From Coulomb's Law:

$$f = final \qquad\qquad o = original$$

$$q_{1f} = 2q_{1o} \qquad q_{2f} = 2q_{2o} \qquad r_f = 2r_o$$

$$\frac{F_f}{F_o} = \frac{k\frac{q_{1f} q_{2f}}{r_f^2}}{k\frac{q_{1o} q_{2o}}{r_o^2}} = \frac{q_{1f} q_{2f}}{r_f^2} \cdot \frac{r_o^2}{q_{1o} q_{2o}} = \frac{2q_{1o} 2q_{2o}}{(2r_o^2)} \cdot \frac{r_o^2}{q_{1o} q_{2o}} = \frac{2 \cdot 2 \cdot q_{1o} \cdot q_{2o} \cdot r_o^2}{4 \cdot r_o^2 \cdot q_{1o} \cdot q_{2o}} = \frac{4}{4} = 1$$

$$\frac{F_f}{F_o} = 1$$

$$F_f = F_o.$$

Or, by reasoning from Coulomb's Law that since force is directly proportional to the product of the charges, the doubling of each charge would increase the force by a factor of $(2)(2) = 4$.  Since force is proportional to the inverse square of the separation, the increase in separation decreases the force by $(\frac{1}{2})^2 = \frac{1}{4}$.  Multiplying these factors together to get the net change as $(4)(\frac{1}{4}) = 1$ or no change.

QUESTION #14   (Answer:  c)  From Coulomb's Law:

$$F \propto 1/r^2$$

QUESTION #15   (Answer:  c)  From Coulomb's Law:

$$f = final \qquad\qquad o = original$$
$$q_{1f} = 2q_{1o} \qquad\qquad q_{2f} = 3q_{2o}$$

$$\frac{F_f}{F_o} = \frac{k\frac{q_{1f} q_{2f}}{r^2}}{k\frac{q_{1o} q_{2o}}{r^2}} = \frac{q_{1f} q_{2f}}{q_{1o} q_{2o}} = \frac{(2q_{1o})(3q_{2o})}{(q_{1o})(q_{2o})} = \frac{2 \cdot 3}{1} = 6$$

$$F_f = 6F_o$$

Or, by reasoning from Coulomb's Law that since force is directly proportional to the product of the charges, since this product is increased $(2)(3) = 6$ times so the force must be also.

QUESTION #16   (Answer:  d)  From Coulomb's Law:

$$F = k(q_1 q_2 / r^2) = k(+2)(-4)/(2)^2 = -2k \text{ nts}$$

Since the sign is negative, the force is attractive.

QUESTION #17   (Answer: d)  This problem may be solved by the symmetry of the system, Coulomb's Law and geometry.  The forces (vectors) and their components exerted by $q_A (F_A)$ and $q_B (F_B)$ on $q_C$ are:

the forces            components of forces

The x-components ($F_{A_x}$ and $F_{B_x}$) cancel (because they are equal and opposite by the symmetry of the system) and the y-components sum to a vertically downward force.  So, by elimination the answer is (d).
OR, first by applying Coulomb's Law:

$$F_A = k(q_A q_C / r^2) = k\left[(+2)(+1)/(2)^2\right] = k/2$$

$$F_B = k(q_B q_C / r^2) = k\left[(-2)(+1)/(2)^2\right] = -k/2$$

the r = 2 m (meters) is derived by:

the side opposite the 30° angle is ½ the hypotenuse (which must then be 2 m)

The x-components still cancel and the y-components are:

$$F_{Ay} = -(1/2)F_A = -1/2(k/2) = -k/4$$
$$F_{By} = (1/2)F_B = 1/2(-k/2) = -k/4$$
$$F_y = F_{Ay} + F_{By} = -k/4 - k/4 = -k/2 \text{ nts}$$

the minus sign means the $F_y$ is directed down the y-axis.

QUESTION #18   (Answer:  c)  The formula for the electric field (E) is:

$$E = F/q_o = kq/r^2; \text{ hence, } E \propto 1/r^2.$$

QUESTION #19   (Answer:  c)  Eq = force generated by E on q.

QUESTION #20   (Answer: c) The directions of the lines of an electric field is the direction a positive charge would move if placed in it.  To move a positive charge in the opposite direction requires energy, and this energy is stored as the potential energy which increases.  The potential energy of the system may be used to move any charge along the direction of the field lines.

QUESTION #21 (Answer: c) The direction of the field lines of an electric field is the direction a positive charge would move if placed in it. So, a negative charge would normally move in the opposite direction or against the field. When a charge moves in the expected direction in an electric field, the potential energy of the charge system decreases. This is like the potential energy of a rock decreasing as it fell toward the earth, because this is its expected direction to move in the gravitational field.

QUESTION #22 (Answer: c) The formula for V is:

$$V = kq/r = k(+4/1) = +4k \text{ volts.}$$

QUESTION #23 (Answer: d) Since the electric potential (V) is a scalar, the V contribution by each charge is determined separately and added algebraically to get the net potential at point A:

For $q_1$: $V_1 = k(q_1/r_1) = k(+4/1) = +4k$ volts
For $q_2$: $V_2 = k(q_2/r_2) = k(-16/2) = -8k$ volts
Total: $V_A = V_1 + V_2 = +4k - 8k = -4k$ volts.

QUESTION #24 (Answer: c) The work done in this instance can be calculated by using the following formulations:

$W =$   $q_1 (V_B - V_A) = q_1 (PD)$
      $V_B = k(q/r_A) = k(+8/3) = (+8/3) k$ volts
      $V_A = k(q/r_A) = k(+8/2) = +4 k$ volts

for both the q is generating the potential
PD (Potential difference) $= V_B - V_A = (8/3)k - 4k = (8-12/3)k = -4k/3$ volts

$W =$   $q_1 (PD) = (-2)(-4k/3) = (+8/3)k$ Joules.

The positive sign means that work must be put into (done to) the system.

5.7.5      <u>VOCABULARY, CONCEPTS, ETC. CHECKLIST FOR ELECTROSTATICS</u>

| | |
|---|---|
| ____ charges | ____ volts |
| ____ conductors | ____ dipole moment |
| ____ insulators | ____ potentials |
| ____ Coulomb's Law | ____ potential |
| ____ electrical forces | differences |
| ____ electric field | ____ electrical dipoles |

5.8      **DC Circuits**

5.8.1      <u>REVIEW OF DC CIRCUITS</u>

<u>DC</u> (direct current) electricity is generated similarly to AC (Section 5.9.1) with one important exception. The AC electricity is converted to DC by substituting a split ring commutator for the slip

rings. This causes the connections to the brush to reverse twice per revolution to coincide with the current change in the armature. The current that is carried away is all in one direction; however, it still pulsates (Fig. 5.12).

**Fig. 5.12 - DC Electricity**

The main elements in a DC circuit are the emf source (V) and the resistors (R). The current (I) results from their interaction. These three quantities are interrelated in Ohm's Law as:

$$V = IR.$$

V, I, R are the total of each in the circuit. Capacitors may also be used in DC circuits.

Circuit elements are either in series or in parallel. Two components are in series when they have only one point in common; that is, the current traveling from one of them back to the emf source must pass through the other. In a complete series circuit, or for individual series loops of a larger mixed circuit, the current (I) is the same over each component and the total voltage ($V_T$ is the sum of all the emf sources) is the sum of voltages across each resistor (including the internal resistances of emf sources--see below). Two components are in parallel when they are connected to two common points in the circuit; that is, the current traveling from one such element back to the source of emf (assume current started at source of emf) need not pass through the second component because there is an alternate path. In a parallel circuit, the total current is the sum of currents for each path (i.e. each path has a different current), and the voltage is equal for all paths and thus equals V.

Electromotive force (V) maintains a constant potential difference and thereby maintains a continuous current. The emf source replaces energy lost by the moving electrons. Sources of emf are batteries (conversion of chemical energy to electrical energy) and generators (conversion of mechanical energy to electrical energy). A source of emf is symbolized in a circuit as in Fig. 5.13.

arrows show normal current direction

**Fig. 5.13 - EMF**

The source of emf does work on each charge to raise it from a lower potential to a higher potential. Then as the charge flows around the circuit (naturally from higher to lower potential) it loses energy which is replaced by the emf source again, etc. Therefore work (energy) must be supplied at the rate energy is lost by the current flowing through the circuit,

energy supplied = energy lost.

Energy is lost whenever a charge (as current) passes through a resistor.

The units of emf (E) are volts (Section 5.7.1). The actual voltage delivered to a circuit is not equal to the V value of the source.

388

This is reduced by an Ir which represents the voltage loss by the internal resistance (r) of the source itself.  The net voltage is called the terminal voltage ($V_t$) and is:

$$V_t = V-Ir = IR_T$$
$$I, R_T = \text{totals for the whole circuit}$$
$$V = \text{maximal voltage output of emf source.}$$

The $V_t$ is the voltage delivered to the circuit by that emf source.

Normally, a charge gains energy as it flows through a source of emf. But when two sources of emf are connected in opposition (positive pole to positive pole), the charge flows from the higher emf source to the lower emf source.  In this instance, it loses energy when passing through the smaller emf because it passes in the opposite direction to normal.  If there is more than one source of emf in a curcuit, the total emf is a sum of these by taking into account the differences in polarity (i.e., reversed emf's are negative):

$$V_t \text{ (total)} = \textstyle\sum V_{ti}, i = 1, 2,\dots.$$

A voltmeter is used to measure voltages (potential differences) in circuits and is symbolized as:

Resistance (R) is the opposition to the flow of electrons in a substance. Resistivity ($\rho$) is an inherent property of a substance and is directly related to resistance. Resistivity varies directly as resistance and cross-sectional area, and indirectly as length.

Resistance has a fixed value for a given material and depends on the size, shape and temperature but not on the emf or current.  Note these relations ($R \propto 1/A$):

    R increases as l increases
    R increases as A decreases
    R increases as temperature increases.

Resistance increases with temperature because the thermal motion of atoms (molecules) increases and results in more collisions with electrons which impede their flow.  The units of resistance are ohms symbolized by $\Omega$ (omega).  From Ohm's Law, an ohm = volt/ampere.

When a +I (current) flows across a resistor, there is a voltage decrease and an energy loss:

    energy loss = Vq = VIt = Joules
    power loss (P) = VIt/t = VI = watts = volt-amperes =
                                        Joules/sec.

The energy loss may be used to perform work.  These relations hold for power (P),

$$P = VI = (IR)(I) = I^2R = V(V/R) = V^2/R.$$

Resistance in a circuit is symbolized by,

A variable resistance (as with a rheostat) is symbolized by:

Resistance in a series circuit is:

$$R = R_1 + R_2 + R_3 + ...$$

Resistance in a parallel circuit is,

$$1/R = 1/R_1 + 1/R_2 + 1/R_3 + ...$$   The R's are the total resistances.

Current (I) is the amount of charge (Q) that flows past a point in a given amount of time (t),

$$I = Q/t = amperes = coulombs/sec.$$

Current is caused by the movement of electrons. The velocity (not current) of electrons is slowed by impurities in the conductor and by the thermal motion of atoms. A transient current is set up when a capacitor discharges (below). A continuous current is set up when a source of emf is present to replace the energy lost by moving electrons (see above). The direction of current is taken as the direction a positive charge moves, by convention. It is represented on a circuit diagram by arrows. Ammeters are used to measure the flow of current and are symbolized as:

Capacitance (C) is an inherent property of a conductor and is formulated as:

$$C = charge/electric \ potential = Q/V = farad = coulomb/volt.$$

This means that C is the number of coulombs that must be transferred to a conductor to raise its potential by one volt. The amount of charge that can be stored is determined by the size, shape and surroundings of the conductor. A smaller conductor usually has a smaller capacitance. A greater degree of curvature (or more pointed) usually means a greater capacity to store charge. The higher the dielectric strength (i.e. the electric field strength at which a substance ceases to be an insulator and becomes a conductor) of the medium, the greater the capacitance of the conductor.

A capacitor is two or more conductors with opposite but equal charges placed near each other. A common example is the parallel plate capacitor. The formulas of importance for capacitors are:
  (1) $C = Q/V$
       V = potential difference between the plates
  (2) $V = Ed$
       E = electric field strength
       d = distance between the plates
  (3) C is directly proportional to the area of the plates
       C is inversely proportional to the distance between the plates; ie: $C_0 = E_0 A/d$ for air (as the medium) between the plates.
  (4) $K = C/C_0$ = dielectric constant
       $K = V_0/V = E_0/E$ also
       $C = KC_0$.

The dielectric substances set up an opposing electric field to that of the capacitor which decreases the net electric field and allows the capacitance of the capacitor to increase (C = Q/Ed). The molecules of the dielectric are dipoles which line up in the electric field (Fig. 5.14).

E = electric field
D = dielectric
C = capacitor
N = net

without dielectric        with dielectric.

**Fig. 5.14 – Capacitors and Dielectrics**

The C's are the total capacitances.

The <u>energy associated with each charged capacitor</u> is:

$V_{avg} = \frac{1}{2}V$

Potential Energy (PE) = W = $(\frac{1}{2}V)(Q)$ = $\frac{1}{2}QV$ = $\frac{1}{2}(CV)(V)$ = $\frac{1}{2}CV^2$
$= \frac{1}{2}Q(Q/C)$ = $\frac{1}{2}Q^2/C$.

The <u>symbol for a capacitor</u> is:

In a <u>DC circuit, the capacitor</u> charges up until the charge ($Q_{max}$) equals $V_T C$ and then the current stops. If the $V_T$ is then removed, the capacitor will discharge. In an <u>AC circuit</u>, there is an alternating surge of charge onto and off the capacitor, and a current exists there even though there is no transfer of charge between the plates. The behavior of a capacitor in a circuit is derived from calculus. Some of the key results are as follows:

  (1) When a C is combined in series with an R:
     $V_T$ = IR + Q/C
  (2) RC = time constant $\tau$ = (ohms)(farads) = seconds
    (a) The capacitor takes about $5\tau$ to become fully charged
       ($Q_{max}$ = $CV_T$).
    (b) In one $\tau$, the capacitor is 63% charged and has 37% of
       its final current ($V_T$/R) delivered to it (these
       numbers arise from the solution and the base of the
       natural logs which is e = 2.7183, ∴ 1/e = 0.37, 1 -1/e
       = 0.63)
    (c) The capacitor will be nearly fully discharged after
       $5\tau$.
    (d) The capacitor will have discharged down to 37% of $Q_{max}$
       after one $\tau$.

(1)   In a DC circuit:

(a) if series, the currents are different for each component
    (e.g., registers, capacitors);
(b) if series, the voltages are the same for each component;
(c) if parallel, the currents are equal for all paths (of the
    circuit);
(d) if parallel, the voltages are equal for all paths.

(2)   The following graph represents which type of current(s)?

(a) AC only                    (b) DC only
(c) AC or DC                   (d) neither AC nor DC

(3)   Ohm's Law is:
(V = potential difference, I = current, R = resistance, C =
capacitance, Q = charge, L = inductance, t = time):

(a) $C = Q/V$                    (b) $L = -\Delta V/(\Delta I/\Delta t)$
(c) $V = IR$                     (d) $V = QLt$

(4)   The actual voltage output of an electromotive source

(a) may be equal to, less than, or greater than the expected
    voltage of the source;
(b) is always equal to the expected voltage;
(c) is always more than the expected voltage;
(d) is always less than the expected voltage.

(5)   All are correct concerning electromotive force (emf) sources
except:

(a) the units of emf are microfarads
(b) maintains constant potential differences in a circuit
(c) replaces energy lost by the moving electrons in a circuit
(d) sources include both batteries and generators

(6)   A source of emf (electromotive force):

(a) generates positive and negative charges
(b) decreases the resistance an electron faces in moving
    through a circuit
(c) does work on each charge to raise it from a lower potential
    (electrical) to a higher potential
(d) changes the sign of the charge during each transit of the
    circuit

(7)   Normally, a charge gains energy as it moves through a source of
emf, but it can lose energy if

(a) the emf source has an internal resistance;
(b) the emf source has a reversed polarity;
(c) the emf source is a generator;
(d) the emf source is of low voltage.

(8)   Resistance, as used in electricity, is

(a) the opposition to flow of electrons in a substance;
(b) the opposition to the generation of emf;
(c) the location of storage of energy of electrons;
(d) has the units of farads.

(9)   Resistance, as used in electricity, is

(a) inversely proportional to the density of the conductor;
(b) inversely proportional to the resistivity of the conductor;
(c) directly proportional to the cross-sectional area of the conductor;
(d) directly proportional to the length of the conductor.

(10)  Resistance (electrical) has a fixed value for a given material and depends on all except:

(a) size of a conductor          (b) current in a conductor
(c) shape of a conductor         (d) temperature

(11)  The resistance of a substance can be expected to increase for all the following situations except:

(a) increasing cross-sectional area
(b) increasing length
(c) increasing temperature
(d) increasing resistivity of materials

(12)  The unit of power is the:

(a) Joule    (b) volt    (c) ampere    (d) watt

(13)  Current is:

(a) time/charge              (b) charge/time
(c) (charge)(time)           (d) none of these

(14)  An ampere is:

(a) coulombs/secs            (b) (coulombs)(secs)
(c) (volts)(ohms)            (d) ohms/volts

(15)  Current is:

(a) caused by the movement of positive charge
(b) increased by the thermal motion of atoms
(c) decreased by impurities in the conductor
(d) all of the above

(16)  To set up a continuous current, as opposed to a transient current, in a circuit, one may use a(n):

(a) source of emf            (b) capacitor
(c) capacitor and resistor   (d) capacitor and inductor

(17)  Capacitance is:

(a) charge/potential         (b) (charge)(potential)
(c) (resistance)(current)    (d) charge/resistance

393

(18) The farad is a unit of capacitance and is equal to:

    (a) coulombs/volts         (b) (volts)(coulombs)
    (c) amperes/ohms          (d) (amperes)(ohms)

(19) All of the following are associated with increased capacitance of a conductor except

    (a) increased inducibility     (b) increased size
    (c) increased curvature      (d) increased dielectric
                                 strength of the medium

(20) In a parallel plate capacitor,

    (a) both plates are the same charge;
    (b) capacitance is directly proportional to the distance between the plates;
    (c) capacitance is independent of the medium between the plates;
    (d) capacitance is directly proportional to the area of the plates.

(21) A capacitor will charge up to a certain point and then will cause the current to stop in a(n):

    (a) DC circuit              (b) AC circuit
    (c) both DC and AC       (d) neither DC nor AC

(22) In an AC circuit with a capacitor in series with a resistor, the voltage of the battery (neglecting internal resistance) is:

    (a) (capacitor voltage)(resistor voltage)
    (b) voltage across the capacitor minus voltage across the resistor
    (c) voltage across the resistor minus voltage across the capacitor
    (d) voltage across the resistor plus voltage across the capacitor

(23) If total resistance is 9 ohms and total voltage is 3 volts the current is:

    (a) 1/27 ampere         (b) 1/3 ampere
    (c) 3 amperes           (d) 27 amperes

(24) A current of 2 amperes and a resistance of 8 ohms requires what voltage (in a circuit):

    (a) 1/16 volt           (b) 1/4 volt
    (c) 4 volts            (d) 16 volts

(25) If it requires 20 volts to cause a current of 5 amperes in a wire, the resistance of the wire is:

    (a) 1/100 ohm          (b) 1/4 ohm
    (c) 4 ohms            (d) 100 ohms

(26) Assuming internal resistances of circuit elements is negligible, a charge would lose the most energy when it passes through a(n):

(a) capacitor
(b) inductor
(c) resistor
(d) battery

(27) A battery has a voltage of 6V marked on it and an internal resistance of 0.5 ohm. If it is placed in the circuit below, what is the actual voltage it is producing in that circuit?

R = 5 ohms

? $V_T$    ↑ I = 1 ampere

(a) 10 volts
(b) 8.5 volts
(c) 5.5 volts
(d) 5 volts

(28) Calculate the internal resistance of the 20-volt battery in the following circuit:

R = 4 ohms

↑ I = 2 amperes

(a) 16 ohms
(b) 10 ohms
(c) 3 ohms
(d) 2 ohms

(29) Determine the total emf (electromotive force) in the following circuit:

I    $V_2$ = 5V

$V_1$ = 10V         V = volts
                    I = current
$V_3$ = 7V    I

(a) 2 volts
(b) 8 volts
(c) 12 volts
(d) 22 volts

(30) All are formulations of power (P) in a circuit with an emf (V) source and a resistor (R) with a current (I), except:

(a) $P = VI$
(b) $P = IR/V$
(c) $P = I^2R$
(d) $P = V^2/R$

(31) A circuit has a current of 2 amperes and a resistance of 4 ohms. The maximal power that can be delivered is:

(a) 16 watts
(b) 8 watts
(c) 2 watts
(d) 1/2 watt

(32) If the cross-sectional area of a conductor is quadrupled (x4), the resistance:

(a) increases by a factor of 16
(b) increases by a factor of 4
(c) decreases by a factor of 1/4
(d) decreases by a factor of 1/16

(33) If the length of a conductor is doubled, the resistance:

(a) is not affected
(b) decreases by a factor of 1/2
(c) decreases by a factor of 1/4
(d) increases by a factor of 2

(34) In a circuit with a voltage of 10 volts and a resistance of 10 ohms and a current passing for 10 secs, the maximum possible number of Joules of heat produced is:

(a) 100 Joules      (b) 1000 Joules
(c) 1 Joule      (d) 10 Joules

$P = I^2 R t$
$= \frac{V^2}{R} t = \frac{100}{10} \cdot 10$

(35) Determine the current (I) in the following circuit:

V = 5 volts     $R_1 = 5$ ohms     $R_2 = 4$ ohms     I = ?

(a) 5/9 amperes      (b) 1.8 amperes
(c) 2.25 amperes      (d) 45 amperes

$\frac{5}{20} + \frac{4}{20} = \frac{9}{20}$
$\frac{20}{9}$   $\frac{5 \cdot 9}{20} = \frac{45}{20}$

(36) The voltage (V) of the following battery is (neglect internal resistance of battery):

V=?     $R_1 = 3$ ohms     $R_2 = 10$ ohms     I = 10 amperes

$R_3 = 5$ ohms

18·10

(a) 180 volts      (b) 18 volts
(c) 1.8 volts      (d) 0.55 volts

(37) A current of 8 amperes will deliver what charge in 4 seconds?

(a) 2 statcoulombs      (b) 2 coulombs
(c) 32 statcoulombs      (d) 32 coulombs

$8 amp = \frac{C}{sec}$
$8 an$

(38) If 10 coulombs pass a point in 2 seconds, the current is:

(a) 0.20 amps      (b) 5 amps
(c) 20 amps      (d) 200 amps

(39) A conductor discharges (i.e., cannot hold any more charge) when 40 coulombs is placed on it at a voltage of 10 volts. What is its capacitance?

(a) 4000 farads      (b) 400 farads
(c) 0.25 farads      (d) 4 farads

(40) The capacitance of a parallel plate capacitor in air is 20 farads. This capacitor is placed in a medium with a dielectric constant equal to 5. What is the capacitance now?

(a) still 20 farads      (b) 4 farads
(c) 400 farads      (d) 100 farads

(41) In air, a parallel plate capacitor has a capacitance of 4 farads. In medium A, the capacitance is 32 farads. What is the dielectric constant of medium A?

(a) 1/8      (b) 8
(c) 128      (d) need the dielectric constant of air

(42)   The units of resistance times capacitance is:

      (a) voltage               (b) amperes
      (c) henries               (d) seconds


## 5.8.3     ANSWERS TO QUESTIONS IN SECTION 5.8.2

| ( 1) | d | (2) | b | (3) | c | (4) | d | (5) | a | (6) | c | (7) | b |
|------|---|-----|---|-----|---|-----|---|-----|---|-----|---|-----|---|
| ( 8) | a | (9) | d | (10) | b | (11) | a | (12) | d | (13) | b | (14) | a |
| (15) | c | (16) | a | (17) | a | (18) | a | (19) | a | (20) | d | (21) | a |
| (22) | d | (23) | b | (24) | d | (25) | c | (26) | c | (27) | c | (28) | c |
| (29) | b | (30) | b | (31) | a | (32) | c | (33) | d | (34) | a | (35) | c |
| (36) | a | (37) | d | (38) | b | (39) | d | (40) | d | (41) | b | (42) | d |


## 5.8.4     DISCUSSION OF ANSWERS TO QUESTIONS IN SECTION 5.8.2

QUESTIONS #1 to #22:  Adequately discussed in Section.

QUESTION #23  (Answer:  b)  From Ohm's Law:

$$V = IR$$

$$I = V/R = 3 \text{ volts}/9 \text{ ohms} = 1/3 \text{ amp.}$$

QUESTION #24  (Answer:  d)  Solve using Ohm's Law:

$$V = IR = (2 \text{ amps})(8 \text{ ohms}) = 16 \text{ volts.}$$

QUESTION #25  (Answer:  c)  Use Ohm's Law:

$$V = IR$$
$$R = V/I = \frac{20 \text{ volts}}{5 \text{ amps}} = 4 \text{ ohms}$$


QUESTION #26  (Answer:  c)  Energy is lost when a charge passes through a resistance.

QUESTION #27  (Answer:  c)  The terminal voltage ($V_t$) of an emf source is determined by taking into account the internal resistance:

$$V_t = V - Ir = IR_T \quad \text{(see Section)}$$
$$R_T = R + r = 5 + 0.5 = 5.5 \text{ ohms (series circuit)}$$
$$V_t = (1 \text{ amp})(5.5 \text{ ohms}) = 5.5 \text{ volts.}$$

QUESTION #28  (Answer:  c)  See Section for an explanation of the formula:

$$V - Ir = IR_T$$
$$R_T = R + r = 4 + r \quad \text{(series circuit)}$$
$$20 - 2r = 2(4 + r) = 8 + 2r$$
$$12 = 4r$$
$$3 = r.$$

QUESTION #29  (Answer:  b)  The total emf's around the loop of the circuit is:

$$V_{total} = \xi V = V_1 + V_2 - V_3 = 10 + 5 - 7 = 8$$

$V_3$ is negative because the current is moving through it in the reverse direction.

The internal resistances of the batteries have been neglected.

QUESTION #30  (Answer:  b)  Try to remember how to convert it to the others using Ohm's Law, although this is not explicitly required for the test.

QUESTION #31  (Answer:  a)  The appropriate formula is:

$$P = I^2 R = (2)^2 (4) = 16 \text{ watts}$$

The units are arrived at as follows:

$$P = (\text{amperes})^2 (\text{ohms}) = (\text{amps})^2 (\text{volts/amps}) = (\text{amps})(\text{volts})$$
$$= (\text{coulomb/sec}) \text{volts} = \text{volt-coulomb/sec} = \text{Joules/sec} = \text{watts}$$

Remember: Joule = volt - coulomb.

QUESTION #32  (Answer:  c)  Resistance (R) $\propto$ 1/Area(A).  Then if A increases by a factor of 4, the R decreases by 1/4.
OR:
$$R_2/R_1 = (\rho \ell /A_2)/(\rho \ell /A_1) = (1/A_2)/(1/A_1) = (1/A_2)(A_1/1) = A_1/A_2$$
$$= A_1/(4A_1) = 1/4 \qquad\qquad (A_2 = 4A_1)$$
$$\therefore R_2 = 1/4\, R_1.$$

QUESTION #33  (Answer:  d)  Resistance (R) $\propto$ length ($\ell$).  So, if length doubles, the R is doubled.
OR:
$$R_2/R_1 = (\rho \ell_2/A)/(\rho \ell_1/A) = \ell_2/\ell_1 = 2\ell_1/\ell_1 = 2$$
$$\therefore R_2 = 2R_1. \qquad\qquad (\ell_2 = 2\ell_1)$$

QUESTION #34  (Answer:  a)  $P = V^2/R$  (see Section)
$$P = (10)^2/10 = 10 \text{ watts}$$
$$(\text{Power})(\text{time}) = \text{Joules} = (10)(10) = 100 \text{ Joules.}$$

QUESTION #35  (Answer:  c)  $R_1$ and $R_2$ are in parallel.  Then:

$$1/R_T = 1/R_1 + 1/R_2 = 1/5 + 1/4 = 4/20 + 5/20 = 9/20$$
$$\therefore R_T = 20/9 \text{ ohms.}$$

Then using Ohm's Law:  V = IR
$$I = V/R = 5 \text{ volts}/(20/9 \text{ ohms}) = 5(9/20) = 9/4 = 2.25 \text{ amps.}$$

QUESTION #36  (Answer:  a)  This is a series circuit because the current (I) must pass through each resistor (R) before returning to the voltage source (V).  The total resistance ($R_T$):
$$R_T = R_1 + R_2 + R_3 = 3 + 10 + 5 = 18 \text{ ohms.}$$

Calculate V using Ohm's Law:  V = IR = (10 amps)(18 ohms)
$$= 180 \text{ volts.}$$

QUESTION #37  (Answer:  d)

$$I = q/t$$
$$q = (I)(t) = (8 \text{ amps})(4 \text{ seconds}) = 32 \text{ coulombs.}$$

QUESTION #38  (Answer:  b)

$$I = q/t = 10 \text{ couls}/2 \text{ secs} = 5 \text{ amps}$$

QUESTION #39    (Answer:  d)  $C = q/V = 40$ coulombs/10 volts = 4 farads

QUESTION #40    (Answer:  d)  $C = K\, Co$         $Co$ = capacitance in air
                              $C = (5)(20) = 100$ farads.

QUESTION #41    (Answer:  b)  $C = K\, Co$
                              $K = C/C_o = 32/4 = 8.$

QUESTION #42    (Answer:  d)

    resistance (R) = ohms = volts/amperes = volts/(coulombs/sec)
                                               = (volt-sec)/couls
    capacitance (C) = farads = couls/volt

Then:   (R)(C) = (volt-sec/coul)(coul/volt) = secs.


## 5.8.5    VOCABULARY, CONCEPTS, ETC. CHECKLIST FOR DC CIRCUITS

| | | |
|---|---|---|
| ____ current | ____ DC electricity | |
| ____ battery | ____ series circuits | |
| ____ internal resistance | ____ parallel circuits | |
| ____ Ohm's Law | ____ emf | |
| ____ resistors | ____ volts | |
| ____ resistivity | ____ farad | |
| ____ resistance | ____ ohm | |
| ____ capacitors | ____ dielectric constant | |
| ____ capacitance | ____ dielectrics | |


## 5.9    AC Circuits


## 5.9.1    REVIEW OF AC CIRCUITS

AC (alternating current) electricity constitutes 99% of that used in
the U.S.  It is made by converting mechanical energy to electrical
energy.  An armature which is a loop of wire is rotated in a magnetic
field using mechanical energy.  A current is induced (see inductance
below) in the wire of the armature.  This current changes direction
because the direction of the velocity of the loop and the magnetic
field changes.  Slip rings are fused to each end of the wire loop and
rotate with it.  Since the direction of the current alternates, the
slip rings alternate in conducting the current away from the loop
(hence AC).  Graphite brushes are on the slip rings and these brush
against conducting materials which carry the current away from the
generator.  AC looks like a sine wave (Fig. 5.15).

Fig. 5.15 - AC Electricity

Note that the maximum voltages (V) are not the same as $V_{eff}$
(effective voltage, or root-mean square voltage).  Similarly, the

399

maximum current is not the effective (root—mean square) current delivered ($I_{eff}$). These relations are,

$$V_{eff} = 0.707 \, V_{max}$$
$$I_{eff} = 0.707 \, I_{max}.$$

One effective volt of AC will develop one effective ampere of current through a resistance of one ohm. The frequency of alternation of the cycle is also important in determining the V and I values. A typical frequency is 60 cycles/second.

## 5.9.2 QUESTION TO REVIEW AC CIRCUITS

(1) In an AC circuit, the effective value of the current is

(a) equal to the maximum value of the AC current;
(b) greater than the maximum value of DC current;
(c) less than the maximum value of AC current;
(d) greater than the maximum value of DC current.

## 5.9.3 ANSWERS TO QUESTIONS IN SECTION 5.9.2

( 1)  c

## 5.9.4 DISCUSSION OF ANSWER TO QUESTION IN SECTION 5.9.2

QUESTION #1:  Adequately discussed in Section.

## 5.9.5 VOCABULARY, CONCEPTS, ETC. CHECKLIST FOR AC CIRCUITS

____ AC circuits
____ AC electricity
____ root mean-square current

5.10.1    REVIEW OF GENERAL WAVE CHARACTERISTICS

A wave is a disturbance in a medium such that each particle in the medium vibrates about an equilibrium point in a simple harmonic motion (below). If the direction of vibration is perpendicular to the direction of propagation of the wave, the wave is called a transverse wave (e.g., light). If the direction of vibration is in the same direction as propagation of the wave, the wave is called a longitudinal wave (e.g., sound). Longitudinal waves are characterized by condensations (regions of crowding of particles) and rarefactions (regions where particles are far apart) along the wave in the medium (Fig. 5.17).

**Fig. 5.16 - Transverse and Longitudinal Waves**

The wavelength ($\lambda$) is the distance from crest to crest (or valley to valley) of a transverse wave. It may also be defined as the distance between two particles with the same displacement and direction of displacement. In a longitudinal wave, the wavelength can be taken as the distance from one rarefaction (or condensation) to another. The amplitude (A) is the maximum displacement of a particle in one direction from its equilibrium point. Frequency (f) is the number of wavelengths (cycles) that pass a point per unit time. Period (T) is the time required for one wavelength to pass a point. Speed (v) of a wave refers to its propagation through the medium. Speed increases as the inertia of the medium decreases (e.g., as density decreases). Phase ($\phi$) is the difference in displacement and direction of a particle due to two different waves. Two waves are in phase if each particle has the same displacement and direction of motion ($\phi = 0$) (Fig. 5.18):

$$V = \lambda f = \lambda/T \qquad (f=1/T)$$
$2\pi$ corresponds to one $\lambda$
$\pi$ corresponds to one-half $\lambda$.

**Fig. 5.17 – Some Characteristics of Waves**

The superposition principle states that the effect of two or more waves on the displacement of a particle are independent. This means the displacement of a particle by simultaneous waves in a medium are algebraically additive. Interference is the summation of the displacements of different waves in a medium. Constructive interference is when the waves add to a larger resultant wave than either original. This occurs maximally when the phase difference ($\phi$) is a whole wavelength ($\lambda$) which corresponds to multiples of 360° ($2\pi$). So, this occurs at $\phi = 0$, $2\pi$, $4\pi$, etc. Since $0 = 2\pi \Delta L/\lambda$, where $\Delta L$ equals the difference in path to a point of two waves (of equal wavelength), these waves interfere constructively when $\Delta L = 0$, $\lambda$, $2\lambda$, $3\lambda$, etc. Destructive interference is when the waves add to a smaller resultant wave than either original wave. This occurs maximally when $\phi = \pi$, $3\pi$, $5\pi$, etc., which are multiples of one-half wavelengths (180° = $\pi$ corresponds to 1/2 $\lambda$). This occurs when $\Delta L = \lambda/2$, $3\lambda/2$, $5\lambda/2$, etc. (Figs. 5.19, 5.20, 5.21.)

( $\Delta L = 0$, $\lambda$, $2\lambda$, etc.)

Waves (1) and (2) begin at the points shown, have the same $\lambda$ but different A's.
The summation wave is maximal since $\Delta L = \lambda$ in this example.

**Fig. 5.18 – Maximal Constructive Interference**

( $\Delta L = \lambda/2$, $3\lambda/2$, $5\lambda/2$, etc.)

Waves (1) and (2) begin as shown, have the same $\lambda$ and the same A's.
The summation wave is the horizontal line (or the minimum) since $\Delta L = \lambda/2$ in this example.

**Fig. 5.19 – Maximal Destructive Interference**

$L_1$, $L_2$ are distances from origins of waves to point A
$\Delta L = \left| L_2 - L_1 \right|$ (absolute value).

**Fig. 5.20 – Schematic for $\Delta L$**

402

Standing waves result when waves are reflected off a stationary object back into the oncoming waves of the medium, and superimposition (see above) results. Nodes are points where there is no particle displacement, which are similar to points of maximal destructive interference (above). Nodes occur at fixed end points (points that cannot vibrate). Antinodes are points that undergo maximal displacements and are similar to points of maximal constructive interference. Antinodes occur at open or free end points (Fig. 5.22).

closed end — open end

(a) = antinodes
(n) = nodes

PIPE

STRING - fixed at both ends

**Fig. 5.21 – Standing Waves**

The particles that are undergoing displacement when a wave passes through a medium undergo motion called simple harmonic motion (SHM) and are acted upon by a force described by Hooke's Law. SHM is caused by an inconstant force (called a restoring force) and as a result has an inconstant acceleration. The force is proportional to the displacement (distance from the equilibrium point) but opposite in direction (Figure 5.23),

$$F = -kx$$
$$k = \text{constant}$$

Hooke's Law
x = displacement from equililbrium

maximal
displacement = A

particle

equilibrium point

**Fig. 5.22 – Simple Harmonic Motion**

Features of SHM and Hooke's Law are:

(1) Force and acceleration are always in the same direction.
(2) Force and acceleration are always in the opposite direction of the displacement.
(3) Force and acceleration have their maximal values at +A and −A; they are zero at the equilibrium point.
(4) Velocity direction has no constant relation to displacement or acceleration.
(5) Velocity is maximum at equilibrium and zero at A and −A.

The electromagnetic spectrum has the sequence below from long wavelength ( $\lambda$ ) and low frequency (f) to short wavelength and high frequency. Many regions overlap,

Long $\lambda$                                                                 Short $\lambda$

Radiowaves/Microwaves/Infrared/Visible/Ultraviolet/x-rays/gamma rays

Low f                                                                          High f

The visible light is broken down into colors remembered by the mnemonic, ROY G. BIV:

Red, Orange, Yellow, Green, Blue, Indigo, Violet

Planck developed the relation between energy (E) and the frequency ($\nu$) of electromagnetic radiation,

$$E = h\nu$$
$$h = \text{Planck's Constant}$$

Since, $\nu \propto 1/\lambda$, then, $E \propto 1/\lambda$. That is, high frequencies but short wavelengths correspond to high energy and vice versa. See Section 5.11.1 for resonance and beats.

### 5.10.2 QUESTIONS TO REVIEW GENERAL WAVE CHARACTERISTICS

(1) If the direction of vibration of particles of a medium is in the direction of propagation of a wave, the wave is called:

(a) longitudinal        (b) transverse
(c) both                (d) neither

(2) Condensations and rarefactions would be found in

(a) light waves         (b) electromagnetic radiation
(c) transverse waves    (d) longitudinal waves

(3) "The effect of two or more waves on the displacement of a particle are independent" is a statement of:

(a) Interference Principle      (b) Huyghens Principle
(c) Correspondence Principle    (d) Superposition Principle

(4) At the node of a wave:

(a) the displacement is maximal
(b) there is no displacement
(c) there may be an open or a free point
(d) both (a) and (c)

(5) Select the incorrect relationship between the energy (E) of a wave and the parameters given:
(f = frequency, $\lambda$ = wavelength, A = amplitude)

(a) $E \propto f$        (b) $E \propto A^2$
(c) $E \propto 1/\lambda$    (d) all are correct

(6) The restoring force that causes an object to undergo simple harmonic motion is

(a) a constant force;
(b) inversely proportional to the displacement (from equilibrium) and in the same direction;
(c) directly proportional to the displacement but opposite in direction;
(d) both (a) and (b).

(7)  All of the following are true about simple harmonic motion **except:**

(a) Force and acceleration have their maximum values at the equilibrium point.
(b) Force and acceleration are always in the same direction.
(c) Velocity direction has no constant relation to displacement or acceleration.
(d) Velocity is maximal at the equilibrium point.

(8)  Which of the following colors of visible light has the shortest wavelength?

(a) green     (b) blue     (c) yellow     (d) red

(9)  Which of the following colors of visible light has the longest wavelength?

(a) yellow     (b) orange     (c) blue     (d) green

(10)  If f = frequency and $\lambda$ = wavelength of light, then the speed of light (c) is:

(a) $c = 1/f$                    (b) $c = \lambda/f$
(c) $c = f/\lambda$              (d) $c = f\lambda$

(11)  The relation, $E = h\nu$ , was put forth by

(a) Planck                       (b) Einstein
(c) Newton                       (d) Maxwell

(12)  Constructive interference occurs when:

(a) phase differences are 0, $2\pi$ , $4\pi$ , etc.
(b) path differences are 0, $\lambda$ , $2\lambda$ , $3\lambda$, etc.
(c) neither
(d) both

(13)  If the frequency of a wave is 10,000 hertz and it is travelling at 5000 m/sec, then its wavelength is:

(a) 5 m                          (b) 2m
(c) 0.5 m                        (d) 0.2 m

(14)  The speed of light (c) is $3.0 \times 10^{10}$ cm/sec.  If the wavelength ( $\lambda$) of red-light is approximately 400 nm (nm = $10^{-9}$m), then the frequency (f) of red-light is:

(a) $7.5 \times 10^{12}$/sec            (b) $7.5 \times 10^{14}$/sec
(c) $1.2 \times 10^{4}$/sec             (d) $1.2 \times 10^{6}$/sec

(15)  Electromagnetic radiation (e.g., light) with frequency (f) of 50,000 hertz (hertz = 1 cycle/sec) would have a wavelength ( $\lambda$ ) of:

(a) 1/50,000 cms                 (b) $6.0 \times 10^{-5}$ cms
(c) $6.0 \times 10^{5}$ cms             (d) cannot be determined

(16) In a vibrating column of air

    (a) open ends can only have nodes;
    (b) nodes can occur at open or closed ends;
    (c) open ends can only have antinodes;
    (d) antinodes may occur at closed ends.

**Use the following data for Questions #18 through #23**

The particle of mass = 2 kg below is moving about the fixed point 0 as shown. Given are some values of the force on the particle at different values of displacement (X) from 0. The maximal displacement from 0 in any one direction is $\pm$A and A = 5 m.

| X (meters) | +3 | +1 | -2 | -4 |
|------------|------|------|------|------|
| F (newtons) | -0.6 | -0.2 | +0.4 | +0.8 |

(17) This type of motion is called:

    (a) uniform linear motion     (b) simple harmonic motion
    (c) projectile motion     (d) free fall motion

(18) The force is described by:

    (a) Faraday's Law     (b) Newton's First Law
    (c) Hooke's Law     (d) none of the above

(19) If the above motion and force follow Hooke's Law, the value of k (neglect the units) is:

    (a) 0.1     (b) 0.2     (c) 0.5     (d) 1.0

(20) The value of F at A = -5m is:

    (a) 0.2 nts     (b) 0.5 nts
    (c) 1.0 nts     (d) 5 nts

(21) The force has a value of zero at x = ?

    (a) 0 m     (b) +5 m     (c) -5 m     (d) $\pm$2m

(22) At x = -2 m, the acceleration (a) is (in m/sec$^2$):

    (a) 4.0     (b) 2.0     (c) 1.0     (d) 0.2

(23) A standing wave is established in a string fixed at both ends between two points 1m apart. Which of the following is not a possible wavelength of waves for this system?

    (a) 4 m     (b) 2 m     (c) 1.0 m     (d) 0.5 m

(24) A standing wave is established in a pipe which is open at one end and is 2m long. All of the following are possible wavelengths of waves for this system except:

    (a) 8 m     (b) 6 m
    (c) 2 2/3 m     (d) all are possible

( 1)  a  ( 2)  d  ( 3)  d  ( 4)  b  ( 5)  d  ( 6)  c  ( 7)  a
( 8)  b  ( 9)  b  (10)  d  (11)  a  (12)  d  (13)  c  (14)  b
(15)  c  (16)  c  (17)  b  (18)  c  (19)  b  (20)  c  (21)  a
(22)  d  (23)  a  (24)  b


## 5.10.4    DISCUSSION OF ANSWERS TO QUESTIONS IN SECTION 5.10.2

QUESTIONS #1 to #11, #16:  Adequately discussed in the text.

QUESTION #12  (Answer:  d)  It takes one whole cycle ($2\pi = 360^\circ$) for a sine wave to completely repeat itself.  So, for two waves to add constructively at every point, their phase must differ by multiples of $2\pi$, i.e.,

$$2n\pi \text{ where } n = 0,1,2,3, \text{ etc.}$$

The phase difference ($\phi$) for any given path difference to a given point is $\phi = 2\pi(\Delta L/\lambda)$ for a given wave with wavelength = $\lambda$. This is reasoned from the graph below:

W$_1$ and W$_2$ are two waves out of phase
L$_1$, L$_2$ are distances from O (origin).
the phase difference is $\phi$
the path difference is $\Delta L$
the following ratio holds because the corresponding distances
   are equal in the diagram above:

part/whole = $\phi/2\pi = \Delta L/\lambda$
then:   $\phi = 2\pi(\Delta L/\lambda)$

For constructive interference:

$\phi = 2n\pi = 2\pi(\Delta L/\lambda)$
$n = \Delta L/\lambda$
$\Delta L = n\lambda$  where n = 0,1,2,3 etc.

QUESTION #13  (Answer:  c)

$v = \lambda f$
$\lambda = v/f = 5,000/10,000 = 0.5$ m

QUESTION #14  (Answer:  b)

$c = f\lambda$
$f = c/\lambda = (3.00 \times 10^{10} \text{cm/sec})/4 \times 10^{-5} \text{cm} = 0.75 \times 10^{15}/\text{sec} = 7.5 \times 10^{14}/\text{sec}$
   ($\lambda = 400 \times 10^{-9} = 4.0 \times 10^{-7}\text{m} = 4 \times 10^{-5}\text{cm}$)

QUESTION #15   (Answer:  c)

$c = f \lambda = 3.00 \times 10^{10}$ cm/sec
$f = 50{,}000$/sec $= 5.0 \times 10^{14}$/sec
$\lambda = c/f = 3.00 \times 10^{10}/5.0 \times 10^4 = 0.60 \times 10^6$ cms
$\lambda = 6.0 \times 10^5$ cms.

QUESTION #17   (Answer:  b)  The particle is oscillating about a fixed point (0) which is called simple harmonic motion.

QUESTION #18   (Answer:  c)  The force is a restoring force and the motion is SHM.  This is described in Hooke's Law as F = -kx.

QUESTION #19   (Answer:  b)  The motion follows Hooke's Law: F = -kx.

So, to find the k, any set of F and x may be substituted in the equation:

$k = -(F/x) = -(-0.6$ nts$/+3$m $= +0.2$ nt/m
$k = -(F/x) = -(-0.2$ nts$/+1$m$) = +0.2$ nt/m
etc.

QUESTION #20   (Answer:  c)  Use the data from #20:
$$F = -kx$$
$$F = -(0.2)(-5) = +1.0 \text{ nts}$$
Note at +A, the F has its maximal value.

QUESTION #21   (Answer:  a)      F = -kx = 0
                                   -kx = 0
                                     x = 0 because k is not equal
                                            to zero.

QUESTION #22   (Answer:  d)  Can use F = +0.4 nts from chart at x = -2,
                        OR:  F = -kx from Hooke's Law
                             F = ma from Newton's 2nd Law (Section
                                  5.3.1)
                             ma = -kx
                             $a = -kx/m = -(0.2)(-2)/2 = +0.2$m/sec$^2$.

QUESTION #23   (Answer:  a)  If the string is fixed at both ends, then only nodes can occur at these points.  Then the smallest part of a wave that can exist between these points is 1/2 $\lambda$ which then equals 1 m:

Then the $\lambda$ of the above situation is 2 m as shown.  This is the maximal allowed $\lambda$ for this set-up.  Other $\lambda$ s are possible as follows:

the next node after ½ $\lambda$ is  2 $\lambda$ away and the next node after that is  another ½ $\lambda$ away.  These then are n(½ $\lambda$) where n = 0,1,2,3 etc., are the possible ½ $\lambda$'s that can fit into the distance ( $\ell$ = 1m)
then:  n(½ $\lambda$)  = 1m = $\ell$
           n$\lambda$/2 = $\ell$
              $\lambda$ = 2 $\ell$/n = allowable $\lambda$'s
Then, the 1.0m and 0.5m are allowable $\lambda$'s:
   n = 2 $\ell$/$\lambda$ = (2)(1)/0.5 = 4 for $\lambda$ = 0.5m
   n = 2 $\ell$/$\lambda$ = (2)(1)/1  = 2 for $\lambda$ = 1.0m

Also, the $\lambda = 4m$ is not allowable because it does not give a value
of n that is a whole number:

$n = 2\ell/\lambda = (2)(1)/4 = 0.5$ which is not acceptable.

Note that the allowable frequencies (f) are:

$f = v/\lambda = v/(2\ell/n) = nv/2\ell$

$v$ = velocity of wave proportion.

QUESTION #24   (Answer:  b)   At the closed end of the pipe there must
be a node and at the open end there must be an antinode.   The
shortest fraction of a wave that has a node and antinode in sequence
is $1/4\,\lambda$ which must equal the 2m:

$\frac{1}{4}\,\lambda = 2m$

$\lambda = 8m$ as the longest possible allowable $\lambda$ .   The next
antinode occurs $\frac{1}{2}\,\lambda$ beyond $\frac{1}{4}\,\lambda$ and then the next is $\frac{1}{2}\,\lambda$ beyond
that, etc.  (Only worry about next antinode because these go at
the open end of the pipe.)   The sequence of possible fractions
of $\lambda$'s for this system is:

$1/4\,\lambda$
$1/4\,\lambda + 1/2\,\lambda = 3/4\,\lambda$
$3/4\,\lambda + 1/2\,\lambda = 5/4\,\lambda$
$5/4\,\lambda + 1/2\,\lambda = 7/4\,\lambda$ etc.

or to generalize this:  $n\lambda/4$ where n = 1,3,5,7,9 etc.
(note that only the odd numbers are possible.)

Then each of these fractional $\lambda$ s must fit into the $2m = \ell$ :

$n\lambda/4 = 2m = \ell$
$n\lambda/4 = \ell$
$\lambda = 4\ell/n$   n = 1,3,5,7 etc.

Then any $\lambda$ is possible as long as it gives n = 1,3,5,7, etc., when
substituted in the above equation:

$n = 4\ell/\lambda$

for $\lambda = 8m$: $n = (4)(2)/8 = 1$   $\therefore$ possible
for $\lambda = 6m$: $n = (4)(2)/6 = 4/3$   $\therefore$ not possible
for $\lambda = 8/3\,m$: $n = (4)(2)/(8/3) = 8 \cdot 3/8 = 3$ $\therefore$ possible
Note that the frequencies (f) in this case are

$f = v/\lambda = v/(4\ell/n) = vn/4\ell$   n = 1,3,5

$v$ = velocity of wave propagation.

5.10.5        VOCABULARY, CONCEPTS, ETC. CHECKLIST FOR GENERAL WAVE
              CHARACTERISTICS

____  simple harmonic motion          ____  phase
____  constructive interference       ____  period
____  destructive interference        ____  Hooke's Law

_____ frequency          _____ wavelength
_____ velocity           _____ standing waves
_____ amplitude          _____ nodes
_____ transverse waves   _____ antinodes
_____ longitudinal waves _____ radiowaves
_____ superposition of waves _____ microwaves
_____ electromagnetic radiation _____ infrared
_____ energy of waves    _____ visible
_____ gamma rays         _____ ultraviolet
_____ ROY G. BIV         _____ x-rays
                         _____ E = hv


**5.11      Sound**


**5.11.1      REVIEW OF SOUND**


Sound is a longitudinal (Section 5.10.1) mechanical wave which travels through an elastic medium. Sound is thus produced by vibrating matter. There is no sound in a vacuum (because there is no matter). Compressions (condensations) are regions where particles (of matter) are close together and are high pressure regions. Rarefactions are regions where particles are sparse and are low pressure regions of sound waves.

The speed (v) of sound is proportional to the square root of the elastic restoring force and inversely proportional to the square root of the inertia of the particles (e.g., density, $\rho$, is a measure of inertia),

$$v \propto \sqrt{F}$$
$$v \propto 1/\sqrt{\text{inertia}}.$$

The speed in various substances is as follows (See Section 5.6.1):
      wire or rod:           $v = \sqrt{Y/\rho}$      Y = Young's modulus
      fluid (gas or liquid)  $v = \sqrt{B/\rho}$      B = Bulk modulus.
The speed of sound also increases with temperature.

Forced vibrations occur when a series of waves impinge upon an object and cause it to vibrate. Natural frequencies are the intrinsic frequencies of vibration of a system. If the forced vibration causes the object to vibrate at one of its natural frequencies, the body will vibrate at maximal amplitude. This situation is called resonance. Note also that energy and power are proportional to the amplitude squared, so these two are also at a maximum.

Hearing is subjective but its characteristics are closely tied to the physical characteristics of sound. These relations are:

      SENSORY: loudness        PHYSICAL: intensity (I)
               pitch                     frequency (f)
               quality                   waveforms.

The quality depends on the number and the relative intensity of the overtones of the waveforms. Frequency, and, therefore, pitch, are perceived by the ear from 20 to 20,000 Hz (Hertz = cycles/second). Frequencies below 20 Hz are called infrasonic. Frequencies above 20,000 Hz are called ultrasonic. Sound intensity (I) is the rate of

410

energy (power) propagation through space:

$$I = \text{Power/area} \propto f^2A^2$$
$$f = \text{frequency and } A = \text{amplitude.}$$

The loudness varies with the frequency. The ears are most sensitive (hear sounds of lowest intensity) at approximately 2,000 to 4,000 Hz. $I_o$ is taken to be 10-12 watts/cm$^2$, is barely audible and is assigned a value of 0(zero) dB(decibels).

Then the intensity level(I) of a sound wave in dB is,

$$db = 10 \log (I/I_o)$$
$$I = \text{intensity at a given level}$$
$$I_o = \text{threshold intensity.}$$

Examples of some values of db's are: whisper (20), normal conversation (60), subway car (100), pain threshhold (120) and jet engine (160). Continual exposure to sounds greater than 90 db can lead to hearing impairment.

When sounds of different frequencies are heard together, they interfere (Section 5.10.1). Constructive interference results in beats. The number of beats per second is the absolute value of the difference of the frequencies ( $|f_1-f_2|$ ). Hence, the new frequencies heard include the original frequencies and the absolute differences between them.

The Doppler effect is the effect upon the observed frequency caused by the relative motion of the observer (o) and the source (s). If the distance is decreasing between them, there is a shift to higher frequencies and shorter wavelengths, (to higher pitch for sound and toward the blue-violet for light). If the distance is increasing between them, there is a shift to longer wavelengths and lower frequencies (to lower pitch for sound and toward red for light). The summary equation of the above in terms of frequency (f) is:

$$fo/(V \pm v_o) = fs/(V \pm v_s)$$
$$fo = fs (V \pm v_o)/(V \pm v_s)$$
$$V = \text{speed of wave}$$
$$v = \text{speed of observer (o) or source (s).}$$

Choose the + or - such that the frequency varies as you would predict. If the o or s is moving toward the other the f should increase and vice versa. Predict the results and select the sign for the s and o independently of the motion of the other.

5.11.2      QUESTIONS TO REVIEW SOUND

(1)   Sound waves:

    (a) are transverse waves
    (b) are produced by vibrating matter
    (c) may be transmitted in a vacuum
    (d) all of the above

411

(2)  The speed of sound is:

(a) proportional to the square root of the elastic restoring force of the medium
(b) inversely proportional to the square root of the inertia of the particles of the media
(c) neither
(d) both

(3)  The speed of sound is _____ by an increase of temperature.

(a) decreased    (b) increased    (c) does not change

(4)  When an object is forced to vibrate at one of its natural frequencies of vibration,

(a) resonance exists;
(b) energy is a minimum;
(c) work is a minimum;
(d) the amplitude of vibration is a minimum.

(5)  Which sensory (as interpreted by the brain) aspect of sound is incorrectly paired with its physical correlate of sound?

(a) loudness-intensity
(b) pitch-frequency
(c) quality-waveforms
(d) all are correctly paired

(6)  A human with normal hearing probably could not hear sound at:

(a) 100,000 hz                    (b) 20,000 hz
(c) 5,000 hz                      (d) 20 hz

(7)  The intensity (pressure per unit area) of a sound is

(a) inversely proportional to the square of the frequency;
(b) directly proportional to the square of the frequency;
(c) inversely proportional to the frequency;
(d) directly proportional to the frequency.

(8)  Decibels are used in describing:

(a) light                         (b) sound
(c) electricity                   (d) magnetism

(9)  The effect upon the frequency of sound observed when the source of the sound is moving relative to the observer is explained by the:

(a) Doppler Effect                (b) Compton Effect
(c) Theory of Relativity          (d) none of the above

(10)  If the density of a gas is quadrupled (x4), the speed (v) of sound through it is:

(a) decreased by a factor of ½
(b) increased by a factor of 2
(c) increased by a factor of 4
(d) not changed

412

(11) If the elasticity (restoring force) of medium #1 is four times the elasticity of medium #2, then sound will travel

(a) twice as fast in #1 as in #2;
(b) twice as fast in #2 as in #1;
(c) four times as fast in #1 as in #2;
(d) four times as fast in #2 as in #1.

(12) If the tension (F) in a string is increased by a factor of 4, the speed (v) of a wave in that string will be:

(a) quadrupled (x4)
(b) doubled
(c) reduced by 1/2
(d) reduced to 1/4 the original

(13) Three notes of 128, 256, and 512 are sounded; the frequencies heard are:

(a) 128, 256, 384, 512, 640, 768
(b) 512, 640, 768
(c) 128, 256, 384, 512
(d) 128, 256, 512

(14) A sound has an intensity 100 times that of the standard intensity. How many decibels is it?

(a) 10     (b) 20     (c) 50     (d) 100

(15) If a source which is emitting sound is moving toward an observer, the frequency of sound heard by the observer is _____ the frequency emitted by the source.

(a) the same as     (b) less than     (c) greater than

(16) If a source which is emitting light is moving away from an observer, the wavelength of light seen by the observer is _____ the wavelength emitted by the source.

(a) the same as     (b) shorter than     (c) longer than

(17) An observer is moving toward a source at 170 m/sec. The source is moving toward the observer at 130 m/sec and is emitting sound at a frequency of 10,000 hertz. The frequency of sound heard by the observer (assume speed of sound is 330 m/sec) is:

$$f_o = f_s \frac{(v \pm v_o)}{(v \mp v_s)}$$

(a) 15,000 hertz                    (b) 7,500 hertz
(c) 25,000 hertz                    (d) 5,000 hertz

5.11.3     ANSWERS TO QUESTIONS IN SECTION 5.11.2

( 1) b   (2) d   (3) b   (4) a   (5) d   (6) a   (7) b
( 8) b   (9) a   (10) a   (11) a   (12) b   (13) c   (14) b
(15) c   (16) c   (17) c

QUESTIONS #1 to #9:  Adequately discussed in Section.

QUESTION #10   (Answer:  a)

$$v \propto 1/\sqrt{\rho} \qquad\qquad \rho = \text{density}$$

$$\frac{v_2}{v_1} = \frac{1/\sqrt{\rho_2}}{1/\sqrt{\rho_1}} = \frac{1}{\sqrt{\rho_2}} \cdot \frac{\sqrt{\rho_1}}{1} = \frac{\sqrt{\rho_1}}{\sqrt{\rho_2}} = \sqrt{\frac{\rho_1}{\rho_2}} = \sqrt{\frac{\rho_1}{4\rho_1}} = \sqrt{\frac{1}{4}} = \frac{1}{2}$$

$$\frac{v_2}{v_1} = \frac{1}{2}$$

$$v_2 = \frac{1}{2} v_1. \qquad\qquad\qquad \rho_2 = 4\rho_1$$

QUESTION #11   (Answer:  a)

Speed of sound (v) $\propto \sqrt{\text{restoring force}} = F$

$$\frac{v_2}{v_1} = \frac{\sqrt{F_2}}{\sqrt{F_1}} = \sqrt{\frac{F_2}{F_1}} = \sqrt{\frac{F_2}{4F_2}} = \sqrt{\frac{1}{4}} = \frac{1}{2}$$

$$\frac{v_2}{v_1} = \frac{1}{2} \qquad\qquad F_1 = 4F_2$$

$$2v_2 = v_1$$

QUESTION #12   (Answer:  b)

$$v \propto \sqrt{F}$$
$$F_2 = 4F_1$$
$$v_2/v_1 = \sqrt{F_2}/\sqrt{F_1} = \sqrt{F_2/F_1} = \sqrt{4F_1/F_1} = \sqrt{4} = 2$$
$$v_2 = 2v_1$$

QUESTION #13   (Answer:  c)  The frequencies heard are the original frequencies plus all new frequencies resulting from the differences of the original frequencies:

512-128 = 384   (This is the only new frequency.)

QUESTION #14   (Answer:  b)   $db = 10 \log I/I_O = 10 \log(100/1)$
$= 10 \log 100 = 10(2) = 20$
$(\log 100 = 2).$

QUESTION #15   (Answer:  c)  As the observer and source move together the observed frequency increases.

QUESTION #16   (Answer:  c)  If the distance between observer and source is increasing, the wavelength observed increases as the frequency decreases.

QUESTION #17   (Answer:  c)  Use Doppler's relation as given in the Section:

$$f_O = f_S (V \pm v_O)/(V \pm v_S).$$

since the source (s) is moving toward the observer (o), this tends to increase the $f_O$ over the $f_S$; for the $f_O > f_S$ must use $V - v_S$ because as the denominator decreases the fraction increases and this makes $f_O > f_S$

since the o is moving toward the s, this tends to increase the $f_O$ over the $f_S$; for the $f_O > f_S$ need $V + v_O$ because as the numerator increases the fraction increases and this makes $f_O > f_S$.

Then:

$$f_O = f_S(V + v_O)/(V - v_S) \text{ for this problem}$$
$$f_O = (10,000)(330 + 170)/(330 - 130) = (10,000)(500/200) =$$
$$f_O = (10,000)(5/2) = 25,000 \text{ hertz.}$$

## 5.11.5    VOCABULARY, CONCEPTS, ETC. CHECKLIST FOR SOUND

____ production of sound          ____ pitch
____ intensity                    ____ decibel scale
____ speed of sound               ____ resonance
____ beats                        ____ Doppler effect
____ loudness

## 5.12    Optics

## 5.12.1    REVIEW OF OPTICS

## 5.12.1.1    Reflection

Reflection is the process by which light rays (imaginary lines drawn perpendicular to advancing wave fronts) bounce back into a medium from a surface with another medium (versus being refracted or absorbed). The Laws of Reflection are: (1) The angle of incidence (I) equals the angle of reflection (R) at the normal (N, perpendicular to surface), and (2) the I, R, N all lie on the same plane.

Mirrors may have a plane surface or a nonplane surface; only spherical nonplane mirrors will be discussed. For a plane mirror, all incident light is reflected in parallel off it and therefore all images seen are virtual, erect, left-right reversed and appear to be just as far (perpendicular distance) behind the mirror as the object is in front of the mirror. A virtual image has no light rays passing through it and cannot be projected upon a screen. A real image has light rays passing through it and can be projected upon a screen.

Spherical mirrors may have the reflecting surface convex (diverges light) or concave (converges light). Note the images formed by a converging mirror (concave) are like those for a converging lens (convex); and diverging mirrors (convex) and diverging lens (concave) also form similar images. The terminology for spherical mirrors (see Fig. 5.24) is:

```
R = radius of curvature
C = center of curvature
F = focal point
V = vertex (center of mirror itself)
axis = line through C and V
f = focal length (distance from F to V)
i = image distance (distance from V to object along axis)
o = object distance (distance from V to object along axis)
AB = linear aperature (chord connecting ends of mirror, larger
     aperature means better resolution).
```

CONCAVE (CONVERGING)          CONVEX (DIVERGING)

**Fig. 5.23 - Reflection by Spherical Mirrors**

With <u>concave mirrors (spherical)</u> the incident light is converged
(toward the axis). The path of light rays is as follows:

(1) incident rays parallel to the axis reflect through F;
(2) incident rays along a radius (of curvature) reflect back
    on themselves (rays through C);
(3) incident rays through F reflect parallel to the axis.

The image formed by an object depends on the position of the image
relative to the F and C (or f and R). General rules for image
formation are:

(1) if $o < f$, then image is virtual and erect;
    if $o > f$, then image is real and inverted;
(2) if $o = f$, then no image if formed;
(3) if $o < R$, then image is enlarged in size;
    if $o > R$, then image is reduced in size;
    if $o = R$, then image is same size.

These relations are similar to those for a converging lens (convex).

With <u>convex (spherical) mirrors,</u> the incident light is diverged
(from the axis) after reflection. It is the backward extension
(dotted lines above) that may pass through the F. The path of light
rays are as follows:

(1) incident rays parallel to the axis have backward extension
    of their reflections through F (see above);
(2) incident rays along a radius (that would pass through C if
    extended) reflect back along themselves;
(3) incident rays that pass through F (if extended) reflect
    parallel to the axis.

The image formed for a convex mirror is always virtual, erect and
smaller than the object.

416

The mirror equation and derivations from it allow the above relations between object and image to be calculated instead of memorized. The equation is valid for convex and concave mirrors:

$$1/i + 1/o = 1/f$$
$$f = R/2$$
$$M = \text{magnification} = -i/o$$

conventions:      for i and o, positive values mean real, negative values mean virtual,

for R and f, positive means converging, negative is diverging,

for M, positive means erect, negative is inverted.


## 5.12.1.2    Refraction


Refraction is the bending of light as it passes from one transparent medium to another and is caused by the different speeds of light in the two media. If $\theta_1$ is taken as the angle (to the normal) of the incident light and $\theta_2$ is the angle (to the normal) of refracted light, where 1 and 2 represent the different media, the following relations hold (Snell's Law) (Fig. 5.25):

$$\frac{\sin\theta_1}{\sin\theta_2} = \frac{v_1}{v_2} = \frac{n_2}{n_1} = \frac{\lambda_1}{\lambda_2}$$

v=velocity   $\lambda$=wavelength

n=index of refraction=

$$\frac{\text{speed in free space}}{\text{speed in medium}} = \frac{C}{V}$$

(C=$3\times10^{10}$cm/sec or 181,000 mi/sec)

n=1.0 for air  n=1.33 for $H_2O$
n=1.5 for glass  (at $\lambda$=589 nm)

**Fig. 5.24 – Refraction**

Note that the $\theta$ is smaller (closer to the normal) in the more optically dense (higher n) medium. Also the smaller the wavelength of the incident light (i.e., toward the violet end), the closer is $\theta_2$ to the normal (i.e., it is smaller than $\theta$). This means longer wavelengths travel faster in a medium than shorter wavelengths. This leads to dispersion which is the separation of white light (all colors together) into the individual colors by this differential refraction. For example, a prism disperses white light. The Laws of Refraction are:

(1) The incident ray, the refracted ray and the normal ray all lie in the same plane.
(2) The path of the ray (incident and refracted parts) is reversible.

When light passes from a more optically dense (higher n) medium into a less optically dense medium, there exists an angle of incidence such that the angle of refraction ($\theta_2$) is 90°. This special angle of incidence is called the critical angle ($\theta_c$). This is because when the angle of incidence is less than $\theta_c$ refraction occurs. If the angle of incidence is equal to $\theta_c$, then neither refraction nor reflection occur. And if $\theta_1 > \theta_c$, then <u>internal reflection</u> (ray is reflected back into the more dense medium) occurs. The $\theta_c$ is found from Snell's Law:

$$n_1 \sin \theta_c = n_2 \sin \theta_2$$

$$n_1 \sin \theta_c = n_2(1) \qquad \text{(Since } \theta_2 = 90° \text{ and } \sin 90° = 1)$$

$$\sin \theta_c = n_2/n_1$$

e.g., $\theta_c = 42°$ for glass.

When looking at an object under water from above the surface, the object appears closer than it actually is. This is due to refraction. In general:

apparent depth/actual depth $= n_2/n_1$

$n_2$ = medium of observer
$n_1$ = medium of object.

A <u>lens</u> is a transparent material which refracts light. Converging lenses refract light toward the axis, and diverging lenses refract the light way from the axis. A converging lens is wider at the middle than at the ends, and a diverging lens is thinner at the middle than at the ends (Fig. 5.26).

CONVERGING (CONVEX) LENS              DIVERGING (CONCAVE) LENS

R = radius of curvature
If the surface (note) is convex, the R is positive ($R_1$, e.g.).
If the surface is concave the R is negative ($R_2$, e.g.).
Subscript 1 refers to the incident side, subscript 2 refers
  to the refracted side.

C = center of curvature
F = focal point
V = optical center of the lens
axis = line through C and V
f = focal length is distance between V and F
i = image distance (from V to image)
o = object distance (from V to object).

**Fig. 5.25 - Lens**

418

The path of rays through a lens is:

(1) incident rays parallel to the axis refract through $F_2$ of a converging lens, and appear to come from $F_1$ of a diverging lens (backward extensions of the refracted ray, see dotted line on diverging diagram);
(2) an incident ray through $F_1$ of a converging lens or through $F_2$ of a diverging lens (if extended) are refracted parallel to the axis;
(3) incident rays through V are not deviated (refracted).

For a <u>converging lens</u> (biconvex, e.g.) the image formed depends on the object distance relative to the focal length (f). The relations (note similarity to a converging mirror) are:

(1) if $o < f_1$, the image is virtual and erect,
    if $o > f_1$, the image is real and inverted,
(2) if $o = f_1$, no image is formed,
(3) if $o < 2f_1$(R), image is enlarged in size,
    if $o > 2f_1$, image is reduced in size
    if $o = 2f_1$, image is the same size.

For a <u>diverging lens</u> (biconcave, e.g.), the image is always virtual, erect and reduced in size as for a diverging mirror.

The above relations can be calculated rather than memorized by the use of the <u>lens equation</u> (similar to the mirror equation) and derivations from it,

(1) $1/o + 1/i = 1/f$ (lens equation, same as mirror equation)
(2) $f = (n - 1)(1/R_1 + 1/R_2)$, (lens maker's equation)
(3) <u>dioptres</u> (D) = $1/f$ where f is in meters
    Measures the refractive power of the lens, the larger the dioptres (D) the stronger the lens. It has a +D for converging lens and a -D for diverging lens. To get the refractive power (D) of lenses in series just add the dioptres which can then be converted into focal length:

$$D_T = D_1 + D_2 = 1/f_T \qquad\qquad T = total$$

(4) Note that you cannot add focal lengths except as reciprocals:
$$1/f_T = 1/f_1 + 1/f_2.$$
(5) M = magnification = $-i/o$
    $M = M_1M_2$ for lens in series.

Conventions:

(1) for i and o, positive values are real, negative values are virtual,
(2) for R, see above,
(3) for f, positive means converging, negative is diverging,
(4) for M, positive means erect, negative is inverted.

The lens equation holds only for thin lenses--the thickness is small relative to other dimensions.

For a combination of lenses not in contact with each other, the image is found for the first lens (nearer the object) and then this image is used as the object of the second lens to find the image formed by it (see questions for examples).

(1)  Using the diagram below, select the <u>incorrect</u> statement of the Laws of Reflection of light from surfaces

$\longrightarrow$ = light ray

surface

(a)  $\theta_I = \theta_R$
(b)  $\theta_I + \theta_R = 90^\circ$
(c)  I, N and R all lie in the same plane
(d)  both (a) and (c)


(2)  All are true of images seen in plane (flat) mirrors <u>except</u>:

(a)  they are always virtual
(b)  they appear at a distance behind the mirror equal to the distance (perpendicular) of the object in front of the mirror
(c)  they are right-left reversed
(d)  they are inverted


(3)  A virtual image:

(a)  cannot be projected onto a screen
(b)  has light rays passing through it
(c)  cannot be formed by plane (flat) mirrors
(d)  all are correct

(4)  The reflected light rays from a smooth concave mirror:

(a)  converge                    (b)  diverge
(c)  are parallel                (d)  are diffuse


(5)  The reflected rays from a convex mirror:

(a)  diverge                     (b)  converge
(c)  are parallel                (d)  are diffuse


(6)  In terms of the reflected light and images, concave mirrors are most like:

(a)  triangular prisms           (b)  square prisms
(c)  concave lens                (d)  convex lens


(7)  In terms of reflected light and images, a convex mirror is most like a(n):

(a)  convex lens                 (b)  concave lens
(c)  triangular prism            (d)  square prism

(8) For the spherical convex mirror below:
($f_1 = f_2$; $R_1 = R_2$; f = focal length; R = radius of curvature)

mirror surface          ←——←—— incident light

$-\!-\!-\!•\!-\!-\!-\!•\!-\!-\!)\!-\!-\!-\!-\!-\!•\!-\!-\!-\!•\!-\!-\!-\!-\!-\!-\!-\!-\!-\!-\!-$ AXIS(A)
$R_2$   $f_2$           $f_1$   $R_1$

(a) incident rays parallel to A reflect through $f_1$
(b) incident rays passing through $R_1$ reflect through $R_2$
(c) the forward extensions of incident rays that reflect through $f_2$ pass through $f_1$
(d) the backward extensions of reflected rays that result from incident rays parallel to A pass through $f_2$

(9) For the spherical concave mirror below:
mirror surface

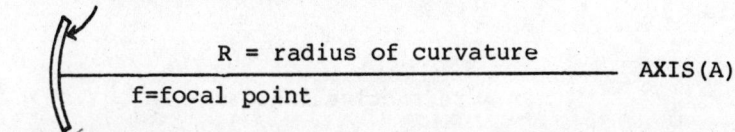

R = radius of curvature
———————————————————————— AXIS(A)
f=focal point

(a) incident rays parallel to A reflect through f
(b) incident rays passing through R reflect parallel to A
(c) incident rays through f reflect through R
(d) all of the above are correct

(10) For a convex mirror with f = focal length, R = radius of curvature, and o = object distance (along the axis) from the mirror, then

(a) images are always virtual, erect and reduced in size;
(b) if o > f, the image is virtual and inverted;
(c) if o = R, the image and object are the same size;
(d) if o > R, the image is larger than the object.

(11) For a concave mirror with f = focal length, R = radius of curvature and o = distance (along the axis) of the object from the mirror, then

(a) if o < f, then the image is real and inverted;
(b) if o = f, then no image is formed;
(c) if o > f, then the image is virtual and erect;
(d) if o > R, then the image is larger than the object.

(12) The mirror equation is:
(f = focal length, o = object distance, i = image distance)

(a) f = o + i                    (b) f = 1/o + 1/i
(c) 1/f = o + i                  (d) 1/f = 1/o + 1/i

(13) If f = focal length, R = radius of curvature of a spherical mirror, then:

(a) f = 2R                       (b) f = R/2
(c) $f = R^2$                    (d) $f = \sqrt{R}$

(14) If i = image distance and o = object distance from a mirror, then linear magnification (m) is:

(a) $m = -i/o$

(b) $m = (i)(o)$

(c) $m = -o/i$

(d) $m = 1/(i)(o)$

(15) The phenomenon of refraction ("bending" of light rays) is attributable to

(a) the particle character of light;

(b) the varying speeds of light in different media;

(c) the longitudinal wave character of light;

(d) none of the above.

(16) Given the diagram below for refraction of light, the correct relationship between the angles ( $\theta$ ) shown and the velocities (v) of light in the media is:

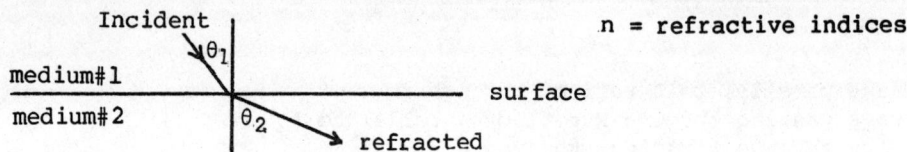

Incident    $\theta_1$                    n = refractive indices

medium#1 _____ surface

medium#2    $\theta_2$

refracted

(a) $n_2 \sin \theta_1 = n_1 \sin \theta_2$

(b) $n_1 v_1 = n_2 \theta_2$

(c) $\sin \theta_1 / \sin \theta_2 = n_2/n_1$

(d) $\theta_1 / \theta_2 = n_1/n_2$

(17) The index of refraction of a medium is

(a) the speed of light in free space divided by the speed of light in that medium;

(b) the density of the medium divided by the density of air;

(c) the absorption of light in the medium divided by the absorption of light in water;

(d) none of the above.

(18) Dispersion of white light into its component colors (as in a prism) occurs by the process of:

(a) diffraction

(b) polarization

(c) refraction

(d) reflection

(19) A critical angle of incidence ( $\theta_c$ )

(a) is reached when light passes from a lower optically dense medium into a higher optically dense medium;

(b) means that the angle of refraction is 90°;

(c) means that at all angles of incidence less than $\theta_c$, light is reflected;

(d) all of the above.

(20) A converging lens should be

(a) of equal width at the middle and ends;

(b) wider at the ends than at the middle;

(c) wider at the middle than at the ends;

(d) may be any of the above.

(21) A concave lens:

    (a) diverges light         (b) converges light
    (c) both                 (d) neither

(22) Select the correct statement concerning the lens below:
    V = vertex; F = focal point; C = center of curvature

Incident light

$C_1$    $F_1$    V    $F_2$    $C_2$      Axis

    (a) If the incident rays are parallel to the axis, the
        backward extensions of the refracted rays pass through $C_1$;
    (b) If the forward extension of an incident ray would pass
        through $F_2$, then the backward extension of the refracted
        ray would pass through $F_1$;
    (c) Incident rays through V are not refracted;
    (d) All of the above are correct.

(23) Select the correct statement concerning the lens below:
    F = focal points; C = center of curvature; V = vertex

$C_2$      V          $C_2$
       $F_1$        $F_2$      Axis

    (a) Incident rays parallel to the axis refract through $C_2$;
    (b) Incident rays through $F_1$ refract parallel to the axis;
    (c) Incident rays through V refract along the axis;
    (d) All of the above are correct.

(24) Concerning the image formed by a converging lens, select the
    <u>incorrect</u> statement:
    (f = focal length, o = object distance from lens)

    (a) If $o < f$, the image is virtual and erect;
    (b) If $o = f$, no image is formed;
    (c) If $o > f$, the image is real and inverted;
    (d) If $o < 2f$, the object is reduced in size.

(25) Select the correct statement concerning the image formed by a
    diverging lens:
    (f = focal length, o = object distance)

    (a) If $o > f$, the image is virtual and inverted;
    (b) If $o < 2f$, the image is real and reduced;
    (c) All images are virtual, erect and reduced;
    (d) All images are real, inverted and enlarged.

(26) Dioptres:

    (a) the number of degrees of visual acuity
    (b) a type of lens that corrects astigmatism
    (c) the refractive power of a lens
    (d) the reflective power of a mirror

(27) A concave mirror with a focal length (f) = 4 cms forms an image (i) of an object (o) placed 10 cms from it. The magnification (M) of this image is:

(a) 1/3 of the object      (b) 2/3 of the object
(c) 5/2 times the object      (d) 3 times the object

(28) An object (o) is place 10 cms from a concave mirror with focal length (f) = 2 cms. The image is:

(a) real, inverted, reduced and 2.50 cms from the mirror
(b) virtual, erect, enlarged and 8 cms from the mirror

(29) An image formed by a concave mirror is 5 cms from the mirror, erect and virtual. If the focal length of the mirror is 3 cms, the object is how far from the mirror?

(a) 5/3 cms          (b) 2 cms
(c) 10/7 cms        (d) 3/5 cms

(30) Optically dense media have high indices of refraction. From the diagram below, select the correct statement:

interface ———————— $n_1$

$n_1 > n_2$

$\theta_1$

$\theta_2$   $n_2$

(light ray)

$\frac{n_2}{n_1} = \frac{\sin \theta_1}{\sin \theta_2}$

(a) $\theta_1 < \theta_2$          (b) $\theta_1 = \theta_2$
(c) $\theta_1 > \theta_2$          (d) need more information

(31) The index of refraction (n) for water is 1.5. The speed of light in water is:

(a) $4.5 \times 10^{10}$ cm/sec
(b) $2 \times 10^{10}$ cm/sec
(c) $3 \times 10^{10}$ cm/sec
(d) need the frequency of light in water to determine the speed

(32) If violet light and red light both have the same angle of incidence, which statement is correct concerning the angles of refraction?

(a) the angles of refraction are equal
(b) the angle of refraction of the violet light is larger
(c) the angle of refraction of the red light is larger
(d) need velocities in the media to evaluate

(33) A ray of light passing from a type of glass into air has a critical angle ($\theta_c$) of:
(n = index of refraction, n of air = 1.00 and n of glass = 2.00)

(a) $5^\circ$      (b) $15^\circ$      (c) $30^\circ$      (d) $45^\circ$

(34) A fish is 8 meters from the surface in a tank of water. Looking from the air surface, the fish would appear to be how deep?
(n of air = 1.00, n of water = 1.33)

(a) 6 m
(c) 10.67 m

(b) 8 m
(d) need the angles of incidence and refraction

(35) An object is 15 cms from a converging lens with a focal length of 5 cms. The image formed is:

(a) no image is formed
(b) virtual, erect, reduced
(c) real, erect, enlarged
(d) real, inverted, reduced

(36) An object is placed 8 cms from a biconcave lens with a focal length of 10 cms. The image formed is:

(a) virtual, erect, reduced
(b) real, inverted, reduced
(c) real, erect, enlarged
(d) virtual, inverted, reduced

(37) An object is placed 5 cms from a diverging lens with a focal length of 10 cms. The image formed is:

(a) virtual, inverted, enlarged
(b) virtual, erect, reduced
(c) real, inverted, enlarged
(d) real, erect, reduced

(38) A 20 cm tall object is placed 5 cms from a convex lens with a focal length of 10 cms. The image is:

(a) real, erect, 2.5 cms from lens and 10 cms tall
(b) virtual, erect, 10 cms from lens and 40 cms tall
(c) real, inverted, 10 cms from lens and 40 cms tall
(d) virtual, inverted, 2.5 cms from lens and 10 cms tall

$$\frac{1}{i} + \frac{1}{o} = \frac{1}{f}$$

$$\frac{1}{i} + \frac{1}{5} = \frac{1}{10}$$

$$\frac{1}{i} = -\frac{1}{10}$$

$$i = -10$$

(39) An object 10 cms tall is placed 20 cms from a concave lens with a focal length of 5 cms. The image is:

(a) virtual, inverted, 40 cms from lens and 20 cms tall
(b) virtual, erect, 4 cms from lens and 4 cms tall
(c) real, inverted, 40 cms from lens, 20 cms tall
(d) real, erect, 4 cms from lens and 4 cms tall

$$\frac{1}{i} + \frac{1}{20} = \frac{-1}{5}$$

$$i = -4$$

(40) A lens with a focal length of 10 cms is how many dioptres?

(a) 0.10    (b) 1    (c) 10    (d) 100

(41) A lens of 2 dioptres has a focal length equal to:

(a) 50 cms
(c) 4 cms

(b) 25 cms
(d) 0.5 cms

(42) A diverging lens of focal length (f) 20 cms is placed in contact with a converging lens of focal length (f$_2$) 10 cms, the focal length (f) of the combination is:

(a) 10/3 cms          (b) 10 cms

(c) 20 cms           (d) 30 cms

(43) Which of the following is not a converging lens?

(a)    (b)    (c)    (d)

### 5.12.3  ANSWERS TO QUESTIONS IN SECTION 5.12.2

| ( 1) b | (2) d | (3) a | (4) a | (5) a | (6) d | (7) b |
|--------|-------|-------|-------|-------|-------|-------|
| ( 8) d | (9) a | (10) a | (11) b | (12) d | (13) b | (14) a |
| (15) b | (16) c | (17) a | (18) c | (19) b | (20) c | (21) a |
| (22) c | (23) b | (24) d | (25) c | (26) c | (27) b | (28) a |
| (29) c | (30) a | (31) b | (32) c | (33) c | (34) a | (35) d |
| (36) a | (37) b | (38) b | (39) b | (40) c | (41) a | (42) c |
| (43) d | | | | | | |

### 5.12.4  DISCUSSION OF ANSWERS TO QUESTIONS IN SECTION 5.12.2

QUESTIONS #1 to #26: Adequately discussed in the Section.

QUESTION #27   (Answer: b) Use the mirror equation:

$$1/f = 1/o + 1/i$$

f = +4 cm because of converging mirror

1/4 = 1/10 + 1/i
20i(1/4) = 20i(1/10) + 20i(1/i)
(note 20i is the least common denominator)
5i = 2i + 20
3i = 20
i = 20/3 cms from the mirror and is real

m = -i/o = (-20/3)/10 = (-20/3)(1/10) = -2/3 of the object

The image is inverted (because it is negative).

QUESTION #28   (Answer: a) Use the mirror equation:

$$1/f = 1/o + 1/i$$

f = +2 cm because of converging mirror

1/2 = 1/10 + 1/i
10i(1/2) = 10i(1/10) + 10i(1/i)
5i = i + 10
4i = 10
i = 10/4 = +5/2 = 2.50 cms from the mirror

Since, o (10 cms) > f (2cms), the image is real and inverted.
Since, o (10 cms) > R (4cms), the image is reduced
         R = 2f = 2·2 = 4.

426

QUESTION #29  (Answer:  c)  Use the lens equation:

$$1/f = 1/o + 1/i$$
$i = -5$cm because it is virtual
$f = +2$cm because the mirror is converging
$$1/2 = 1/o - 1/5$$
$$10o(1/2) = 10o(1/o) - 10o(1/5)$$
$$5o = 10 - 2o$$
$$7o = 10$$
$$o = 10/7 \text{ cms.}$$

QUESTION #30  (Answer:  a)  The angle to the normal is smaller in the more optically dense medium for refraction of light.

QUESTION #31  (Answer:  b)

$n$ = speed in free space/speed in medium (s)
$$1.5 = (3.0 \times 10^{10} \text{ cm/sec})/s$$
$$s = (3.0 \times 10^{10})/1.5 = (2)(10^{10} \text{ cm/sec})$$

QUESTION #32  (Answer:  c)  For light, the smaller the wavelength, the closer the refracted ray to the normal.  Since violet light has a shorter wavelength than red, red light will be refracted through a larger angle.

QUESTION #33  (Answer:  c)

$$\sin \theta_c = n_2/n_1 = 1.00/2.00 = 0.5$$
$n_2$ = less optically dense (glass)
$n_1$ = more optically dense (air)
$$\theta_c = 30^\circ$$

You should remember that $\sin 30^\circ = 1/2$ or recall that in a $30^\circ$-$60^\circ$ right triangle the following is true:

$$\sin 30^\circ = 1/2$$

QUESTION #34  (Answer:  a)  apparent depth (Da)/actual depth $= n_2/n_1$

$n_2$ = of observer = 1.00
$n_1$ = of object = 1.33
$$Da/8 = 1.00/1.33 = 1/(4/3) = 3/4$$
$$Da = (3/4)(8) = 6 \text{ meters.}$$

QUESTION #35  (Answer:  d)  Since the object distance is greater than the focal length, the image is real and inverted.  Since the object distance is more than twice the focal length, the image is reduced in size.

QUESTION #36  (Answer:  a)  A biconcave lens is a diverging lens. The image is always virtual, erect and reduced in size.

QUESTION #37  (Answer:  b)  All images formed by diverging lenses are virtual, erect and reduced.

QUESTION #38  (Answer:  b)  Use the lens equation:

$$1/f = 1/o + 1/i$$
f = +10cm because of converging lens
$$1/10 = 1/5 + 1/i$$
$$10i(1/10) = 10i(1/5) + 10i(1/i)$$
$$i = 2i + 10$$
$$-i = 10$$
$$i = -10 \text{ cm}$$
    this means the object is virtual (negative sign) and
    10 cms from the mirror
M = magnification = $-i/o$ = $-(-10)/5$ = $+2$
∴ the image is erect (positive sign) and is 2(20) = 40 cms tall.


QUESTION #39  (Answer:  b)  A concave lens is a diverging lens.  Use
the lens equation:

$$1/f = 1/o + 1/i$$
f = -5 cms because of diverging lens
$$1/-5 = 1/20 + 1/i$$
$$20i(1/-5) = 20i(1/20) + 20i(1/i)$$
$$-4i = i + 20$$
$$-5i = 20$$
  i = -4cms (negative means virtual)
  m = magnification = $-i/o$ = $-(-4)/10$ = 4/10 = 2/5
    positive M means the object is erect;
    the image is (2/5)(10) = 4 cms tall.


QUESTION #40  (Answer:  c)

dioptres = 1/focal length in meters = $1/(1/10)$ = (1)(10/1) = 10
10 cms = 1/10 meter

QUESTION #41  (Answer:  a)

dioptres (d) = 1/focal length in meters (f)
$$d = 1/f$$
$$f = 1/d = 1/2m$$
$$1/2m = (1/2m)(100 \text{ cms}/1m) = 50 \text{ cms.}$$


QUESTION #42  (Answer:  c)  The focal length of lenses in contact is
found by:

dioptres:  lens #1:  20 cm  = 1/5m
                    $D_1$   = -5 (because diverging)
          lens #2:  10 cm  = 1/10m
                    $D_2$   = 10

Total dioptres:  $D_T$ = $D_1 + D_2$ = -5 + 10 = +5
          Then $f_T$ = f = $1/D_T$ = 1/5m or 20 cm


QUESTION #43  (Answer:  d)  A converging lens is smaller at the
edges than the middle--this holds for (a), (b) and (c).  The lens in
(d) is larger at the ends than in the middle.

| | | | |
|---|---|---|---|
| ____ | reflection | ____ | diverging lens |
| ____ | virtual image | ____ | dioptres |
| ____ | real image | ____ | plane mirror |
| ____ | combinations of lenses | ____ | lens equation |
| ____ | spherical mirror | ____ | mirror equation |
| ____ | Snell's Law | ____ | focal length |
| ____ | total internal reflection | ____ | converging lens |
| ____ | center of curvature | | |

## 5.13      Nuclear Structure, and Atomic and Quantum Physics

### 5.13.1      REVIEW OF NUCLEAR STRUCTURE

An atom is made of a nucleus containing protons (mass = 1 a.m.u., charge +1) and neutrons (mass = 1 a.m.u., charge = -1). The atomic number (AN) is the number of protons in the nucleus of an atom. An element is a group of atoms with the same AN; i.e., it is the number of protons that make elements different from each other. The mass number (MN) is the sum of protons and neutrons in a given atom (not element!). Isotopes are atoms of the same element with different MNs, i.e., they have the same number of protons but different numbers of neutrons. The atomic weight (AW) is the weighted average of all naturally occurring isotopes of an element. Note that it is the number of protons that distinguishes one element from another, and it is the electron configuration (Section 3.1.1) of a given element that determines its chemical reactivity.

Coulomb repulsive force (between protons) in the nuclei are overcome by nuclear forces. The nuclear force is a nonelectrical type of force that binds nuclei together and is equal for protons and neutrons. The nuclear binding energy ($E_b$) is a result of the Coulomb and nuclear binding forces. Einstein derived the relation between energy and mass changes associated with nuclear reactions,

$$\Delta E = \Delta mc^2 = \text{ergs if m = grams and c = cm/sec}$$
$$\Delta E = \text{energy released or absorbed}$$
$$\Delta m = \text{mass lost (mass deficit) or gained, respectively}$$
$$c = \text{speed of light} = 3.0 \times 10^{10} \text{ cm/sec}$$

conversions:

$$1 \text{ gram} = 9 \times 10^{20} \text{ ergs}$$

$$1 \text{ amu (atomic mass unit)} = 931.4 \text{ MeV}$$

$$1 \text{ amu} = 1/12 \text{ the mass of } _6C^{12}$$

The above is a statement of the Law of Conservation of Mass and Energy. The value of $E_b$ depends upon the mass number (MN) as follows,

$E_b/MN$ = binding energy per nucleon; this is the energy released by the formation of a given nucleus.

Note that the peak $E_b/MN$ is at MN = 60. Also, the $E_b/MN$ is relatively constant after MN = 20. Fission is when a nucleus splits into smaller nuclei. Fusion is when smaller nuclei combine to form a larger nucleus. Energy is released from a nuclear reaction (see diagram above) when nuclei with MN $\gg$ 60 undergo fission or nuclei $\ll$ 60 undergo fusion.

Not all combinations of protons are equally likely or stable. An even number of protons or an even number of neutrons, in general, means the nuclei are more stable. The most stable nuclei are those with an even number of protons and an even number of neutrons. The least stable nuclei are those with an odd number of protons and an odd number of neutrons. Also, as the atomic number (AN) increases, there are more neutrons (N) needed for the nuclei to be stable (Fig. 5.27).

Fig. 5.26 - Stability of Atoms

Up to AN = 20 (Calcium) the protons equal the neutrons, after this there are more neutrons. If an atom is in region #1 above, it has too many protons or too few neutrons and must decrease its protons or increase its neutrons to become stable. The reverse is true for region #2. Also all nuclei after AN = 84 (Polonium) are unstable.

Unstable nuclei can become stable nuclei by fission (splitting) to smaller nuclei or by absorbing or emitting small particles. Spontaneous fission is rare. Spontaneous radioactivity (emitting particles) is common. The common particles are (1) alpha ($\alpha$) particle $_2He^4$ (helium nucleus); (2) beta ($\beta$) particle $_{-1}e^0$ (an electron); (3) a positron $_{+1}e^0$; (4) gamma ($\gamma$) ray—no mass, just energy; and (5) orbital electron capture—nucleus takes electrons from K shell and converts a proton to a neutron. If there is a flux of particles such as neutrons ($_0n^1$), the nucleus can absorb these also.

Nuclear reactions are reactions in which changes in nuclear composition occur. An example of nuclear reactions and the terminology is:

$$_{92}U^{238} + {_1}H^2 \longrightarrow {_{93}}Np^{238} + 2{_0}n^1$$

Note:

$$_{92}U^{238} \xleftarrow{\text{mass number}} {^{238}}U \longrightarrow {^{238}}U$$
$$_{92} \xleftarrow{\hspace{1cm}} \text{atomic number} \xrightarrow{\hspace{1cm}} 92$$

the sum of the lower (higher) numbers on one side of the equation equals the sum of the lower (higher) numbers on the other side.

Another way of writing the above reaction is:

$$_{92}U^{238}\left({_1}H^2, \; 2{_0}n^1\right) {_{93}}Np^{238}$$

Spontaneous radioactive decay is a <u>first order process</u>. This means that the rate of decay is directly proportional to the amount of material present:

$$\Delta m / \Delta t \propto M$$

$\Delta M$ = change in mass
$\Delta t$ = change in time
$M$ = mass present at a given time
$\Delta M / \Delta t$ = rate of decay.

This relation is equalized by adding a proportionality constant called the <u>decay constant</u> (k),

$$\Delta m / \Delta t = -km \quad \text{(equation \#1)}$$

The minus sign indicates that mass is disappearing. The meaning of k is:

$$k = -(\Delta m/m) / \Delta t = \text{fraction of the mass that decays with time.}$$
$$\text{(equation \#2)}$$

Note that $k = 1/\text{time}$. If time is seconds, then $k = 1/\text{secs}$. This means that if $k = 0.1/\text{sec}$, then 1/10 of the substance (that is present at that time) will disappear in the next second.

The <u>half-life</u> ($T_{\frac{1}{2}}$) of a radioactive atom is the time required for one-half of it to disintegrate. The $T_{\frac{1}{2}}$ is related to k as follows,

$$T_{\frac{1}{2}} = 0.693/k.$$

This is derived from equation #1 by calculus. Although not exactly correct, the amount left after n half-lives is:

amount left = $(1/2)^n M$
    $M$ = mass began with
    $n$ = number of half-lives = elapsed time/$T_{\frac{1}{2}}$

Or, the amount that has disappeared can be calculated using k from equation #2 and is:

$$\text{amount decayed} = \Delta M = (k)\ (\Delta t)\ (M)$$
$$k = \text{decay constant}$$
$$\Delta t = \text{elapsed time}$$
$$M = \text{mass began with.}$$

5.13.1.2     REVIEW OF ATOMIC AND QUANTUM PHYSICS

The energy that an electron contains is not continuous over the whole range of possible energies. Rather, electrons in an atom may contain only discrete energies and occupy certain orbits. Electrons of each atom are restricted to these discrete energy levels. These levels have an energy below zero. This means energy is released when an electron moves from infinity into these energy levels. A representative set of energy levels of an electron in an atom may be:

If there is one electron in the atom above, its ground state will be in the n = 1, or lowest energy level available. Any other energy level, n = 2 or n = 3, e.g., is considered an excited state for that electron. The difference in energies (E) between the levels gives the energy and, hence, frequency (f) of light necessary to cause the excitation (absorption, electron A):

$$E_3 - E_1 = hf$$
$$E_1 = \text{energy level one}$$
$$E_2 = \text{energy level two}$$
$$h = \text{Planck's Constant}$$
$$f = \text{frequency of light absorbed.}$$

So, if light is passed through a substance (gas, e.g.), certain wavelengths (since $\lambda = c/f$, c = speed of light, $\lambda$ = wavelength) will be absorbed, which corresponds to the energy needed for the electron transitions. An absorption spectrum will result that has dark lines against a light background. Multiple lines result because there are possible transitions from all quantum levels occupied by electrons to any unoccupied levels (e.g., n = 1 to n = 2, n = 3, etc., n = 2 to n = 3, n = 4, etc.).

An emission spectrum results when an electron is excited to a higher level by another particle or by an electric discharge, for example. Then, as the electron falls from the excited state to lower states, light is emitted that has wavelength (frequency) corresponding to the energy difference between the levels. As an example (emission, electron B):

$$E_1 - E_4 = hf$$

The resulting spectrum will have light lines against a dark background.

The absorption and emission spectrums should have the same number of lines but often will not. This is because in the absorption spectrum, there is rapid radiation of the absorbed light in all directions, and transitions are generally from the ground state initially. These factors result in fewer lines in the absorption than in the emission spectrum.

Fluorescence is an emission process that occurs after light absorption excites electrons to higher electronic and vibrational levels. The electrons spontaneously lose excited vibrational energy to the electronic level and then emit light as they fall to the ground vibrational and electronic states. There are certain molecular types that possess this property, e.g., some amino acids (tryptophan).

The fluorescence process is depicted as follows:

Step 1 - absorption light
Step 2 - spontaneous deactivation of vibrational levels to zero vibrational level for electronic state
Step 3 - fluorescence with light emission (longer wavelength than absorption).

5.13.2    QUESTIONS TO REVIEW NUCLEAR STRUCTURE, AND ATOMIC AND QUANTUM PHYSICS

(1)    A proton is _____ charged and has a mass of _____ amu(s).

    (a) positively, one                    (b) negatively, 1/1845
    (c) neutral, one                       (d) none of the above

433

(2)    The sum of protons and neutrons in a nucleus is called the:

    (a) electron number       (b) atomic number
    (c) atomic weight        (d) mass number

(3)    Isotopes have the _____ atomic numbers and _____ mass numbers.

    (a) same, same         (b) same, different
    (c) different, same     (d) different, different

(4)    The particles that distinguish one element from another are the:

    (a) neutrons           (b) protons
    (c) electrons          (d) mesons

(5)    The particle of the nucleus which has mass, energy and can be charged or neutral is called the:

    (a) neutron           (b) proton
    (c) neutrino          (d) meson

(6)    Which particle has no mass?

    (a) neutron           (b) meson
    (c) neutrino          (d) electron

(7)    The nuclear binding energy of nuclei depends on:

    (a) coulomb forces      (b) nuclear forces
    (c) both              (d) neither

(8)    If $\Delta E$ = the energy change, $\Delta m$ = mass change and c = the speed of light, the correct relation between these for describing the conversion of mass and energy is

    (a) $\Delta E = \Delta m/c$      (b) $\Delta E = c^2/\Delta m$
    (c) $\Delta E = \Delta mc$       (d) $\Delta E = \Delta mc^2$

(9)    Which of the following statements is correct concerning binding energy ($E_b$)?

    (a) binding energy depends on protons only
    (b) binding is relatively constant at all mass numbers
    (c) the peak in binding energy per nucleon is at mass number = 60
    (d) none of the above

(10)   Which of the following particles is emitted by nuclei in spontaneous radioactivity?

    (a) $\propto$ -particle       (b) $\beta$ -particle
    (c) $\gamma$ -ray         (d) all of the above

(11)   The particle composed of two protons and two neutrons is the:

    (a) $\gamma$ -ray         (b) $\propto$ -particle
    (c) neutrino         (d) positron

(12)    The rate of radioactive decay

    (a) is independent of the amount of material present;
    (b) is inversely proportional to the amount of material present;
    (c) varies unpredictably but does depend on the amount of material present;
    (d) is directly proportional to the amount of material present.

(13)    The radioactive decay constant

    (a) is the fraction of mass that decays in a given amount of time;
    (b) is the amount of mass that decays in one half-life;
    (c) is not related to the half-life;
    (d) none of the above.

(14)    The atomic number is the number of ____ contained in the nucleus.

    (a) neutrons                    (b)  electrons
    (c) protons                     (d)  positrons

(15)    The atomic weight of an element is

    (a) the weighted average of naturally occurring isotopes;
    (b) the sum of protons and neutrons;
    (c) twice the number of protons;
    (d) none of the above.

(16)    Carbon has an atomic number (AN) of 6. One of its isotopes has a mass number (MN) of 13. The number of neutrons in this isotope is:

    (a)  6     (b)  7      (c)  13      (d)  19

(17)    An isotope of boron has 5 protons and 6 neutrons. The atomic number (AN) of boron is:

    (a) 11      (b)  10      (c)  6      (d)  5

(18)    Suppose the natural abundance of the isotopes of berylium (atomic number = 4) is 90% of mass number = 8; 10% of mass number = 9. The atomic weight (AW) is:

    (a) 9.00                        (b)  8.50
    (c) 8.10                        (d)  8.00

(19)    An atom has an atomic number (AN) = 18 and a mass number (MN) = 38. Letting P = # of protons and N = # neutrons, which atom below is an isotope of this atom?

    (a) P = 18, N = 19              (b)  P = 20, N = 18
    (c) P = 19, N = 18             (d)  none of the above

(20)    A nuclear reaction proceeds with a mass deficit (mass loss) of $5 \times 10^{-5}$ gms. The amount of energy released is:

    (a) $1.5 \times 10^6$ ergs              (b)  $4.5 \times 10^{16}$ ergs
    (c) $9.0 \times 10^{20}$ ergs           (d)  none of the above

(21)  The radioactive decay of a substance has a half-life ($T_{\frac{1}{2}}$) of 10 secs, the decay constant (k) is:

(a) 1.4 secs$^{-1}$
(b) 0.069 secs$^{-1}$
(c) 6.9 secs$^{-1}$
(d) none of the above

(22)  After 20 days, how much of a substance with a half-life of 5 days is left if there were 10 gms initially?

(a) 2.50 gms
(b) 2 gms
(c) 5/8 gm
(d) none of the above

(23)  How much of 5 gms of radioactive substance with a half-life of 10 secs has decayed in 2 seconds?

(a) 1.38 gms
(b) 1.0 gms
(c) 0.69 gms
(d) none of the above

(24)  What is the missing particle in the following reaction?

$$_{27}Co^{59} + ? \longrightarrow _{27}Co^{60}$$

(a) proton
(b) electron
(c) neutron
(d) none of the above

(25)  What is the missing particle in the following reaction?

$$_{92}U^{238} + ? \longrightarrow _{94}Pu^{239} + 3\ n$$

(a) $\beta$ –particle
(b) proton
(c) $\gamma$ –ray
(d) none of the above


5.13.3       ANSWERS TO QUESTIONS IN SECTION 5.13.2


( 1)  a  ( 2)  d  ( 3)  b  ( 4)  b  ( 5)  d  ( 6)  c  ( 7)  c
( 8)  d  ( 9)  c  (10)  d  (11)  b  (12)  d  (13)  a  (14)  c
(15)  a  (16)  b  (17)  d  (18)  c  (19)  a  (20)  b  (21)  b
(22)  c  (23)  c  (24)  c  (25)  d


5.13.4       DISCUSSION OF ANSWERS TO QUESTIONS IN SECTION 5.13.2

QUESTIONS #1 to #15:  Adequately discussed in Section.

QUESTION #16   (Answer:  b)  MN = protons (P) + neutrons (N)
                             13 = 6 + N   (AN=P)
                              7 = N.

QUESTION #17   (Answer:  d)  The AN is the number of protons.

QUESTION #18   (Answer:  c)  The AW is the weighted average of the naturally occurring isotopes.  This is simply found by multiplying the percent abundance (as a decimal) of each isotope times the mass number of that isotope and adding all of these together:
          AW = (0.90)(8) + (0.10)(9) = 7.2 + 0.9 = 8.1

QUESTION #19   (Answer:  a)   The AN = the number of protons and this must be the same because isotopes are of the same element. Therefore, the answer is (a).

QUESTION #20   (Answer:  b)

$$\Delta E = \Delta mc^2 = (5 \times 10^{-5} \text{ gms})(3.0 \times 10^{10} \text{cm/sec})^2$$
$$= (5 \times 10^{-5})(9 \times 10^{20}) = 45 \times 10^{15} = 4.5 \times 10^{16} \text{ ergs.}$$

QUESTION #21   (Answer:  b)

$$k = 0.693/T_{\frac{1}{2}} = 0.693/10 \text{ secs} = 0.0693 \text{ secs}^{-1}$$

QUESTION #22   (Answer:  c)

$$\text{amount left} = (1/2)^n m = (1/2)^{20/5}(10) = (1/2)^4(10)$$
$$= (1/16)(10) = 10/16$$
$$= 5/8 \text{ gms}$$

QUESTION #23   (Answer:  c)   One may use $T_{\frac{1}{2}}$ or k to find the amount left.  In this case it is easier to use k:

$$k = 0.693/T_{\frac{1}{2}} = 0.693/10 \text{ secs} = 0.069 \text{ secs}^{-1}$$

$$\text{amount left} = (k)(\Delta t)(m)$$
$$= (0.069)(2)(5) = (0.069)(10) = 0.69 \text{ gms}$$

QUESTION #24   (Answer:  c)   Adding the top numbers (the sum of protons and neutrons):
$$59 + x = 60$$
$$x = 1$$
Adding the bottom numbers (the number of protons):
$$27 + y = 27$$
$$y = 0.$$

The particle is then: $_0?^1$
which fits the neutron; $_0n^1$.

QUESTION #25   (Answer:  d)   See question #30 for steps:

top numbers
$$238 + x = 239 + 3(1) = 242$$
$$x = 242-238 = 4$$
bottom numbers
$$92 + y = 94 + 3(0) = 94$$
$$y = 94-92 = 2.$$

The particle is:  $_2?^4$

which fits the $\alpha$-particle (or helium nucleus):  $_2He^4$.

5.13.5    VOCABULARY, CONCEPTS, ETC. CHECKLIST FOR NUCLEAR
          STRUCTURE

_____ atomic number                 _____ $\Delta E = \Delta mc^2$
_____ atomic weight                 _____ mass number
_____ binding energy (nuclear)      _____ isotopes
_____ neutrons                      _____ electrons
_____ protons                       _____ $\beta$ -particle
_____ half-life                     _____ nuclear reactions
_____ decay constant                _____ $\alpha$ -particle
_____ mass deficit


5.14       References for Review of Physics

Halliday, D., and Resnick, R. Fundamentals of Physics. John Wiley
    and Sons, Inc., 1970.

Tippins, P. E. Applied Physics. McGraw-Hill Book Company, 1973. A
    very good, well-written and concise book for review of physics.

White. H. E. Modern College Physics, 5th ed. D. Van Nostrand
    Company, Inc., 1966.